MINDFULNESS AND ACCEPTANCE

Mindfulness and Acceptance

Expanding the Cognitive-Behavioral Tradition

Edited by
STEVEN C. HAYES
VICTORIA M. FOLLETTE
MARSHA M. LINEHAN

THE GUILFORD PRESS
New York   London

© 2004 The Guilford Press
A Division of Guilford Publications, Inc.
72 Spring Street, New York, NY 10012
www.guilford.com

Paperback edition 2011

Printed in the United States of America

This book is printed on acid-free paper.

Last digit is print number: 9 8 7 6 5 4

Library of Congress Cataloging-in-Publication Data

Mindfulness and acceptance : expanding the cognitive-behavioral tradition /
edited by Steven C. Hayes, Victoria M. Follette, Marsha M. Linehan.
    p. cm.
 Includes bibliographical references and index.
 ISBN 978-1-59385-066-1 (hardcover)
 ISBN 978-1-60918-989-1 (paperback)
 1. Cognitive therapy. 2. Behavior therapy. I. Hayes, Steven C. II. Follette,
Victoria M. III. Linehan, Marsha.
 RC489.C63M55 2004
 616.89'142—dc22

                                                              2004007843

To my friend and mentor, John D. Cone
—S. C. H.

To everyone who has taught me so well:
my clients, my students, and my mentors
—V. M. F.

To Pat Hawk, Zen Master in the Diamond Sangha,
a wonderful friend and mentor
—M. M. L.

About the Editors

Steven C. Hayes, PhD, is Nevada Foundation Professor at the Department of Psychology at the University of Nevada. Author of 34 books and over 470 scientific articles, his career has focused on the analysis of the nature of human language and cognition and the application of this to the understanding and alleviation of human suffering. Dr. Hayes has been President of Division 25 of the American Psychological Association, of the American Association of Applied and Preventive Psychology, of the Association for Contextual Behavioral Science, and of the Association for Behavioral and Cognitive Therapies. His work has been recognized by several awards including the Exemplary Contributions to Basic Behavioral Research and Its Applications from Division 25, the Impact of Science on Application award from the Society for the Advancement of Behavior Analysis, and the Lifetime Achievement Award from the Association for Behavioral and Cognitive Therapies.

Victoria M. Follette, PhD, is Foundation Professor of Psychology and Chair of the Department of Psychology at the University of Nevada. She heads the Trauma Research Institute of Nevada, using a contextual behavioral approach to understanding the sequelae of trauma. Dr. Follette's areas of interest include taking science into applied treatment and mindfulness- and acceptance-based approaches to treatment.

Marsha M. Linehan, PhD, is Professor of Psychology and Adjunct Professor of Psychiatry and Behavioral Sciences at the University of Washington and Director of the Behavioral Research and Therapy Clinics, a consortium of research projects developing new treatments and evaluating their efficacy for persons with severe mental disorders and multiple diagnoses. Dr. Linehan's primary research is in the application of behavioral models to suicidal behaviors, drug abuse, and borderline personality disorder. She was president of the Association for Advancement of Behavior Therapy and is currently a Fellow of the American Psychological Association and the American Psychopathological Association, as well as a Diplomate of the American Board of Behavioral Psychology. Dr. Linehan has written two treatment manuals, *Cognitive-Behavioral Treatment of Borderline Personality Disorder* (1993, The Guilford Press) and *Skills Training Manual for Treating Borderline Personality Disorder* (1993, The Guilford Press), and has published extensively in scientific journals. She also serves on a number of editorial boards.

Contributors

Michael Addis, PhD, Department of Psychology, Clark University, Worcester, Massachusetts

Arthur W. Blume, PhD, Department of Psychology, University of Texas at El Paso, El Paso, Texas

Madelon Bolling, PhD, Department of Psychology, University of Washington, Seattle, Washington

T. D. Borkovec, PhD, Department of Psychology, Pennsylvania State University, University Park, Pennsylvania

Sarah W. Bowen, BA, Department of Psychology, University of Washington, Seattle, Washington

Andrew Christensen, PhD, Department of Psychology, University of California, Los Angeles, California

Rick Crutcher, BA, Northwest Vipassana Center, Ethel, Washington

Tiara M. Dillworth, BA, Department of Psychology, University of Washington, Seattle, Washington

Sona Dimidjian, MSW, Department of Psychology, University of Washington, Seattle, Washington

Victoria M. Follette, PhD, Department of Psychology, University of Nevada, Reno, Nevada

Alan E. Fruzzetti, PhD, Department of Psychology, University of Nevada, Reno, Nevada

Krista S. Gattis, MA, Department of Psychology, University of California, Los Angeles

Mandra L. Rasmussen Hall, MA, Department of Psychology, University of Nevada, Reno, Nevada

Steven C. Hayes, PhD, Department of Psychology, University of Nevada, Reno, Nevada

Kate M. Iverson, BA, Department of Psychology, University of Nevada, Reno, Nevada

Jonathan W. Kanter, PhD, Department of Psychology, University of Wisconsin–Milwaukee, Milwaukee, Wisconsin

Robert J. Kohlenberg, PhD, Department of Psychology, University of Washington, Seattle, Washington

Mary E. Larimer, PhD, Department of Psychiatry and Behavioral Sciences, University of Washington, Seattle, Washington

Jennifer Block Lerner, PhD, Department of Psychology, Skidmore College, Saratoga Springs, New York

Marsha M. Linehan, PhD, Department of Psychology, University of Washington, Seattle, Washington

Heather S. Lonczak, PhD, Department of Psychology, University of Washington, Seattle, Washington

Laura Marie Macpherson, MS, Department of Psychology, University of Washington, Seattle, Washington

G. Alan Marlatt, PhD, Department of Psychology, University of Washington, Seattle, Washington

Christopher Martell, PhD, private practice and Department of Psychology, University of Washington, Seattle, Washington

Amy R. Murrell, MA, Department of Psychology, University of Mississippi, University, Mississippi

Susan M. Orsillo, PhD, Women's Health Sciences Division, Boston Veterans Affairs Healthcare System, Boston, Massachusetts

Kathleen M. Palm, MA, Psychological Services, Brown University, Providence, Rhode Island

Chauncey Parker, BS, Department of Psychology, University of Washington, Seattle, Washington

George A. Parks, PhD, Department of Psychology, University of Washington, Seattle, Washington

Clive J. Robins, PhD, Department of Psychiatry and Behavioral Sciences, Duke University Medical Center, Durham, North Carolina

Lizabeth Roemer, PhD, Department of Psychology, University of Massachusetts, Boston, Massachusetts

Henry Schmidt III, PhD, Behavioral Affiliates, Inc., Seattle, Washington

Zindel V. Segal, PhD, Department of Psychiatry and Psychology, University of Toronto, Toronto, Ontario, Canada

Mia Sevier, MA, Department of Psychology, University of California, Los Angeles, California

Brian Sharpless, MS, MA, Department of Psychology, Pennsylvania State University, University Park, Pennsylvania

Lorelei E. Simpson, MA, Department of Psychology, University of California, Los Angeles, California

Tracy Simpson, PhD, Department of Psychiatry, University of Washington, and Women's Trauma Recovery Clinic, VA Puget Sound Health Care System, Seattle, Washington

John D. Teasdale, DPhil, Medical Research Council Cognition and Brain Sciences Unit, Cambridge, United Kingdom

Mavis Tsai, PhD, private practice, Seattle, Washington

Matthew T. Tull, MA, Department of Psychology, University of Massachusetts, Boston, Massachusetts

Reo Wexner, MS, Department of Psychology, University of Washington, Seattle, Washington

Katie Witkiewitz, MA, Department of Psychology, University of Washington, Seattle, Washington

J. Mark G. Williams, DPhil, Department of Psychology, Oxford University, Oxford, United Kingdom

G. Terence Wilson, PhD, Graduate School of Applied and Professional Psychology, Rutgers University, Piscataway, New Jersey

Kelly G. Wilson, PhD, Department of Psychology, University of Mississippi, University, Mississippi

Preface

The cognitive-behavioral therapy tradition (defined very broadly to include traditional behavior therapy, cognitive therapy, cognitive-behavioral therapy, clinical behavior analysis, and so on) began in the 1950s and blossomed in the 1960s. In its lifetime, this tradition has been through many changes, yet has maintained its core commitments to science, theory, and good practice. In the last 10 years, a set of new behavior therapies has emerged that emphasizes issues that were traditionally less emphasized or even off limits for behavioral and cognitive therapists, including mindfulness, acceptance, the therapeutic relationship, values, spirituality, meditation, focusing on the present moment, emotional deepening, and similar topics. These have emerged from the most behavioral wings and the most cognitive wings of the tradition. They differ from what is more common in the behavior therapy tradition not only in their focus but also in their technology, which often seems unexpectedly experiential, involving second-order change strategies, as well as more direct ones. Some involve sophisticated philosophy of science considerations. All are hard to characterize using the traditional distinctions between behavior therapy and other traditions, or those within the behavioral and cognitive tradition.

This is the first volume to try to examine that set of new developments and to ask some basic questions about it. Leading authors, researchers, and clinicians were brought together for a 3-day conference in Reno, Nevada, in the summer of 2002 to discuss all of these issues. They were asked to characterize their approaches clinically, and to consider how the focus of their approaches relates to the broader set of issues embraced by the new behavior therapies. They were asked to articulate their theoretical models, and examine their similarities and differences with other models both inside and outside of behavior therapy. Authors were encouraged to characterize briefly the research in support of their approaches, both outcome and process, and to try to look ahead at the implications of these data for the field. When they returned home, they were asked to react to the kinds of things they heard from other leaders in this set of new approaches.

What results is this volume: a wide-ranging exploration of a field in a phase of rapid development. The data and concepts in these chapters are challenging, exciting, and hopeful. These new developments seem to be broadening behavioral and cognitive therapy, and emboldening therapists to take on some of the most difficult clinical issues and challenges. It is not possible to know where this will lead, but it is clear that we are witnessing a significant expansion of the cognitive-behavioral tradition that is opening up new avenues of exploration for researchers and clinicians alike.

The book is organized such that the first few chapters look at more general technologies and issues, then gradually move toward technologies and issues that become more focused on specific populations. There is no hard and fast line between the two, and there is a great deal of interconnection between these treatments; thus, we did not attempt formal sections.

We would like to thank the sponsors of the Nevada Conference on Mindfulness, Acceptance, and Relationship; The Guilford Press; the Change Companies; the University of Nevada, Reno; and Context Press. Don Kuhl, of the Change Companies, is especially thanked for his generous support. The student assistants for the conference are also thanked, particularly Alethea Smith and Casey Sackett.

STEVEN C. HAYES
VICTORIA M. FOLLETTE
MARSHA M. LINEHAN

Contents

1

Acceptance and Commitment Therapy and the New Behavior Therapies

Mindfulness, Acceptance, and Relationship

Steven C. Hayes

Beyond their existence in the behavior therapy tradition broadly defined, no single factor unites the methods presented in this volume more than how hard it is to classify them using existing terms within empirical clinical psychology. Many are venturing boldly into areas outside the behavior therapy tradition, such as dialectics, spirituality, relationship, and mindfulness. The methods are unusually flexible, including means that are direct and indirect, didactic and experiential, instructional and metaphorical. Cognitively rationalized approaches are questioning the primacy of changes in cognitive content. Behaviorally rationalized approaches are embracing cognitive topics. What is going on here?

When many new approaches emerge that are difficult to classify, it is possibly a sign that the field itself is reorganizing. This has happened before in behavior therapy. It seems to be happening again (Hayes, in press).

FIRST- AND SECOND-GENERATION BEHAVIOR THERAPY

Behavior therapy (referring to the entire range of behavioral and cognitive therapies, from clinical behavior analysis to cognitive therapy) emerged as an approach committed to the development of well-specified and rigorously tested applied technologies based on scientifically well-established basic principles (Franks & Wilson, 1974). It rejected existing clinical theories and technologies that were poorly specified, vaguely argued, and little researched. Behavior therapists criticized (e.g., Bandura, 1969, pp. 11–13; Wolpe & Rachman, 1960) the amazing flights of psychoanalytic fancy that could be occasioned by the simplest of phobias or other clinical disorders (e.g., Freud, 1909/1955). As a form of instructive ridicule, behavior therapists trained simple actions by direct shaping in the chronically mentally ill, and then watched with amusement as psychoanalytic colleagues concocted bizarre symbolic interpretations of behaviors that had known and simple histories (e.g., Ayllon, Haughton, & Hughes, 1965). The alternative presented by behavior therapy was direct, humble, rational, and empirical. Abandoning an interest in hypothesized unconscious fears and desires, behavior therapists focused instead on direct symptom relief. The psychoanalytic worry that this would result only in superficial behavioral gains (e.g., Bookbinder, 1962; Schraml & Selg, 1966) was criticized (e.g., Yates, 1958), puzzled over (Bandura, 1969, pp. 48–49), and shown empirically to be largely unfounded (Nurnberger & Hingtgen, 1973).

The rejection of existing clinical concepts and methods had several collateral effects, beyond the inclusion of science and well-established basic principles. It became unfashionable in behavior therapy to dabble in clinical issues that were too subtle, complex, or broad in scope. Clinical targets generally involved "first-order" change. If an anxious child was not going to school, going to school or anxiety about going to school was the target, not unconscious interests or conflicts. The approach was not only first order but also often direct. Perhaps because the products of science are sets of verbal rules, the clinical approaches themselves tended to be presented to clients in relatively straightforward or didactic ways. If social skills were poor, attempts were made to specify verbally the various components of "good social skills" and then train them directly, often including such methods as instructions and feedback.

This first generation of behavior therapy changed dramatically with the advent of cognitive methods. Both stimulus–response associationism and behavior analysis had failed to provide an adequate account of human language and cognition, and early behavior therapists soon learned that they needed to deal with thoughts and feelings in a more direct and central way. The cognitive therapy movement (e.g., Beck, Rush, Shaw, & Emery, 1979; Mahoney, 1974; Meichenbaum, 1977) attempted to do so. The objections of early founders that cognition had been dealt with all along (e.g.,

Wolpe, 1980) were largely ignored, because it was the centrality of cognition and the ability to deal with it in a natural way that was more at issue. In the absence of adequate basic accounts, early cognitive-behavioral therapies approached cognition in a direct and clinically relevant way. In this work, "cognition" generally referred to the commonsense categories of thoughts, ideas, beliefs, or suppositions. Through the use of questionnaires and clinical interviews focused on such targets, clinicians learned to identify cognitive errors in particular patient populations, and direct means were developed to correct these problems.

Some of the leaders of these new approaches sought to overthrow behavior therapy, as was reflected in Beck's well-known challenge: "Can a fledgling psychotherapy challenge the giants in the field—psychoanalysis and behavior therapy?" (1976 , p. 333), but the behavior therapy tradition proved more flexible than that. What made a relatively smooth transition to the second generation of behavior therapy possible was the first-order change focus of the cognitive movement: "Cognitive therapy is best viewed as the application of the cognitive model of a particular disorder with the use of a variety of techniques designed to modify the dysfunctional beliefs and faulty information processing characteristic of each disorder" (Beck, 1993, p. 194). This first-order change focus comported so well with the overall approach of the first wave of behavior therapy that a second generation of behavior therapy could be created simply by expanding the scope, models, and methods of the tradition. "Cognitive-behavioral therapists" added irrational thoughts, pathological cognitive schemas, or faulty information-processing styles to the list of direct targets for change, along with new methods appropriate for these targets. In the second wave of behavior therapy, undesirable thoughts would be weakened or eliminated through their detection, correction, testing, and disputation, much as anxiety was to be replaced by relaxation in the first wave.

All of this happened 25–30 years ago. In the years that have followed, cognitive-behavioral therapy (CBT) has seen unprecedented success. The empirical basis of the field has been enormously strengthened, and in problem area after problem area, empirical clinicians have shown that CBT is helpful. Behavior therapy dominates lists of empirically supported treatments (Chambless et al., 1996) and clinical practice guidelines based on effective approaches (Hayes, Follette, Dawes, & Grady, 1995; Hayes & Gregg, 2001).

CONTEXTS SUPPORTING A NEW GENERATION OF BEHAVIOR THERAPY

Long periods of normal science occur when adherents have interesting work to do, rewards for doing that work, and when the organizational narrative seems to be coherent and progressive. In such phases, it is what is implicit, not what is explicit, that is most powerful. Assumptions about the questions, issues, methods, and forms of evidence appropriate to a field are often more important to maintaining a dominant paradigm than are specific theories, studies, principles, or technologies. Eventually, however, things change. Anomalies emerge that undermine the dominant paradigm. Patterns of support shift, and lines of research become less fruitful. Young professionals enter the field without being as bound to underlying assumptions. Questions that were never resolved reemerge. As a result, new questions dare to be asked and new methods and principles are developed. As the assumptive base of a dominant paradigm weakens or diversifies, this process can accelerate, particularly if new ideas are productive and help remove or resolve previously encountered roadblocks and anomalies. Sometimes change of this kind occurs in a deliberate way, with a political or an even revolutionary quality to it, but more commonly it happens in a humble and entirely natural way. Researchers simply begin to think outside the largely implicit box, and interesting findings emerge. That seems to be exactly what has happened with most of the methods discussed in this volume.

The contexts supporting the emergence of the new behavior therapies are several. First, a number of empirical anomalies have emerged. Clinical improvement in CBT often occurs before the presumptively key features have been adequately implemented (Ilardi & Craighead, 1994). Despite challenges (Tang & DeRubeis, 1999), this disturbing finding has not been adequately explained (Ilardi & Craighead, 1999; Wilson, 1999). Changes in cognitive mediators often fail to explain the impact of CBT (e.g., Burns & Spangler, 2001; Morgenstern & Longabaugh, 2000), particularly in areas that are causal and explanatory rather than descriptive (Beck & Perkins, 2001; Bieling & Kuyken, 2003). Component analyses of CBT (e.g., Gortner, Gollan, Dobson, & Jacobson, 1998; Jacobson et al., 1996; Zettle & Hayes, 1987) have led to the disturbing conclusion that there is "no additive benefit to providing cognitive interventions in cognitive therapy" (Dobson & Khatri, 2000, p. 913).

Second, the underlying treatment development model is showing signs of wear. Effect sizes have largely stagnated for technologies that are rigidly adherent to second-generation assumptions (Öst, 2002). Researchers, who are largely dependent for their funding on a technological model of treatment development (Rounsaville, Carroll, & Onken, 2001), are facing a proliferation of similar treatment manuals (Hayes, 2002b) in the absence of methods for their distillation. The federal funds that fed the rise of the second wave of behavior therapy increasingly have emphasized the need for innovative theory and a link to basic science (Rounsaville et al., 2001), which is leading to new models and to more focus on the empirical anomalies of the second generation. Because some research areas are well-plowed fields, researchers have tended to focus on unusual populations and subpopulations that can be examined within the existing model—but this has sometimes led to the development of new methods that do not fully comport with second-generation assumptions.

Third, the rise of constructivism and similar postmodernist (and post-postmodernist) theories, have weakened the mechanistic assumptions that have dominated in some wings of behavior therapy (Hayes, Hayes, Reese, & Sarbin, 1993). Instead, more pragmatic and contextualistic assumptions have come to the fore (Biglan & Hayes, 1996; Jacobson, 1997). Even the thinking of leaders of second-generation behavior therapy show the assumptive changes (e.g., cf. Beck, Rush, Shaw, & Emery, 1979, with Emery & Campbell, 1986; or Mahoney, 1974, with Mahoney, 2002). This change is subtle, but it is pervasive and powerful, and we discuss it extensively shortly.

THE THIRD WAVE

Contextual changes are not enough to change a field. New ideas are also needed. As the present volume shows, these new ideas have emerged and greatly strengthened over the last decade (cf. Hayes, Jacobson, Follette, & Dougher, 1994, with this volume). On the behavioral side, as exposure-based therapies focused on internal events (Barlow, 2002), it became clearer that it was the *function* of these events that was most at issue, not their form, frequency, or situational sensitivity per se. The positive outcomes for dialectical behavior therapy (DBT; Linehan, 1993; see Hayes, Masuda, Bissett, Luoma, & Guerrero, 2004, for a recent outcome review) provided strong support for mindfulness and both acceptance and change in the treatment of complex clinical problems. Mindfulness and acceptance are radical additions to behavior therapy, because they challenge the universal applicability of first-order change strategies. Within the cognitive wing, similar changes have occurred. Attentional and metacognitive perspectives (e.g., Wells, 1994) began to make clear that it was the function of problematic cognitions, not their form, that was most relevant. More emphasis began to be given to contacting the present moment (e.g., Borkovec & Roemer, 1994; see Borkovec & Sharpless, Chapter 10, this volume) and mindfulness (Segal, Williams, & Teasdale, 2001; Teasdale et al., 2002), strengthening that shift in focus.

The third generation of behavior therapy has been defined in the following way (Hayes, in press):

> Grounded in an empirical, principle-focused approach, the third wave of behavioral and cognitive therapy is particularly sensitive to the context and functions of psychological phenomena, not just their form, and thus tends

to emphasize contextual and experiential change strategies in addition to more direct and didactic ones. These treatments tend to seek the construction of broad, flexible and effective repertoires over an eliminative approach to narrowly defined problems, and to emphasize the relevance of the issues they examine for clinicians as well as clients. The third wave reformulates and synthesizes previous generations of behavioral and cognitive therapy and carries them forward into questions, issues, and domains previously addressed primarily by other traditions, in hopes of improving both understanding and outcomes.

Defined in that way, the new behavior therapies carry forward the behavior therapy tradition, but they (1) abandon a sole commitment to first-order change, (2) adopt more contextualistic assumptions, (3) adopt more experiential and indirect change strategies in addition to direct strategies, and (4) considerably broaden the focus of change.

Acceptance and commitment therapy (ACT, said as one word, not as A-C-T; Hayes, Strosahl, & Wilson, 1999) is in line with all of these features of the new behavior therapies. ACT is neither simple behavior therapy nor classic CBT. It is a contextualistic behavioral treatment that sits squarely among the set of third-generation treatments described in this volume. As such, an explication of ACT may help reveal commonalities and connections among some of these other treatments.

ACCEPTANCE AND COMMITMENT THERAPY

Underlying Philosophy

ACT emerged from behavior analysis, one of the more misunderstood wings of modern psychology. It is not by accident that several of the new behavior therapies are most closely linked to this wing of behavior therapy, which only recently has developed sufficiently to impact adult psychotherapy in a powerful way.

Behavior analysis is much easier to understand when its philosophical foundations are understood. Although mechanistic forms of behavior analysis exist, by far the more dominant strand of modern behavior analysis is based on a type of American pragmatism we have termed functional contextualism (Hayes, 1993). A full discussion of contextualism as a philosophy of science is a topic beyond the scope of the present chapter (but see Biglan & Hayes, 1996; Hayes et al., 1993; Hayes, Hayes, & Reese, 1988; Pepper, 1942), but some attention seems warranted for two reasons. First, explicitly (e.g., Jacobson, 1997) or implicitly, several of the new behavior therapies have contextualistic roots. Second, this philosophical difference seems to make more sense of the difference between second-generation behavior therapy and the new forms that have emerged.

The contextualistic wing of the new behavior therapies conceptualizes psychological events as a set of ongoing interactions between whole organisms and historically and situationally defined contexts. The root metaphor of contextualism (Pepper, 1942) is the "ongoing act in context," that is, the commonsense situated action. Contextualists seek to maintain contact with the whole event and its context, and to analyze that event in such a way that its holistic quality is not undermined.

Contextualists are supremely interested in function over form) because formal events literally have no meaning. An event disconnected from its history and current situational context is, in some sense, not an "event" at all: "It is not an act conceived as alone or cut off that we mean; it is an act in and with its setting" (Pepper, 1942, p. 232). Consider an action such as "walking to the store to get food for dinner." If we focus purely on the movements of muscles in the legs, and allow them to be separated from context, a whole action of this kind and its functional nature disappears. As we remove a place to go from and to (e.g., remove "stores" from consideration), the "walk" becomes disorganized and directionless. As we remove both the motivational and situational antecedents (e.g., not having the food needed at home; the approach of dinnertime; food deprivation) and the consequences of this action (e.g., obtaining and ultimately eating the food; entertaining family or friends at dinner), the walk becomes purposeless and ahistorical. Indeed, as we remove behavioral context and its history (e.g., the ongoing set and sequence of microactions involved in lifting one leg and then another; balancing on one foot in transition; the long history of millions of such steps and transitions in a lifetime that included "learning to walk" when those integrated actions were not known), "walking" itself disappears, and we are uncertain whether the muscle movement we are speaking of is twitching, kicking, wiggling, dancing, or any of thousands of other actions.

Mechanists deal with functional events by assembling a composite from the "elementary" pieces of interest. The assumptions of mechanism lead to the idea that the world is preorganized into parts, relations, and forces—one only has to discover the true underlying elements. Thus, an ontological claim underlies mechanism: The parts are already there; we must find them; without them, we cannot understand complexity. Contextualism makes no ontological claims at all. A functional unit is the unit, but it is so for pragmatic purposes brought into the situation by the analyst. Just as "going to the store" can be a functional unit, so too can "analyzing patients behavior into treatment responsive units." Actions are functional, including those of the clinician and scientist.

From the point of view of contextualism, determining the functional nature of a given event requires an ever-widening examination of context. As this process goes on, functional events continuously change their quality: What once was context becomes content, and more context needs to be sought. The movement of a leg that occurs in the context of particular sequences of leg movements is "walking," whereas the same movement in another context is "kicking." Once we are speaking of walking, however, further contextual examination shows that walking in the context of food preparation is different than walking for exercise, functionally speaking. Making a dinner in the context of having one's boss visit is different than making a private dinner to be eaten alone.

This could go on *ad infinitum*. What limits the process of examining context in an ever widening circle is the contextualist's pragmatic view of truth. The truth criterion of contextualism is successful working (Hayes et al., 1988; Pepper, 1942). The process of contextual explication is not thought of as "discovering" the "truth" but as a process of construing the situation so that effective action is possible. Thus, analysis for a contextualist "becomes important in reference to the end" (Pepper, 1942, p. 251). Skinner is quite clear about this: "It is true that we could trace human behavior not only to the physical conditions which shape and maintain it but also to the causes of those conditions and the causes of those causes, almost *ad infinitum*" but we need take analysis only to the point at which "effective action can be taken" (Skinner, 1974, p. 210). Thus, a "proposition is 'true' to the extent that with its help the listener responds effectively to the situation it describes" (p. 235). That stance on truth, built into behavior analysis, has a big impact on treatments that take a functional analytic approach.

It is also this pragmatic approach that makes goals so important in contextualism. In order to know whether one is responding effectively, it is necessary to know what effects are being sought. Thus, goals are foundational in contextualism, and different goals can lead to different types of contextualism (Hayes, 1993). Goals enable analysis by allowing successful working to be assessed, but goals can only be stated, not evaluated. This is because evaluation requires a measuring stick, and in contextualism, it is the analytic goal that is itself the measuring stick.

By far the most dominant form of contextualism is descriptive contextualism (Hayes, 1993). Examples include constructivism, hermeneutics, dramaturgy, narrative psychology, feminist psychology, and Marxism. Analysts in these forms seek an appreciation of the features of a whole event. Their analytic practices often look more like history than experimental science, and indeed, they often challenge the overblown knowledge claims of traditional science. Functional contextualists seek the prediction and influence of ongoing interactions between whole organisms and historically and situationally defined contexts. Analyses are sought that have precision (only certain terms and concepts apply to a given phenomenon), scope (principles apply to a range of phenomena), and depth (they cohere across scientific levels of analysis, such as biology, psychology, and cultural anthropology).

Behavior analysis is the dominant example of functional contextualism, and understanding that demystifies several features of behavior analysis (Hayes & Brownstein, 1986). Consider "environmentalism." If one adopts "prediction and influence" as a unified goal (i.e., if principles and theories should help accomplish both simultaneously), then it is logically necessary for analyses to include manipulable contextual variables. It is not possible to influence psychological events without changing their context. Only contextual variables can be manipulated directly. Thus, while analyses that begin and end in the domain of psychological dependent variables (e.g., emotion, thought, overt action) can achieve good levels of prediction, a gap necessarily exists between these analyses and the actions that might be taken to change psychological events. By understanding the contextualistic nature of behavior analysis, its environmentalism is revealed to be pragmatic, not dogmatic.

Each of these features in the previous discussion (function, context, situated truth, and purpose) is emphasized in ACT and in several of the other of the therapies in this volume. New behavior therapists are not moved very much by form: The issue is function. It is not enough to know that a thought or feeling of a particular form or intensity occurred to know whether this is a problem, for example. One also has to know the context in which it occurred and, through that analysis, the function it serves. Furthermore, once it is known to be a problem, it is not necessarily the case that it will be targeted directly. It is possible that the same event, formally defined, could become functionally inert by changing context rather than content.

This approach is revealed in the embrace of acceptance, defusion, mindfulness, and so on. In ACT, as in many of the new behavior therapies, there is a conscious posture of openness and acceptance toward psychological events, even if they are formally "negative," "irrational," or even "psychotic." What determines whether an event will be targeted for change is not form but function, and there is considerable flexibility about how it will be targeted. A "negative thought" mindfully observed will not necessarily have a negative function, even though it might in other contexts, such as one of literal truth or falsity. A difficult emotion accepted as an emotion will not necessarily have a negative function, even though it might in other contexts, such as one of resistance, suppression, or behavioral compliance.

Underlying an interest in what given psychological events serve is a view that truth is always itself a contextually situated function. We know the world only through our interactions in and with it, and these interactions are always historically and contextually limited. Thus, clients and therapists alike are often encouraged to hold an interest in the literal "truth" of their own thoughts or evaluations lightly. In ACT, this can be seen quite clearly, such as when clients are asked "not to believe a word" of ACT.

Finally, the foundational nature of goals in contextualism is reflected in the emphasis on chosen values as a necessary component of a meaningful life and a meaningful course of treatment. This is seen very clearly in DBT, behavioral activation (Jacobson, Martell, & Dimidjian, 2001), integrated behavioral couple therapy (IBCT; Christensen, Jacobson, & Babcock, 1995; Jacobson, Christensen, Prince, Cordova, & Eldridge, 2000), and ACT. Instead of pursuing truth, clients are encouraged to become passionately interested in how to live according to their own values, that is, how to accomplish their purposes.

Basic Theory: Relational Frame Theory

The second generation of behavior therapy emerged because the first generation failed to deal adequately with cognition. The second generation either adopted a more natural but also a more commonsense approach, or tried to make information processing do the necessary analytic work. A commonsense approach undermined the critically important link between behavior therapy and basic principles, but the information processes approach proved difficult to use as a basis of clinical change. The latter is not surprising, since most information processes analyses do not include clear historical or situational variables. Instead, the "cause" of cognitive function in most information-processing accounts is either in the material basis of cognitive systems (e.g., neurological events) or in the structure of cognitive systems themselves. It is not obvious how to alter either of these directly in therapy. Given current inadequacies in neuroscience, the form of cognitive systems tended to be targeted, but the information-processing theories generally did not specify precisely how contextual events can be changed to alter the structure or function of cognitive systems. This is a problem for therapists, since therapists are, after all, outside of the cognitive system being examined.

Behavior analysts can be interested in the nature of cognition, since private events are explicitly embraced (Skinner, 1945), but the analysis must be contextual: "We cannot account for the behavior of any system while staying wholly inside it" (Skinner, 1953, p. 35). ACT is based on a comprehensive functional contextual program of basic research on language and cognition called relational frame theory (RFT; Hayes, Barnes-Holmes, & Roche, 2001). The presence of such a research program is unique to ACT. ACT is an empirical clinical intervention that is tightly integrated with its own comprehensive basic science program on the nature of human cognition, itself composed of scores of human experimental studies.

RFT research has shown that human beings are extraordinarily able to learn to derive and combine stimulus relationships and to bring them under arbitrary contextual control. These derived stimulus relations, in turn, alter the functions of events that participate in relational networks—a process that is also under contextual control. Together, these features are argued to form the foundation of human language and higher cognition.

Nonarbitrary stimulus relations are those defined by formal properties of related events. Nonarbitrary stimulus relations impact strongly on the behavior of all complex organisms. For example, even insects might learn to approach the darker of two holes (Reese, 1968). Humans, however, can readily learn to relate events that are *not* formally related (Lipkens, Hayes, & Hayes, 1993). For example, having learned that x is "smaller than" X, humans may later be able to apply this stimulus relation to events under the control of arbitrary cues (such as the words *smaller than*). A very young child will know, say, that a nickel is bigger than a dime, but a slightly older child will learn that a nickel is "smaller than" a dime by attribution even though, in a formal sense, it is not.

There are three main properties of this kind of relational learning. First, such relations exhibit "bidirectionality"—a relation learned in one direction entails another in the opposite direction. If a person learns that A relates in a particular way to B in a context (the context is termed "C_{rel}" for "relational context"), then this must entail some kind of relation between B and A in that context. For example, a person who is taught that cold is the same as freezing will conclude that freezing is the same as cold. Second, such relations show combinatorial entailment: If a person learns in a particular context that A relates in a particular way to B, and B relates in a particular way to C, then this must entail some kind of mutual relation between A and C in that context. For example, if a child learns in a given context that a nickel is smaller than a dime, and a dime is smaller than a quarter, then he or she will conclude that a quarter is bigger than a nickel, and a nickel is smaller than a quarter. Finally, such relations enable a transformation of stimulus functions among related stimuli. If a child needs to buy candy and a dime is known to be valuable, in an appropriate context that selects this function (the context is termed "C_{func}" for "functional context"), then he or she will conclude that a nickel will be less valuable and a quarter will be more valuable, without necessarily directly purchasing candy with nickels and quarters. When all three features are established with a given type of relational responding, we call the performance a "relational frame."

What makes relational framing clinically relevant is that functions given to one member of related events tend to alter the functions of other members. Suppose a child has never before seen or played with a cat. After learning "C-A-T" → animal, and C-A-T → "cat," the child can derive four additional relations: animal → C-A-T, "cat" → C-A-T, "cat" → animal, and animal → "cat." Now suppose that the child is scratched while playing with a cat, cries, and runs away. When the child later hears father saying, "Oh, look! A cat," she may cry and run away even though scratches never occurred in the presence of the words "Oh, look! A cat." What brings these situations together is not their formal properties but the derived relations among them.

There are by now scores of studies on RFT (reviewed in Hayes et al.,

2001). The research program has now reached the point that virtually every key feature of the theory has been tested at least to some degree. While hardly "proven," no data currently exist that contradict the tenets of the theory.

RFT focuses ACT not merely on the nature of a relational network in a given situation (hardly a new idea, since in different terms that is what differentiated first- from second-generation behavior therapy) but on the contexts that can alter that network or its function. Thus, ACT has a technical account that can predict and explain the counterintuitive effects of first-order change efforts in the cognitive domain, or the pervasive effects of mindfulness, acceptance, defusion, and so on.

Theory of Psychopathology: Psychological Inflexibility

Even a small set of relational frames allows human beings to talk or think about events that are not present, to compare possible outcomes, and then to have these verbal relations alter how analyzed events function. Consider a simple problem: A door is locked. A human being might literally talk through the problem using only frames of coordination (e.g., naming), time or contingency (if . . . then), and comparison: If I do this, that will happen, which would be good. This process is enormously useful and seems to underlie the tremendous ecological success of human beings, who have become the dominant species on the planet despite being relatively weak, slow, and unprepared for physical combat.

Unfortunately, even such a small set of relational frames is enough to create human misery in the midst of ecological success. A socially anxious person might apply these same frames to a speaking situation: "If I avoid speaking, I won't get anxious, which is good." A depressed person might apply it to self-harm: "If I kill myself, I will stop suffering, which is good." With no more in the cognitive toolset than these kinds of relational behaviors frames, humans can worry about their performance; compare themselves or a partner unfavorably to an ideal, compare the present to a conceptualized past, or compare the present to a feared or favored future.

Although human language enables an explosion of indirect sources of control over human responding (and thus a considerable increase in the flexibility of the human repertoire), several key processes are fostered by relational frames that are repertoire narrowing. Three are described here.

The Ubiquity of Pain

Organisms are naturally especially attuned to aversive stimulation and should be so for evolutionary reasons. Relational frames enormously increase the reach of aversive events. For example, a dog that is kicked by a large man might whimper at the later sight of him, or those who look like him. A verbal human with the same experience could reconstruct that experience in any environmental context. Even formally contradictory events might occasion the relation (e.g., a birthday cake or a beautiful sunset might occasion the thought, "I used to be happy before I was abused"). What this means is that humans have a hugely expanded capacity for aversive stimulation and simultaneously cannot reduce psychological pain through simple situational solutions (e.g., avoid stimuli that are similar to painful events in the past).

Cognitive Fusion

Precisely because verbal events are so useful, language functions dominate over nonverbal functions. Thus, the increased psychological flexibility and creativity purchased by human language in some areas is paid for by the greatly increased inflexibility when responses are needed that are interfered with by literal evaluative rules. A well-established research literature shows that behavior governed by verbal rules tends to be relatively inflexible and rigid (see Hayes, 1989, for a book-length review). There are several known sources of this effect: Verbal rules tend to narrow the range of behavior available to make contact with more direct experiences; they tend to narrow the impact of contingencies themselves; they introduce or augment social compliance or resistance in otherwise less social situations; and, finally, they engage contingencies that strengthen rule generation and rule-following repertoires as such. The end result is that literal, evaluative strategies dominate in the regulation of human behavior, even when less literal and less judgmental strategies would be more effective.

Relational networks are extraordinarily difficult to break up, even with direct, contradictory training (Wilson & Hayes, 1996). Myriad derived relations are available to maintain and reestablish a given relational network. In practical terms, this means that elaborated relational networks continue to be elaborated. Detecting that one is deriving coherent relational networks (e.g., learning that one is "right") or that relating events is leading to effective outcomes (e.g., learning that one has "solved the problem"), and similar processes, in essence provide automatic reinforcement for the action of deriving stimulus relations. This constant generation of reasons and explanations fundamentally alters how psychological events function (see Addis & Jacobson, 1996, for supportive data on this point), yet the broad value of verbal analysis makes it very difficult to slow down language and cognition once it is well established, despite its instrumental nature. This combination of features means that stimulus functions from relational frames typically dominate over other sources of behavioral regulation in humans (what we term "cognitive fusion"), making an individual less in contact with here-and-now experience and direct contingencies, and more dominated by verbal rules and evaluations (Hayes, 1989).

Experiential Avoidance

Experiential avoidance is a nonarbitrary result of the domination of literal and evaluative language. Experiential avoidance is the phenomenon that occurs when a person is unwilling to remain in contact with particular private experiences (e.g., bodily sensations, emotions, thoughts, memories, behavioral predispositions) and takes steps to alter the form or frequency of these events and the contexts that occasion them, even when doing so creates harm. There is a substantial body of evidence that experiential avoidance is harmful in a variety of psychopathological areas (see Hayes, Wilson, Gifford, Follette, & Strosahl, 1996).

As language abilities have evolved, more and more constructs have been applied to private events, and these events have become enmeshed in evaluative verbal regulatory strategies. Originally, these terms were mere metaphors (e.g., being "inclined" to go was metaphorically related to physical objects that were literally "leaning toward going"; "anxiety" referred to a difficulty in breathing; and so on), but eventually they became concrete references to internal "things," and the emotional or cognitive states that were related to evaluated situations themselves acquired evaluative connotations. For example, it is normative to believe that "anxiety is bad," presumably in part because anxiety is a response to events that are themselves construed to be bad.

As a problem-solving repertoire, language and cognition are used to produce positive states of affairs and to avoid negative ones. Once thoughts and feelings themselves become evaluatively entangled, it is an obvious step to do the same thing with these private events, particularly because verbal processes increase the psychological presence of pain and decrease the adequacy of situational solutions to it.

The results are often unhelpful, because private events are historical and verbally entangled. Consider a negatively evaluated thought. In order to avoid a thought deliberately, a verbal rule must be followed specifying the thought to be avoided. Unfortunately, this rule itself contains the avoided thought, and to check on its success, that rule (and thus the thought) must be recontacted. The well-known paradox of thought suppression shows the problem clearly.

Many forms of psychopathology can be thought of as forms of experiential avoidance, yet the processes that give rise to it are inherent in literal language itself. As experiential avoidance takes hold, more stress and arousal are likely, which in turn occasion more evaluative verbal comparisons, and more self-focused avoidance strategies. This is a notably pathological process. Emotion-focused and avoidant strategies predict negative outcomes in depression (DeGenova, Patton, Jurich, & MacDermid, 1994), substance abuse (Ireland, McMahon, Malow, & Kouzekanani, 1994), the sequelae of child sexual abuse (Leitenberg, Greenwald, & Cado, 1992), and many others areas. Deliberate attempts to suppress thoughts and feelings can increase their occurrence and behavioral impact (Cioffi & Holloway, 1993; Clark, Ball, & Pape, 1991; Wegner, Schneider, Carter, & White, 1987), and can greatly complicate exposure-based strategies (Feldner, Zvolensky, Eifert, & Spira, 2003).

Theory of Change: Psychological Flexibility

The goal of ACT is to produce more psychological flexibility: the ability to change or to persist with functional behavioral classes when doing so serves valued ends. Since it is not possible to remove or eliminate language processes that create difficulty for human beings (nor would we want to, since these same processes are essential to human functioning), the goal is to bring these processes under contextual control.

The psychological space within which ACT works is shown in Figure 1.1. Six key processes are shown there. All six are aspects of the same process, which we have termed "psychological flexibility," because all six are linked to an alteration of the core language processes that interfere with such flexibility. ACT interventions can enter into that space through any of the subprocesses and can move through them in any given order. More specifically, ACT increases psychological flexibility by helping clients contact the costs of psychological inflexibility (this is not a specific item in Figure 1.1—rather, it is a process of contacting the costs of alternative psychological patterns), and then (1) establishing psychological acceptance skills; (2) establishing cognitive defusion skills; (3) distinguishing self-as-context from the conceptualized self; (4) contacting the present moment and establishing self-as-process skills; (5) distinguishing choice from reasoned action (necessary to avoid values clarification from becoming excessively rule-governed), clarifying values, and distinguishing them from goals and actions; and (6) teaching committed behavioral persistence and behavioral change strategies linked to choose values. All of this is then brought together into a process of developing larger and larger patterns of psychologically flexible and effective action.

These six processes can be divided into two major groups. The four processes on the left (acceptance, defusion, contact with the present moment, and self-as-context) together delineate acceptance and mindfulness skills from an ACT perspective. The four on the right (contact with the present moment, self-as-context, values, and committed action) together delineate commitment and behavior change skills from an ACT perspective. The reason ACT is called "acceptance and commitment therapy" is that these two larger sets of skills are united into a coherent whole in the ACT approach.

Therapeutic Assumptions and General Approach

ACT is a general clinical approach, not just a specific technology. There are already approximately a dozen specific ACT protocols for specific problems. The specific technologies used to create the psychological functions shown in Figure 1.1 may differ from problem to problem or setting to setting. If they are focused on and move these functions, the total package is ACT.

ACT takes the view that powerful and rapid change is often possible, even in difficult cases. This assumption is in part pragmatic, but it also flows from the underlying theory of change. As a behavior therapy, ACT takes the view that at the level of content, life's difficulties are historical and conditioned (e.g., classically conditioned emotional responding), and highly elaborated and networked in a verbal–cognitive sense. For that reason, psychological *content* tends to change relatively slowly. The *functions*

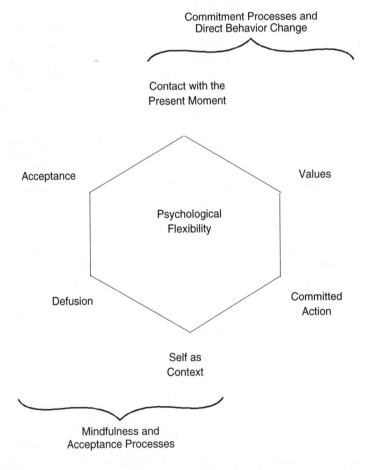

FIGURE 1.1. The facets of psychological flexibility according to the model of change underlying ACT.

example needed for me

of these events are contextual, however. A much smaller set of pivotal events, contextual change can lead to pervasive and rapid functional change.

Human beings will initially focus on difficult content as the core of their problems, but from an ACT perspective, it is the tendency to take these experiences literally and then to fight against them that is viewed as most harmful. This means that "anxiety" is not necessarily the problem in "anxiety disorders"—anxiety embraced is not necessarily a problem at all. A similar point would be made for "depressed mood" or "irrational thoughts," or any private experience supposedly linked mechanically to overt behavior.

This same point applied to the feelings and thoughts of the ACT therapist; ACT encourages therapist to open themselves up to their own difficult thoughts, feelings, memories, and bodily sensations. Thus, the therapeutic relationship in ACT tends to be an equal one: Both the client and therapist are swimming in the same verbal stream.

The key goal of ACT is to support clients in feeling and thinking what they directly feel and think already, as it *is*, not as what it *says it is*, and to help clients move in a valued direction, *with* all of their history and automatic reactions. Because language processes themselves are generally viewed as a source of psychologically rigid repertoires, ACT tends to use a relatively nonlinear form of language. ACT relies heavily on paradox, metaphors, stories, exercises, behavioral tasks, and experiential processes. Direct instruction, logical analysis, and persuasion have a relatively limited role. Even ACT-related concepts are treated in a deliberately flexible manner: The point is not to establish a new belief system, but rather to establish a more flexible repertoire, one that can change when change serves and persist when persistence serves.

ACT techniques are means to establish that kind of psychological flexibility. The process of ACT involves facing the costs of psychological inflexibility and its sources, particularly cognitive fusion (figuring it out, being right, giving reasons, treating oneself as a verbally evaluated object) and avoidance (suppression, passivity in the face of needed action). It also involves learning how to accept and defuse in various areas (emotions, self, thoughts, sensations) in which psychological rigidity has been dominant. It involves a deep interest is what one wants out of life and learning to build larger and larger and larger patterns of effective behavior linked to those goals and values.

similar to psa approaches

Techniques

There are several specific domains of ACT intervention, and each has its own specific methodology, exercises, homework, and metaphors. A book-length version of ACT is available that describes some common ACT technology (Hayes et al., 1999), so only a brief description is needed here. Even that book, however, is only part of what is available, since techniques are the most flexible part of ACT. An ACT protocol for children will differ from that for adults; one for coping with psychotic symptoms will differ from one for quitting smoking. At issue are the core processes: Even techniques created in the spur of the moment are "ACT" if they are focused on and move those processes.

Confronting the System: Creative Hopelessness

If the normal literal context really worked, there would be no need for a technology that fundamentally challenges such normal processes. Thus, often the first stage of ACT—especially for chronic or multiproblem patients—is a detailed examination of the cost of the current contextual situation. In this phase, ACT therapists examine carefully what the client has done to solve the problem and his or her actual experience of how workable those change agendas have been. Their unworkability has been experienced, but instead of generating variability, often it has generated only self-blame and yet another attempt to solve the problem using a direct, literal approach. The ACT therapist asks the client to consider the possibility that maybe the problem is not the techniques but their very purpose. In so doing, the ACT therapists essentially (or sometimes overtly) is asking: "Who do you believe: your mind or your experience?" The process is not so much persuasive as experiential and evocative.

The "person and the hammer" metaphor is an example of an ACT metaphor in this phase of therapy:

> "It would be as if you were to go to the doctor and say that you have a headache, and the doctor looks at you and sort of with your hand out of sight—behind your own back so to speak—you're hitting yourself in the head with a rubber hammer. You may not know that you're hitting yourself, or you might have a very good reason for doing so. It is unlikely that a doctor in that circumstance would want to give you aspirin for a headache, or tell you to wear a hat. What I see in this history you've given me is one attempt after another to reduce the pain, and that's certainly understandable. But what does your experience tell you about that? It seems that this whole effort is just another whack on the head. Now you not only feel bad, you feel bad that you feel bad. That's another whack. And then you've in essence asked other clinicians just what you are asking me now: might they have a really, really strong hat, or a really, really strong aspirin? Well, first, I don't. And, second, I suspect that when you find that out, the hammer will just come down again. 'I can't be helped.' Whack. It's not that you can't be helped. It's that what you've called 'help' are whacks to the head. When you have a headache like that it might be better to put down the hammer."

Control Is the Problem

Deliberate, literal, evaluative problem solving works everywhere except in places that are exacerbated by deliberate, literal, evaluative problem solving. This is hard to see, because in the vast majority of external situations, language can be used to get rid of things and the overarching rule is confirmed: Figure out how to get rid of it and get rid of it. Relational frames can have counterintuitive effects, however. For example, deliberately not thinking of something involves following a rule ("Don't think of x"), contains the avoided item (x), and thus will evoke it. Similarly, if a negative evaluation of anxiety is participating in actions with regard to it, anxiety will be elicited by those action, since anxiety is how humans respond to immanent negative events. In this part of ACT, a simple idea is put on the table: Conscious, deliberate, and purposeful control simply may not work very well with regard to the private experiences the client has been targeting. The following metaphor is designed to expose clients to the hopelessly rigged game deliberate control leads to in the world within:

> "Suppose I tell you right now, 'I don't want you to think about. . . . warm jelly donuts! You know how they smell when they first come out of the oven. . . . The taste of the jelly when you bite into the donut as the jelly squishes out the opposite side into your lap through the wax paper . . . the white flaky frosting on the top of the soft, rounded shape? Now it's very important, DON'T THINK ABOUT ANY OF THIS!' What just happened?"

In processing this metaphor (and similar metaphors or exercises), the client is asked to see whether he or she has been playing into a rigged game in attempts to control automatic thoughts, feelings, and memories.

Cognitive Defusion and Mindfulness Techniques

From an RFT perspective, the literal functions of language and cognition are not automatic or mechanical: They are contextual. Second-generation efforts to change thoughts can have a perverse effect: the C_{rel} events provided (e.g., "Don't think this—instead, think that") also serve as C_{func} events for the very thoughts being targeted (i.e., the change effort underlines and increases the importance of these thoughts themselves). Instead, ACT tends to alter C_{func} events so as to decrease the impact and importance of difficult private events. These cognitive defusion and mindfulness techniques erode the stimulus functions that occur through relational learning (Hayes & Wilson, 1994; Hayes et al., 1999).

The classic ACT defusion technique is the Milk, Milk, Milk exercise, first used by Titchener (1916, p. 425). It consists of an exploration of all of the properties of a single word. For example *milk* is white, creamy, and so on. This word is then said out loud by the therapist and client rapidly for about a minute. In the context of rapid repetition, the word quickly loses all meaning and becomes just a sound. It is clinically powerful to repeat the exercise with a single word variant of a clinical concern or troublesome thought the client may have (e.g., mean, stupid, weak, etc.) (Masuda, Hayes, Sackett, & Twohig, 2004). If later a client is deeply entangled in a negative thought, the ACT therapist might simply say quietly, "Milk, milk, milk," as if to ask the client to notice the process of thinking itself in the moment.

ACT sessions are often begun with mindfulness exercises, and they are used regularly throughout therapy. The Soldiers in the Parade exercise is an example:

> "I want to do a little exercise that will help underline the difference be-
> tween looking *at* thoughts, versus looking *from* thoughts. In a moment,
> I'm going to ask you to let yourself think anything you think. With each
> thought, imagine that there are little soldiers marching out of your ear
> and then in front of you, like a parade in front of a reviewing stand. The
> soldiers are carrying signs, and each thought is printed on a sign in the
> form of words or pictures. The task is simply this: Watch the parade and
> see how long you can go letting it flow by. If it stops for any reason—if
> you join the parade, leave the reviewing stand, become a soldier, or what-
> ever—see if you can catch back up just a moment and see what happened
> right before the observation of the parade stopped."

Clients are allowed a minute or two. For some clients, the parade will never start. For most, it will start and then stop. When either experience is examined, inevitably a thought occurred that the client "bought into" (e.g., the client will remember something that has to be done later and will begin planning or worrying). This exercise if often assigned as homework. The point is to begin to learn how to look at thoughts as thoughts rather than looking at the world through thoughts, and to learn how to detect the difference.

A Transcendent Sense of Self

Difficult thoughts and feelings appear to threaten the self, and in the sense of self as a conceptualize object, they do. For example, anxiety threatens the evaluation, "I'm a calm person." It is not realistic to ask clients to experience private events fully and without defense without providing psychological space within which that is possible. The first published ACT work was focused on how language itself provides a way to solve this problem through the continuity of consciousness that emerges from deictic relational frames such as I–you, here–there, and now–then (Hayes, 1984). RFT research has since begun to confirm the view that these frames create a sense of perspective (Hayes et al., 2001; McHugh & Barnes-Holmes, in press). Perspective taking is psychologically critical because it forms a direct experiential basis for human spirituality (Hayes, 1984). "Here now" is always the perspective from which events are directly experienced and thus cannot be threatened by the difficult nature of psychological content.

Various exercises are used to draw this out in ACT, including the Observer Exercise (a variant of the self-identification exercise developed by Assagioli, 1971, pp. 211–217). A metaphor that helps explain self as context is as follows:

"It's as if there is a chess board that goes out infinitely in all directions. It's covered with different colored pieces, black pieces and white pieces. They work together in teams, like in chess—the white pieces fight against the black pieces. You can think of your thoughts and feelings and beliefs as these pieces; they sort of hang out together in teams too. For example, 'bad' feelings (like anxiety, depression, and resentment) hang out with 'bad' thoughts and 'bad' memories. Same thing with the 'good' ones. Normally, the way the game is played is that we select which side we want to win. We put the 'good' pieces (like thoughts that are self-confident, feelings of being in control, etc.) on one side, and the 'bad' pieces on the other. Then we get up on the back of the white queen and ride to battle, fighting to win the war against our own thoughts and feelings. But there's a problem here. From this posture, huge portions of yourself *are your own enemy*. You've got to win; your life seemingly depends on it. But since time goes in one direction, not two, the pieces don't actually leave the board. You still remember your pain; you still can think scary thoughts. So the battle just goes on and on. But what is you aren't the pieces anyway. Maybe you are more like the board, and if you're the board, maybe its possible to let the game go on without having to live inside it."

Acceptance and Willingness

Etymologically, acceptance means "to take what is offered." In ACT, acceptance is not merely tolerance—it is the active nonjudgmental embracing of experience in the here and now. Acceptance involves undefended "exposure" to thoughts, feelings, and bodily sensations as they are directly experienced to be.

A wide variety of willingness and exposure exercises are used. What is important during these exercises is that the person let go of regulating private events and expose him- or herself to these events without the use of safety behaviors. This is a metaphor to explain the "letting go" quality of acceptance:

"It's like jumping versus stepping down. If you jump from a book, you put yourself in space and let gravity carry you to the ground. The same exact motion would be involved in jumping from a sheet of paper, or the roof of your house, or an airplane. Now stepping down is different. In that case, you never put yourself completely in the hands of gravity. . . . You maintain some degree of control with your leg muscles. But stepping down only works in some situations. You can step down from a book, but you can't step down from the roof of your house. So what we need to do is to practice jumping. We can pick the context, just like we can pick a book or a house to jump from. So we could pick the 7–11 or a big mall to go feel what it feels like to be anxious. Or we could go in for 1 minute or 15. But what we can't do is be willing provided anxiety is below 8 on a scale of 1 to 10. That's not acceptance; it's not willingness; it's not jumping. That's still controlling. It's stepping down."

Values

Values are chosen qualities of action that can be instantiated in behavior but not possessed like an object. ACT therapists ask their clients, "What do you want your life to stand for?" In this phase of treatment, a client is asked to list values in different life domains such as family, intimate relationships, health, spirituality, and so on. Various evocative exercises are used to develop more clarity about fundamental values. For example, the ACT therapist may ask the client to write out what he or she would most like to see on his or her tombstone, or the eulogy he or she would want to hear at his or her own funeral. Once values are clearer, concrete goals (achievable things or events) are identified that instantiate a valued path, and specific behaviors that might lead to these goals are described. Barriers to these actions are also identified. Almost always, these barriers are not so much situational as psychological, and these are dealt with through acceptance, exposure, mindfulness, and defusion. This feature distinguishes ACT from simple evocative therapies. The goal is not endless emotional wallowing. It is acceptance in the service of living a valued life.

Commitment

As in DBT, the "acceptance and change dialectic" (Linehan, 1993) is a focus throughout ACT work. ACT uses concrete homework and behavioral exercises to build larger and larger patterns of effective action. Specific commitments are made in specific areas, generally starting small, but quickly expanding an ever-widening DAVE cycle: defusion, acceptance, values, and engagement. Generally, clients start with small steps, but they continue to watch for emerging larger patterns. The goal is psychological flexibility, which involves taking full responsibility for these behavioral patterns: changing when change is needed, and persisting when persistence is needed. Thus, as its name implies, ACT is as much a change-oriented strategy as an acceptance-oriented one, but change is focused on areas that are readily changeable.

EMPIRICAL FINDINGS OF ACCEPTANCE AND COMMITMENT THERAPY

This chapter is not the place to review a rapidly changing empirical area. However, a brief examination of some of the available process and outcome findings seems warranted.

Process Data

From an ACT–RFT perspective, it is the repertoire-narrowing effects of cognitive fusion and avoidance that produce rigidity, since they prevent new contingency-shaped behavior and undermine healthy forms of extinction. Acceptance and defusion, in particular, have been examined in ACT process work. ACT has been shown to decrease the literal believability of negative thoughts. This seems to occur faster than in traditional CBT (Zettle & Hayes, 1986), and to predict ACT outcomes (e.g., Bach & Hayes, 2002; Hayes, Bissett, et al., in press). Acceptance has also been shown to be improved more rapidly in ACT than in comparison conditions (Bond & Bunce, 2000) and to mediate ACT outcomes (e.g., Bond & Bunce, 2000; Gifford et al., in press; Zettle, 2003).

It is worth noting that this analysis shares features of other accounts, such as Teasdale and colleagues' (2002) analysis of the impact of cognitive therapy (CT) and mindfulness-based cognitive therapy (MBCT), and Bouton, Mineka, and Barlow's (2001) analysis of the mechanisms of conditioning in panic disorder. Indeed, many of the other new behavior therapies also treat thoughts as thoughts, undermine avoidance, and focusing on new behaviors, including Behavioral Activation, DBT, MCBT, and modern interoceptive exposure methods (Barlow, 2002). Furthermore, in the earliest stages of therapy when clinical response is known to be particularly powerful (Ilardi & Craighead, 1994), traditional CT also helps clients distance themselves from their thoughts (cognitive distancing is one of the first steps in traditional CT approaches) and then to behave in different ways toward them (e.g., for purposes of "hypothesis testing"). Thus, the there may be a commonality in some areas among the processes targeted by the new behavior therapies more generally, and a possible partial explanation for some of the empirical anomalies of the second wave behavior therapies.

Outcome Data

A recent review of ACT (and DBT and functional analytic psychotherapy [FAP]) outcomes (Hayes et al., 2004) found effectiveness and efficacy studies in depression, psychosis, substance use disorders, chronic pain, eating disorders, work-related stress, and other problems. The literature is evolving rapidly, with the vast majority of published studies appearing since the publication of the first ACT manual (Hayes et al., 1999). Small randomized, controlled trials have shown ACT to be better than CT (Zettle & Hayes, 1986) or equivalent to group CT (Zettle & Raines, 1989) in depression. It has been found to be better than behavioral workplace modification training for workplace stress management (Bond & Bunce, 2000), and to produce dramatic reductions in rehospitalization among persons coping with positive psychotic symptoms (Bach & Hayes, 2002). It has been shown to be equivalent to systematic desensitization in dealing with math anxiety (Zettle, 2003), and to be superior to methadone alone when used in combination with methadone with polysubstance-abusing opiate-addicted individuals (Hayes, Wilson, et al., in press). It has been shown to be superior to nicotine replacement therapy (NRT) as a method of smoking cessation (Gifford et al., in press) and superior to cognitive-behavioral group therapy with behavioral measures of social anxiety (Block, 2002). A quasi-experimental effectiveness study of ACT has shown that ACT-trained clinicians produce significantly better coping outcomes in the full range of patients normally seen in outpatient settings, and do so more quickly and without as frequent use of medication referrals (Strosahl, Hayes, Bergan, & Romano, 1998). Many of these studies are small and thus preliminary, but the existing data are positive, both on outcomes and the underlying model of psychopathology and therapeutic change.

THE NEW BEHAVIOR THERAPIES

The new behavior therapies have brought a host of new ideas in the behavioral tradition, including mindfulness, acceptance, interoceptive exposure, cognitive defusion, values, focus on the present moment, and so on. It is worth noting that none of these methods is eliminative. Their implicit message is that the literal, evaluative, analytical, avoidant functions that dominate in a normal human mind are just a few of many functions that could occur. Similar to Langer's (1989) analysis of mindfulness, flexibility seems to be a process goal of almost all these new methods.

Although this is new, it echoes the old-fashioned behavioral wisdom of a constructional approach (Goldiamond, 1974), the very basis of early functional, behavioral accounts. Humans are historical organisms. Short of a lobotomy, humans do not get rid of previously established automatic functions so much as they add new ones (Wilson & Roberts, 2002). The language of reduction and elimination seems persuasive only because our conceptual focus and our measurement systems are themselves so narrow.

Mindfulness, acceptance, and defusion are not just different ways of treating traditionally conceptualized problems of depression or anxiety. They imply a redefinition of the problem, the solution, and how both should be measured. As with the even more ancient spiritual traditions from which many of these methods emerged (see Hayes, 2002a), the problem is not the presence of particular thoughts, emotions, sensations, or urges. It is the constriction of a human life.

This change is evolutionary as a matter of process—as all of the chapters in this volume show, behavior therapists are simply following the data. But it may well be revolutionary in its impact. It is truly new for empirical clinical approaches to embrace the kind of deep clinical and human issues that have previously been the province of nonempirical approaches. If the new behavior therapies continue down this road, the entire field of behavioral health seems bound to change in a fundamental way.

REFERENCES

Addis, M. E., & Jacobson, N. S. (1996). Reasons for depression and the process and outcome of cognitive-behavioral psychotherapies. *Journal of Consulting and Clinical Psychology, 64*, 1417–1424.

Assagioli, R. (1971). *The act of will.* New York: Viking.

Ayllon, T., Haughton, E., & Hughes, H. B. (1965). Interpretation of symptoms: Fact or fiction. *Behaviour Research and Therapy, 3*, 1–7.

Bach, P., & Hayes, S. C. (2002). The use of acceptance and commitment therapy to prevent the rehospitalization of psychotic patients: A randomized controlled trial. *Journal of Consulting and Clinical Psychology, 70*, 1129–1139.

Bandura, A. (1969). *Principles of behavior modification.* New York: Holt, Rinehart & Winston.

Barlow, D. H. (2002). *Anxiety and its disorders: The nature and treatment of anxiety and panic* (2nd ed.). New York: Guilford Press.

Beck, A. T. (1976). *Cognitive therapy and the emotional disorders.* New York: International Universities Press.

Beck, A. T. (1993). Cognitive therapy: Past, present, and future. *Journal of Consulting and Clinical Psychology, 61*, 194–198.

Beck, A. T., Rush, A. J., Shaw, B. F., & Emery, G. (1979). *Cognitive therapy of depression.* New York: Guilford Press.

Beck, R., & Perkins, T. S. (2001). Cognitive content-specificity for anxiety and depression: A meta- analysis. *Cognitive Therapy and Research, 25*, 651–663.

Bieling, P. J., & Kuyken, W. (2003). Is cognitive case formulation science or science fiction? *Clinical Psychology: Science and Practice, 10*, 52–69.

Biglan, A., & Hayes, S. C. (1996). Should the behavioral sciences become more pragmatic?: The case for functional contextualism in research on human behavior. *Applied and Preventive Psychology: Current Scientific Perspectives, 5*, 47–57.

Block, J. A. (2002). *Acceptance or change of private experiences: A comparative analysis in college students with public speaking anxiety.* Doctoral dissertation, University at Albany, State University of New York.

Bond, F. W., & Bunce, D. (2000). Mediators of change in emotion-focused and problem-focused worksite stress management interventions. *Journal of Occupational Health Psychology, 5,* 156–163.

Bookbinder, L. J. (1962). Simple conditioning vs. the dynamic approach to symptoms and symptom substitution: A reply to Yates. *Psychological Reports, 10,* 71–77.

Borkovec, T. D., & Roemer, L. (1994). Generalized anxiety disorder. In R. T. Ammerman & M. Hersen (Eds.), *Handbook of prescriptive treatments for adults* (pp. 261–281). New York: Plenum Press.

Bouton, M. E., Mineka, S., & Barlow, D. H. (2001). A modern learning theory perspective on the etiology of panic disorder. *Psychological Review, 108,* 4–32.

Burns, D. D., & Spangler, D. L. (2001). Do changes in dysfunctional attitudes mediate changes in depression and anxiety in cognitive behavioral therapy? *Behavior Therapy, 32,* 337–369.

Chambless, D. L., Sanderson, W. C., Shoham, V., Johnson, S. B., Pope, K. S., Crits-Christoph, P., et al. (1996). An update on empirically validated therapies. *Clinical Psychologist, 49,* 5–18.

Christensen, A., Jacobson, N. S., & Babcock, J. C. (1995). Integrative behavioral couple therapy. In N. S. Jacobson & A. S. Gurman (Eds.), *Clinical handbook of couple therapy* (pp. 31–64). New York: Guilford Press.

Cioffi, D., & Holloway, J. (1993). Delayed costs of suppressed pain. *Journal of Personality and Social Psychology, 64,* 274–282.

Clark, D. M., Ball, S., & Pape, D. (1991). An experimental investigation of thought suppression. *Behaviour Research and Therapy, 29,* 253–257.

DeGenova, M. K., Patton, D. M., Jurich, J. A., & MacDermid, S. M. (1994). Ways of coping among HIV-infected individuals. *Journal of Social Psychology, 134,* 655–663.

Dobson, K. S., & Khatri, N. (2000). Cognitive therapy: Looking backward, looking forward. *Journal of Clinical Psychology, 56,* 907–923.

Emery, G., & Campbell, J. (1986). *Rapid relief from emotional distress.* New York: Rawson.

Feldner, M. T., Zvolensky, M. J., Eifert, G. H., & Spira, A. P. (2003). Emotional avoidance: An experimental test of individual differences and response suppression using biological challenge. *Behaviour Research and Therapy, 41,* 403–411

Franks, C. M., & Wilson, G. T. (1974). *Annual review of behavior therapy: Theory and practice.* New York: Brunner/Mazel.

Freud, S. (1955). Analysis of a phobia in a five-year-old boy. In J. Strachey (Ed. & Trans.), *The standard edition of the complete psychological works of Sigmund Freud* (Vol. 10, pp. 1–149). London: Hogarth Press. (Original work published 1909)

Gifford, E. V., Kohlenberg, B. S., Hayes, S. C., Antonuccio, D. O., Piasecki, M. M., Rasmussen-Hall, M. L., & Palm, K. M. (in press). Applying a functional acceptance based model to smoking cessation: An initial trial of acceptance and commitment therapy. *Behavior Therapy.*

Goldiamond, I. (1974). Toward a constructional approach to social problems. *Behaviorism, 2,* 1–79.

Gortner, E. T., Gollan, J. K., Dobson, K. S., & Jacobson, N. S. (1998). Cognitive-behavioral treatment for depression: Relapse prevention. *Journal of Consulting and Clinical Psychology, 66,* 377–384

Hayes, S. C. (1984). Making sense of spirituality. *Behaviorism, 12,* 99–110.

Hayes, S. C. (Ed.). (1989). *Rule-governed behavior: Cognition, contingencies, and instructional control.* New York: Plenum Press.

Hayes, S. C. (1993). Analytic goals and the varieties of scientific contextualism. In S. C.

Hayes, L. J. Hayes, H. W. Reese, & T. R. Sarbin (Eds.), *Varieties of scientific contextualism* (pp. 11–27). Reno, NV: Context Press.

Hayes, S. C. (2002a). Buddhism and acceptance and commitment therapy. *Cognitive and Behavioral Practice, 9,* 58–66.

Hayes, S. C. (2002b). Getting to dissemination. *Clinical Psychology: Science and Practice, 9,* 424–429.

Hayes, S. C. (in press). Acceptance and commitment therapy, relational frame theory, and the third wave of behavior therapy. *Behavior Therapy.*

Hayes, S. C., Barnes-Holmes, D., & Roche, B. (Eds.). (2001). *Relational frame theory: A post-Skinnerian account of human language and cognition.* New York: Plenum Press.

Hayes, S. C., Bissett, R., Roget, N., Padilla, M., Kohlenberg, B. S., Fisher, G., et al. (in press). The impact of acceptance and commitment training and multicultural training on the stigmatizing attitudes and professional burnout of substance abuse counselors. *Behavior Therapy.*

Hayes, S. C., & Brownstein, A. J. (1986). Mentalism, behavior–behavior relations and a behavior analytic view of the purposes of science. *Behavior Analyst, 1,* 175–190.

Hayes, S. C., Follette, V. M., Dawes, R. M., & Grady, K. E. (Eds.). (1995). *Scientific standards of psychological practice: Issues and recommendations.* Reno, NV: Context Press.

Hayes, S.C., & Gregg, J. (2001). Factors promoting and inhibiting the development and use of clinical practice guidelines. *Behavior Therapy, 32,* 211–217.

Hayes, S. C., Hayes, L. J., & Reese, H. W. (1988). Finding the philosophical core: A review of Stephen C. Popper's *World Hypotheses. Journal of Experimental Analysis of Behavior, 50,* 97–111.

Hayes, S.C., Hayes, L. J., Reese, H. W., & Sarbin, T. R. (Eds.). (1993). *Variety of scientific contextualism.* Reno, NV: Context Press.

Hayes, S. C., Jacobson, N. S., Follette, V. M., & Dougher, M. J. (Eds.). (1994). *Acceptance and change: Content and context in psychotherapy.* Reno, NV: Context Press.

Hayes, S. C., Masuda, A., Bissett, R., Luoma, J., & Guerrero, L. F. (2004). DBT, FAP, and ACT: How empirically oriented are the new behavior therapy technologies? *Behavior Therapy, 35,* 35–54.

Hayes, S. C., Strosahl, K. D., & Wilson, K. G. (1999). *Acceptance and commitment therapy: An experiential approach to behavior change.* New York: Guilford Press.

Hayes, S. C., & Wilson, K. G. (1994). Acceptance and commitment therapy: Altering the verbal support for experiential avoidance. *Behavior Analyst, 17,* 289–303.

Hayes, S. C., Wilson, K. G., Gifford, E. V., Bissett, R., Piasecki, M., Batten, S. V., et al. (in press). A randomized controlled trial of twelve-step facilitation and acceptance and commitment therapy with polysubstance abusing methadone maintained opiate addicts. *Behavior Therapy.*

Hayes, S. C., Wilson, K. G., Gifford, E. V., Follette, V. M., & Strosahl, K. (1996). Emotional avoidance and behavioral disorders: A functional dimensional approach to diagnosis and treatment. *Journal of Consulting and Clinical Psychology, 64,* 1152–1168.

Ilardi, S. S., & Craighead, W. E. (1994). The role of nonspecific factors in cognitive-behavior therapy for depression. *Clinical Psychology: Science and Practice, 1,* 138–156.

Ilardi, S. S., & Craighead, W. E. (1999). Rapid early response, cognitive modification, and nonspecific factors in cognitive behavior therapy for depression: A reply to Tang and DeRubeis. *Clinical Psychology: Science and Practice, 6,* 295–299.

Ireland, S. J., McMahon, R. C., Malow, R. M., & Kouzekanani, K. (1994). Coping style as a predictor of relapse to cocaine abuse. In L. S. Harris (Ed.), *Problem of drug dependence, 1993: Proceedings of the 55th annual scientific meeting* (National Institute on

Drug Abuse Monograph Series No. 141, p. 158). Washington, DC: U.S. Government Printing Office.

Jacobson, N. S. (1997). Can contextualism help? *Behavior Therapy, 28,* 435–443.

Jacobson, N. S., & Christensen, A. (1996). *Integrative couple therapy: Promoting acceptance and change.* New York: Norton.

Jacobson, N. S., Christensen, A., Prince, S. E., Cordova, J., & Eldridge, K. (2000). Integrative behavioral couple therapy: An acceptance-based, promising new treatment for couple discord. *Journal of Consulting and Clinical Psychology, 68,* 351–355.

Jacobson, N. S., Dobson, K. S., Truax, P. A., Addis, M. E., Koerner, K., Gollan, J. K., et al. (1996). A component analysis of cognitive-behavioral treatment for depression. *Journal of Consulting and Clinical Psychology, 64,* 295–304.

Jacobson, N. S., Martell, C. R., & Dimidjian, S. (2001). Behavioral activation treatment for depression: Returning to contextual roots. *Clinical Psychology: Science and Practice, 8,* 255–270.

Langer, E. J. (1989). *Mindfulness.* Reading, MA: Addison-Wesley.

Leitenberg, H., Greenwald, E., & Cado, S. (1992). A retrospective study of long-term methods of coping with having been sexually abused during childhood. *Child Abuse and Neglect, 16,* 399–407.

Linehan, M. M. (1993). *Cognitive-behavioral treatment of borderline personality disorder.* New York: Guilford Press.

Lipkens, G., Hayes, S. C., & Hayes, L. J. (1993). Longitudinal study of derived stimulus relations in an infant. *Journal of Experimental Child Psychology, 56,* 201–239.

Mahoney, M. J. (1974). *Cognition and behavior modification.* Cambridge, MA: Ballinger.

Mahoney, M. J. (2002). Constructivism and positive psychology. In C. R. Snyder & S. J. Lopez (Eds.), *Handbook of positive psychology* (pp. 745–750). London: Oxford University Press.

Masuda, A., Hayes, S. C., Sackett, C. F., & Twohig, M. P. (2004). Cognitive defusion and self-relevant negative thoughts: Examining the impact of a ninety year old technique. *Behaviour Research and Therapy, 42,* 477–485.

McHugh, L., & Barnes-Holmes, Y. (in press). Perspective-taking as relational responding: A developmental profile. *Psychological Record.*

Meichenbaum, D. H. (1977). *Cognitive-behavior modification: An integrative approach.* New York: Plenum Press.

Morgenstern, J., & Longabaugh, R. (2000). Cognitive-behavioral treatment for alcohol dependence: A review of evidence for its hypothesized mechanisms of action. *Addiction, 95,* 1475–1490.

Nurnberger, J. I., & Hingtgen, J. N. (1973). Is symptom substitution an important issue in behavior therapy? *Biological Psychiatry, 7,* 221–236.

Öst, L.-G. (2002, July). *CBT for anxiety disorders: What progress have we made after 35 years of randomized clinical trials?* Keynote address, British Association for Behavioural and Cognitive Psychotherapy, Warwick, UK.

Pepper, S. C. (1942). *World hypotheses: A study in evidence.* Berkeley: University of California Press.

Reese, H. W. (1968). *The perception of stimulus relations: Discrimination learning and transposition.* New York: Academic Press.

Rounsaville, B. J., Carroll, K. M., & Onken, L. S. (2001). A stage model of behavioral therapies research: Getting started and moving from Stage I. *Clinical Psychology: Science and Practice, 8,* 133–142.

Schraml, W., & Selg, H. (1966). Behavior therapy and psychoanalysis. *Psyche, 29,* 529–546.

Segal, Z. V., Williams, J. M. G., & Teasdale, J. D. (2001). *Mindfulness-based cognitive therapy for depression: A new approach to preventing relapse.* New York: Guilford Press.

Skinner, B. F. (1945). The operational analysis of psychological terms. *Psychological Review, 52,* 270–276.

Skinner, B. F. (1953). *Science and human behavior.* New York: Free Press.

Skinner, B. F. (1974). *About behaviorism.* New York: Knopf.

Strosahl, K. D., Hayes, S. C., Bergan, J., & Romano, P. (1998). Assessing the field effectiveness of acceptance and commitment therapy: An example of the manipulated training research method. *Behavior Therapy, 29,* 35–64.

Tang, T. Z., & DeRubeis, R. J. (1999). Reconsidering rapid early response in cognitive behavioral therapy for depression. *Clinical Psychology: Science and Practice, 6,* 283–288.

Teasdale, J. D., Moore, R. G., Hayhurst, H., Pope, M., Williams, S., & Segal, Z. V. (2002). Metacognitive awareness and prevention of relapse in depression: Empirical evidence. *Journal of Consulting and Clinical Psychology, 70,* 275–287.

Titchener, E. B. (1916). *A text-book of psychology.* New York: Macmillan.

Wegner, D. M., Schneider, D. J., Carter, S. R., & White, T. L. (1987). Paradoxical effects of thought suppression. *Journal of Personality and Social Psychology, 53,* 5–13.

Wells, A. (1994). Attention and the control of worry. In G. C. L. Davey & F. Tallis (Eds.), *Worrying: Perspectives on theory, assessment and treatment* (pp. 91–114). Oxford, UK: Wiley.

Wilson, G. T. (1999). Rapid response to cognitive behavior therapy. *Clinical Psychology: Science and Practice, 6,* 289–292.

Wilson, K. G., & Hayes, S. C. (1996). Resurgence of derived stimulus relations. *Journal of the Experimental Analysis of Behavior, 66,* 267–281.

Wilson, K. G. & Roberts, M. (2002). Core principles in acceptance and commitment therapy: An application to anorexia. *Cognitive and Behavioral Practice, 9,* 237–243.

Wolpe, J. (1980). Cognitive behavior: A reply to three commentaries. *American Psychologist, 35,* 112–114.

Wolpe, J., & Rachman, S. (1960). Psychoanalytic "evidence": A critique based on Freud's case of little Hans. *Journal of Nervous and Mental Disease, 131,* 135–148.

Yates, A. J. (1958). Symptoms and symptom substitution. *Psychological Review, 65,* 371–374.

Zettle, R. D. (2003). Acceptance and commitment therapy (ACT) vs. systematic desensitization in treatment of mathematics anxiety. *Psychological Record, 53,* 197–215.

Zettle, R. D., & Hayes, S. C. (1986). Dysfunctional control by client verbal behavior: The context of reason-giving. *Analysis of Verbal Behavior, 4,* 30–38.

Zettle, R. D., & Hayes, S. C. (1987). Component and process analysis of cognitive therapy. *Psychological Reports, 64,* 939–953.

Zettle, R. D., & Raines, J. C. (1989). Group cognitive and contextual therapies in treatment of depression. *Journal of Clinical Psychology, 45,* 438–445.

2

Dialectical Behavior Therapy

Synthesizing Radical Acceptance with Skillful Means

Clive J. Robins, Henry Schmidt III, *and* Marsha M. Linehan

The universe is so constructed that the opposite of a true statement is a false statement, but the opposite of a profound truth is usually another profound truth.
— NIELS BOHR (quoted in Wilber, 1977, p. 27)

Dialectical behavior therapy (DBT) began as a simple application of the standard behavior therapy of the 1970s to treat suicidal individuals (Linehan, 1987). The idea was that individuals who wanted to be dead did not have the requisite skills to build a life worth living. The aim of the treatment was to build these skills. Individuals with multiple suicide attempts were accepted into treatment, and an approach designed to teach requisite skills was attempted. To change the problematic behaviors, DBT began as an application of both social behaviorism (e.g., Skinner, 1974; Staats, 1975; Staats & Staats, 1963) and the traditional practices of clinical behavior therapy (Goldfried & Davison, 1976; O'Leary & Wilson, 1987) that had led to the development of efficacious treatments for many other disorders. Traditional problem-solving strategies such as skills training, exposure, and contingency management were integrated within this framework. In developing the treatment, it quickly became apparent that a treatment focused solely on change would not work. Most of these multiple-suicide attempters were extremely sensitive to criticism and prone to emotion dysregulation. Efforts at change quickly led to increased and at times overwhelming arousal, resulting in either emotional shutdown or, more rarely, storming out of sessions on the one hand, or an attack on the therapist on the other. Dropping the emphasis on change, however, often had equally problematic consequences. Clients interpreted this as the therapist ignoring or treating as of little consequence their palpable suffering. Either extreme hopelessness or rage at the therapist for apparent insensitivity was not infrequent. From either therapeutic stance, an exclusive focus on change or on acceptance, clients experienced their therapist as invalidating not only specific behaviors but also the client as a whole. Research by Swann, Stein-Seroussi, and Giesler (1992) may explain how such perceived invalidation leads to problematic behavior in therapy. Their research revealed that when an individual's basic self-constructs are not verified, the individual's arousal increases. The increased arousal then leads to cognitive dysregulation and the failure to process new information.

To work effectively, keeping both client and therapist in the room working on the problems at hand, the therapist had to somehow figure out how to hold both acceptance and change in the therapy simultaneously, a synthesis that, when found, could engender both new client change and new acceptance. The wish to change every painful experience had to be balanced with a corresponding effort at learning to accept life's inevitable pain for a number of reasons. First, it was impossible to work on changing one set of problems if the client could not at least temporarily tolerate the pain of other problems. Without tolerance, at least for a short time, all problems converged and threatened to overwhelm both the client and the therapy. Second, the inability to accept one's own behavior prohibits any ability to change, because it leads either to withdrawal and avoidance or, alternatively, to emotional responses such as rage or intense shame. Both interfere with the observation and self-understanding necessary for effective change. It was as necessary for the client to hold the synthesis of acceptance and change as it was for the therapist. Although treatment of severe disorders requires the synthesis of many dialectical polarities, that of acceptance and change, the theme of much of this volume, is the most fundamental. It was the necessity of this synthesis that led to considering use of the term "dialectical" as a descriptor of the standard behavior therapy applied in the treatment.

Core elements of DBT (Linehan, 1989) include (1) a biosocial theory of disorder that emphasizes transactions between biological disposition and learning; (2) a developmental framework of stages of treatment; (3) a hierarchical prioritizing of treatment targets within each stage; (4) delineation of the functions that treatment must serve, and treatment modes to fulfill those functions; and (5) sets of acceptance strategies, change strategies, and dialectical strategies. Rather than providing a comprehensive description of each of these aspects of the treatment (e.g., Ivanoff, Brown, & Linehan, 2001; Linehan, Cochran, & Kehrer, 2001; Robins, Ivanoff, & Linehan, 2001; Robins & Koons, 2004), here we focus on the characteristics that most distinguish DBT from more standard behavioral therapies, including (1) a dialectical philosophical framework, (2) the integration of Zen principles and practices within a treatment focused on the application of Western social behavioral principles (Heard & Linehan, in press), and (3) the therapist acceptance strategies of validation, reciprocal communication style, and environmental intervention, which are used in balance with the change strategies of problem solving, irreverent communication style, and consultation with clients about their environment, respectively.

THE DIALECTICS OF DIALECTICAL BEHAVIOR THERAPY

Dialectics has been referred to as the logic of process. Most often associated with Marx and Marxist socioeconomic principles, the philosophy of dialectics actually extends back thousands of years (Bopp & Weeks, 1984; Kaminstein, 1987). Hegel is generally credited with reviving and elaborating the dialectical position. He discerned that specific forms or arguments come and go in a complex interplay, with each argument creating its own contradiction, and each contradiction in turn being negated by a synthesis that often includes or enlarges upon both preceding arguments, beginning the entire process anew. What remains consistent, and thus becomes worthy of study and philosophical explication, is the process of change. Hegel wrote that "appearance is the process of arising and being and passing away again, a process that itself does not arise and pass away, but is per se, and constitutes reality and the life-movement of truth" (cited in Weiss, 1974, p. 8). As such, "the truth of the process is not to be found in any of its single phases, but in its totality (which is no mere plurality), the rational rhythm of the organic whole" (p. 8).

Dialectics has been offered as a coherent system of exploring and understanding our world (Basseches, 1984; Kaminstein, 1987; Levins & Lewontin, 1985; Riegel, 1975; Wells, 1972) and is often given as an alternative to the classificatory logic found in traditional science. After all, "real life operates dialectically, not critically" (Berman, 1981, p. 23). As a worldview, dialectics embodies both static and active principles, or understandings. It speaks to an underlying nature of reality and, as with all good worldviews, a deep understanding of its tenets alters one's experience of the world and activities therein. Thus, it serves as both a description of reality and an articulation of some broad principles found within that description, and as an articulation of the activity of reality. In fact, dialectics articulates the interaction between understanding (knowledge) and action (Linehan & Schmidt, 1995; Reese, 1993).

Briefly, dialectical observations that influence DBT are as follows:

- A whole is a relation of differing parts that hold no independent significance.
- The whole is more than the sum of its parts.
- Parts and wholes are interrelated (and defined in relation to one another).
- Change is an aspect of all systems, and is present at all levels of any given system.

First, it is assumed that a "whole" is a relation of heterogeneous "parts" that hold no intrinsic or previous significance in and of themselves. The parts are important only in relation to one another, and in relation to the whole, which they help to define. (To dispense with the distraction of placing quotation marks around the words *part* and *whole* or the duration of the chapter, we will simply assume that the inherent subjectivity of such a view is noted by the reader.) The two are indivisible within the dialectical reasoning. Levins and Lewotin (1985) point out that the consideration of phenomena as heterogeneously composed has important implications on scientific inquiry. The fact that parts are not merely diverse, but actually are in contradiction or opposition to one another, focuses the observer not on a taxonomical identification of the parts, but rather on the relationship or interaction of the two as they move toward resolution. Also, the fact that wholes comprise heterogeneous parts argues that "there is no basement," no fundamental unit or particle. What is fundamental is the pattern of relationship.

A second tenet of dialectics states that parts acquire properties only as a result of being identified as parts of a particular whole. Thus, the same part may have very different qualities or properties if viewed as an aspect of different wholes. Of course, parts of different wholes will embody different contradictions and dialectical syntheses. A third tenet is that parts and wholes are interrelations, not a mere collision of objects with fixed properties and immutable boundaries. As such, the parts cannot participate in creating the whole without simultaneously being affected themselves by the whole. Thus, it is argued, for instance, that it is not possible for the clients of a particular mental health center not to somehow alter the system within which they interact (and which would not exist without them), and it is certainly the case that they will simultaneously be affected by the system. Nor can there be change within the intrapersonal sphere, in one behavioral response system without a corresponding impact, for or against the client's benefit, upon other systems. This inherent interdependence of behavioral systems argues against any theoretical system that purports that one system (e.g., cognitive or biological) is somehow more important than another.

Fourth, as mentioned already, dialectics recognizes change to be an aspect of all systems, and to be present at all levels of a system. Stability is the rare occurrence, not the idealized goal. However, as Levins and Lewontin (1985) point out, dialectics should not be viewed as some dynamic balance or homeostatic environment; it is neither the careful balance of opposing forces nor the melding of two open currents. Rather, dialectics involves the complex interplay of opposing forces. The white yin and black yang of eastern philosophies do not combine to form a tepid, gray mush, but rather continue to oppose one another, surging here and receding there as they respond to both internal and external forces. Equilibrium among forces, when found, is discovered at a higher level of observation, namely, by looking at the overall process of affirming, negating, and the formation of a new, more inclusive synthesis of the two (Basseches, 1984). What is stable is the continued interplay of forces; there can be no final domination. Thus, change is not the superficial pattern masking some underlying stability; it is the underlying dance of the world, and stasis is our own imposition of convenience based upon societal values (Levins & Lewontin, 1985).

Furthermore, essential in any discussion of dialectics is the commonly known sequence of thesis–antithesis–synthesis, embodying not a static relation of events but rather a complex interplay inherent in the nature of truth, or competing truths. Reality is an activity, not an event, movement rather than repose. In fundamental terms, contradictory truths stand side by side. Apparently opposing events or statements are highly dependent upon each other for existence, and resolvable at further levels of abstraction or across time. A "beginning" is nonexistent without an "end" or "middle." The meaningfulness of life does not negate its meaninglessness, and synthesis may involve acknowledging the huge influence of our actions locally, while distal meanings (in time and space) are inherently unknowable. Notice that the process of thesis–antithesis does not yield a dilution of either, but rather an interplay of both at full force, a shifting of field and ground or black and white that diminishes the intensity or clarity of neither. Life is both intensely meaningful and painfully meaningless (or liberating, to some). Our clients intensely desire change and are often highly fearful of failing or making the attempt. The experience is not the average of mild disinterest, but rather is an interplay of hope and excitement (in some instances) and dread or panic. Changing is both hopeful and terrifying.

An application of the dialectical worldview, dialectical materialism emphasizes that understanding and prediction of the world are, in fact, measured through activity rather than logic (Reese, 1993). A central concept of dialectical materialism is "praxis," defined as action in the world for a specific purpose, or goal-directed activity. Our actions are the employment of our knowledge, and the degree of success of a given action directly reflects the accuracy of our understanding of the world. Yet there is no static variable that constitutes the world, either "out there" or "in here." The world is altered by our actions, and we ourselves are also changed. Thus, a future interaction involves a different context (world and self); this is the wisdom underlying "never stepping into the same stream twice." Neither river nor walker is identical, although many characteristics of each may remain unchanged. Thus, knowledge itself is a process reflected in purposeful action (to distinguish it from theory) and shaped by outcomes. In this way, dialectics articulates a soundly contextual process and understanding of reality. Furthermore, it dictates an active process of knowing by interacting with the data of action rather than spending time developing beliefs about what "should" occur. We work as a manifestation of our knowledge; the outcomes of our actions enhance our knowledge. We are thus changed, as is our world.

In this view, theory is ever in development and not separable from action (as above). Our understanding of how to work with a given client in the midst of his or her dysregulation is informed by the outcomes of our current interactions. Comments followed by a click and dial tone are "failures" when measured by the rule of "helpful and engaging." Comments that are followed by another question from the client, or by statements of intent ("I'll try that") or even appreciation, are "successes" by the same rule, and will likely inform our beliefs about what is "effective" with this particular client when he or she is distressed. This knowledge, in turn, is likely to affect our actions in future similar circumstances. Importantly, however, dialectics articulates a verbal and reflective philosophy rather than strictly operant processes (see Hayes, 1993). "Effectiveness" must be measured by a verbally acknowledged, predefined goal; thus, truth in this sense relies on the ability to articulate a goal and interact with ones environment to achieve it.

Dialectical idealism is the philosophy associated with Hegel, and it reflects a teleological unfolding of Truths occurring within a universe that is nothing but activity, manifesting itself in opposing tensions and resolution (Weissman, 1974). Thus, even in a world devoid of human understanding and reflection, reality has as its basis an ever-changing process, an unfolding in perpetuity. While specific forms may arise and fall away, the process of change is never-ending. DBT makes use of both applications of dialectics, referring clients to the outcomes of their actions (as evaluated by intended or desired outcomes), and also to the more values-oriented analyses of "good" and "bad," "pain" and "pleasure," and so on.

Dialectics, DBT, and Relationship

A dialectical understanding and approach infuses the actions of the therapist in the therapeutic relationship. From a dialectical perspective, the therapeutic relationship is the context in which a more accurate worldview and resulting set of behaviors are fostered. Problematic or maladaptive behaviors are failures to gain or incorporate accurate knowledge of one's environment, or inability to utilize this information to organize purposive behavior. It is within the therapeutic relationship that either or both of these broad issues are addressed. Furthermore, the client comes to treatment with a unique and unstated history and set of assumptions, and it is within the relational context that this history and the complement of expectations are played out.

In DBT, the therapeutic relationship is discussed as a necessarily potent environmental variable. In fact, the early goals of therapy are to establish oneself as a high-valence element of the client's environment, taking steps to quickly identify qualities that increase client behaviors of engaging, revealing, and responding. Understanding the client's goals and agreeing on the goals of therapy (beginning with reduction of suicidality, if that is present) are begun during the pretreatment phase of therapy, and dialectically create a context that allows both client and therapist to evaluate the success of future actions. It further establishes a thesis that will be returned to throughout the course of treatment: the desire to change oneself or one's behavior in clearly articulated ways. As noted earlier, the optimism of this statement will likely be met with fears and judgments concerning change.

As an individual in relationship with the client, the therapist offers both context and response to the client's behavior. As an independent actor in the world, the therapist may stand alongside the client and view the world, examining actions and beliefs, and offering a (we hope more accurate) assessment of validity and effectiveness. To the extent that such messages are delivered in a language, at a point, and with skill such that the client can incorporate them into his or her worldview, the therapeutic relationship becomes a context for interpretation of the world. Rules are made explicit, experiments are carried out (role plays, radically genuine responding, cue removal and/or exposure, etc.) in an environment that can be controlled, and that offers contingencies designed to increase client awareness and effectiveness. In this sense, the therapist must be aware of the "rules of the world" as the client is likely to experience it (given his or her individual characteristics, social norms and practices, etc.), the client's view of the world, and most importantly, be highly sensitive to the client's limitations in terms of tolerating corrective feedback. The meaning of "therapeutic relationship" contextually implies a structuring of experience that facilitates the client's ability to both know and act effectively, improving the skills of recognizing important contextual variables, and modifying behaviors accordingly in order to achieve stated goals.

As actor, the therapist utilizes the qualities and behaviors of him- or herself to increase the likelihood of client contact with reality and effective action. Thus, the high valence and ability to relationally reinforce behavior improves not only the ability to influence client behavior (e.g., through valence, timeliness, intensity of response) but also the generalizability of client behaviors through the use of natural relational versus arbitrary responses. The qualities of warmth, attentiveness and availability, engagement, genuineness, as well as the strategies of reciprocal self-disclosure, environmental intervention, praise or acknowledgment, cheerleading, and so on, are all examples of therapeutic interventions intended to increase client effectiveness and knowledge. Recognizing that the outpatient therapist has a limited window into, and proportional time to influence the client, the therapist seeks to increase effectiveness and "presence" through structuring homework exercises, encouraging telephone contact when needed, and providing tape recordings of sessions, readings, or other means of extending the context of the therapeutic relationship. The principle that the whole is inseparable from its parts, and that each has a mutual influence on the other, dictates that one create a functional environment to support functional behavior (and reduce dysfunctional behavior).

To the extent that treatment is effective in identifying the function of maladaptive behaviors and teaching replacement skills, relational responses can reinforce successively appropriate responses to prompting stimuli and maintain the motivation of the client. Thus, the practice of the client is shaped into increasingly effective behavior, and the therapeutic relationship becomes an integral part of the environmental response. While early treatment responses may include arbitrary and therapeutically manipulated social responses, it is important that the final stages of treatment primarily include responses that are socially appropriate and expectable, with therapy terminating as the client's expectations and behaviors more or less accurately mirror the contingencies found and contextual responding likely to be effective in a broader social context. The therapeutic relationship is both foil and force, reflecting reality and shaping client behavior as action leads to knowledge, which then further shapes action in the never-ending dance of constant change.

CORE MINDFULNESS:
THE SYNTHESIS OF ACCEPTANCE AND SKILLFUL MEANS

Mindfulness is both dictated by dialectics and at the center of DBT. It is both the practice of the therapist and the core skill taught to clients. Mindfulness has to do with the quality of both awareness and participation that a person brings to everyday living. It is a way of living awake, with one's eyes wide open. The roots of mindfulness practice are in the contemplative practices common to both Eastern and Western spiritual disciplines, and the emerging scientific knowledge about the benefits of "allowing" experiences rather than suppressing or avoiding them. Both Eastern and Western psychologies, as well as spiritual practices, are converging on the same insights. As a set of skills, mindfulness practice is the intentional process of observing, describing, and participating in reality nonjudgmentally, in the moment, and with effectiveness (i.e., using skillful means). In formulating these skills, DBT drew primarily from the practice of Zen (e.g., Aitken, 1982), but the skills are compatible with Western contemplative (e.g., Pennington, 1980), and Eastern meditation practices (e.g., Hahn, 1976).

Dialectical theory all but demands mindfulness as a critical element. Distraction, distortion (i.e., judgmentalness, alienation, etc.), and rule-driven behavior each undermine the understanding and practice of dialectics. Mindfulness as observation and mindfulness as engagement (e.g., participating without separation) are pure manifestations of activity directed at knowledge–action. To observe correctly is to intuit the accurate nature of reality, to be aware simultaneously of parts and interrelations of parts in the grand structure and process of unfolding. To be mindfully aware is to open oneself to the activity of exploration and inquiry, to complete the essential function of data collection and evaluation with as clear-eyed an approach as possible. To see clearly is to increase knowledge, later to be exemplified in the "skillful means" of effective action. To observe with judgment is to place a priori value on phenomena and relations, to refuse to allow the parts to interact "as they do" rather than "as they should."

Radical Acceptance

Acceptance is both an outcome and an activity in DBT. The experience of acceptance is one result of understanding the world contextually and dialectically. Of course, our clients act as they do given their learning history, beliefs/expectations, and current experiences. Of course, we respond the way we do given the same. The Zen concept that "all is as it should be" refers not to the snapshot view of reality (we all know that everything is not perfect in this moment), but rather to the dependent unfolding view of reality (given the preexisting conditions, how could things be different?) and the recognition of valuation as human-generated rather than universally intrinsic (perfect for whom, based upon which criteria?). Thus, the experience of acceptance (related to siezing, taking, catching) is that of "getting it," opening oneself to the context, striving to wait for understanding rather than leap in precipitously, acknowledging distress as an understandable outcome in clients and ourselves rather than as a problem to be solved. Indeed, viewing distress as a response to preexisting conditions (antithesis, part of the whole) rather than as a disconnected problem to be solved encourages one to widen one's context of understanding to find the contextually appropriate resolution (synthesis) rather than impulsively jump to reduce it, ignoring the powerful contextual variables that seldom respond to "quick fixes." Thus, acceptance as a state or experience may reflect the wisdom of wanting to gather rather than disperse, catching the context while enduring the moment.

As a practice, acceptance is highly important in working with impulsive, highly sensitive, and reactive clients. Validation is an active acknowledgment, often offered as antithesis or synthesis to a distorted expectation or belief. It jumps the tracks of demand, soothing or defusing the emotional arousal associated with failure, fear, shame, unreasonably blocked goals, or a variety of other stimuli. Acceptance is actively offered both as model and as response, allowing the client to interact with a world perhaps differently ordered than historically experienced, impacting current experience and shaping future expectations. As a response to a worldview that is not highly reflective of structure and contingencies (i.e., distorted), acceptance often points to and highlights a more accurate understanding. It may be the missing element in a too-demanding set of expectations, or the balancing perspective to unwarranted shame. It is certain that, once learned, acceptance is a highly reinforced activity in therapists working with difficult-to-treat clients; its effectiveness in reducing agitation when strategically (and authentically) employed can be remarkable. Its effectiveness in reducing therapist distress when directed toward the self can be equally powerful.

The practice of acceptance includes focusing on the current moment, seeing reality as it is without "delusions," and accepting reality without judgment. The practice also encourages students to let go of attachments that obstruct the path to enlightenment, to use skillful means, and to find a middle way. Zen teaches that each moment is complete by itself, and that the world is perfect as it is. Zen focuses on acceptance, validation, and tolerance instead of change. Finally, in contrast to the experimental evidence required in psychology, Zen emphasizes experiential evidence as a means of understanding the world.

In DBT, clients are taught and encouraged to use skills for accepting life completely and radically, as well as for changing it. Radical acceptance is the fully open experience of what is, entering into reality just as it is, at this moment. Fully open acceptance is without constrictions, and without distortion, without judgment, without evaluation, and without attempts to keep an experience or to get rid of it. What is very important here is this notion of "without adding judgment of good and bad." Accepting is not necessarily evaluating positively. And, in fact, accepting is one thing, and evaluating is another. Nor is acceptance necessarily the same as compassion or love. Another way of thinking about it is that radical acceptance is radical truth. In other words, acceptance is experiencing something without the haze of what one wants and does not want it to be. It is the unrivaled entering into reality as it exists. "This one moment" is the crucial part of the statement. Accepting "at this moment" says nothing, of course, about what is happening in the next. Acceptance "in this moment" is not necessarily saying anything about the next moment. One can radically accept reality in this moment and radically change or let it go completely in the same or the next moment.

Radical acceptance is an act of the total person that allows of "this moment" or "this reality" in this moment. It is without discrimination. In other words, one does not choose parts of reality to accept and parts to reject. The notion of radical acceptance is that of "total allowance now." That means that radical acceptance is not simply a cognitive stance or cognitive activity; it is a total act. It is jumping off a cliff—over and over and over. As discussed by Sanderson and Linehan (1999), the Middle English root for the word *accept* is *kap*, meaning to take, seize, or catch—definitely an active verb, not implying passivity or resignation, as is often mistakenly supposed. Acceptance involves fully entering into and embracing whatever is in the present moment. The capacity to do this rather than to ignore, distract, escape, and so on, is one that can be developed like other skills and capacities.

An act of radical acceptance, particularly when if follows great difficulty, can be experienced as enormously liberating. The experience itself, as with any experience, is difficult to describe. A description of the taste of sugar does not give one the experience of sweetness. It is difficult to understand radical acceptance until some sort of experience in which, possibly out of complete desperation, one simply "gets it." People who have experienced the death of a loved one often speak of not being able to "accept" the death. In many senses, grieving is the process of "radically accepting" the reality that the person has died. Being stuck with a near fatal or fatal illness, or with incurable pain, failure, or loss, may also be the occasion for a person's first experience of "radical acceptance" in its most pure or experienced form.

The idea that the solution to suffering is to increase acceptance of the here and now, and decrease craving and attachment that inevitably keep one clinging to the past, which has changed already, is quite different from behavior therapy's emphasis on developing skills for attaining one's goals. However, the idea that suffering results from things not being the way one strongly wants them to be, or insists they should be, is very compatible with cognitive-behavioral therapies; Albert Ellis is perhaps the clearest, most consistent exponent of this viewpoint.

Skillful Means

The other half of mindful practice is skillful means. As action, mindfulness is synonymous with intense connection with activity. The experience of self as both part and whole, actor and observer, precipitant and respondent in the grand unfolding places one into the heart of the dialectic. Furthermore, the lack of defensiveness or blindness allows one to be aware of how the environment is changed, to quickly assimilate new information (knowledge), and to accurately and sensitively utilize and express these realizations. In the ideal, the path of least resistance and the critical pressure points of an active environment reveal themselves to the mindful participant, who shapes him- or herself as needed (i.e., selflessly) in order to maximize effectiveness. In a reflected understanding of the whole, aligning one's actions with the principles of reality (ever-changing, predicated on previous conditions, etc.) reflects both perfect knowledge and the willingness to allow oneself to be shaped by the rules and laws of experience rather than to require that experience mirror preconceptions. Thus, knowledge as action reflecting understanding of the goals to be attained and the context in which it occurs is definitional of both mindfulness and dialectical understanding.

The theory and strategies outlined in the DBT treatment manual were developed in discussion with graduate students and laboratory affiliates following the viewing of therapist actions in treatment sessions. Those therapist behaviors pulled out of the sessions, highlighted, and aggregated under the term "strategies," were found to be successful or effective in their application to women with borderline personality disorder. As Hayes (1993) noted, the definition of "successful" is dependent entirely upon the stated goals prior to the action. In defining DBT, "success" was identified as accomplishing a specific goal within the treatment hour, or across some other time frame. In some instances, a behavior on the part of the therapist would be highlighted, because it appeared to reduce visible emotion dysregulation on the part of the client, or because it kept the client in the room, or because it took advantage of a given context in order to move the client toward adopting new behavior.

The strategies outlined in the treatment manual were derived from groupings of similarly effective behaviors (i.e., behaviors accomplishing a similar goal in a similar context), and rules–theories were further established contextually. These rules, in turn, were verified (and verifiable) to the extent that therapist decision making about which strategy to employ was informed by them and thereby influenced in such a way as to lead to the employment of a "successful" behavior. The inclusion of a consultation team, whose task it is to bring the therapist back to the theory when drifting, further emphasizes the need to be attending to outcomes and processes, and "reregulating" the therapist, improving consistency between theory, action, and desired outcome.

TREATMENT OUTCOMES

Randomized clinical trials (RCTs) have been conducted to evaluate DBT for treatment of Axis II borderline personality disorder (BPD) and Axis I eating disorders. The trials for BPD conducted in three independent laboratories have found DBT to be more effective than active control conditions. Among suicidal women, it has been shown to reduce the frequency and medical severity of suicidal and other self-injurious behavior, the frequency and total days of psychiatric hospitalizations, and client anger, and to increase treatment retention and social and global adjustment (Koons et al., 2001; Linehan, Armstrong, Suarez, Allmon, & Heard, 1991; Linehan et al., 2002; Verheul et al., 2003). DBT also has been adapted to several other populations and treatment settings. RCTs have supported the efficacy of adaptations of DBT for women with BPD in a community mental health clinic (Turner, 2000), for women with BPD and substance abuse or dependence (Linehan et al., 1999, 2002), for women with binge eating disorder (Telch, Agras, & Linehan, 2001) and bulimia (Safer, Telch, & Agras, 2001), and for depressed elders (Lynch, Morse, Mendelson, & Robins, 2003). Controlled but nonrandomized studies also suggest that adaptations of DBT may have efficacy for clients with BPD in longer term (e.g., 3 months) inpatient settings (Barley et al., 1993; Bohus et al., 2000) and for suicidal adolescents (Rathus & Miller, 2002). These and other treatment outcome studies are summarized in Robins and Chapman (in press), and in Lieb, Zanarini, Linehan, and Bohus (in press).

REFERENCES

Aitken, R. (1982). *Taking the path of zen*. San Francisco: North Point Press.

Barley, W. D., Buie, S. E., Peterson, E. W., Hollingsworth, A. S., Griva, M., Hickerson, S. C., et al. (1993). Development of an inpatient cognitive-behavioral treatment program for borderline personality disorder. *Journal of Personality Disorders, 7*, 232–240.

Basseches, M. (1984). *Dialectical thinking and adult development*. Norwood, NJ: Ablex.

Berman, M. (1981). *The reenchantment of the world*. New York: Bantam Books.

Bohus, M., Haaf, B., Stiglmayr, C., Pohl, U., Bohme, R., & Linehan, M. (2000). Evaluation of inpatient dialectical-behavioral therapy for borderline personality disorder—a prospective study. *Behaviour Reseaarch and Therapy, 38*, 875–887.

Bopp, M. J., & Weeks, G. R. (1984). Dialectical metatheory in family therapy. *Family Process, 23*, 49–61.

Goldfried, M. R., & Davison, G. C. (1976). *Clinical behavior therapy*. New York: Holt, Rinehart & Winston.

Hahn, T. N. (1976). *The miracle of mindfulness: A manual of meditation*. Boston: Beacon Press.

Hayes, S. C. (1993). Analytic goals and the varieties of scientific contextualism. In S. C. Hayes, L. J. Hayes, H. W. Reese, & T. R. Sarbin (Eds.), *Varieties of scientific contextualism* (pp. 11–27). Reno, NV: Context Press.

Heard, H. L., & Linehan, M. M. (in press). Integrative therapy for borderline personality disorder. In J. C. Norcross & A. P. Goldfried (Eds.), *Handbook of integrative psychotherapy*. New York: Oxford University Press.

Ivanoff, A., Brown, M., & Linehan, M. M. (2001). Dialectical behavior therapy for self-mutilating borderline patients. In D. Simeon & E. Hollander (Eds.), *Self-injurious behaviors: Asssessment and treatment* (pp. 149–173). Washington, DC: American Psychiatric Press.

Kaminstein, D. S. (1987). Toward a dialectical metatheory for psychotherapy. *Journal of Contemporary Psychotherapy, 17*, 87–101.

Koons, C. R., Robins, C. J., Tweed, J. L., Lynch, T. R., Gonzalez, A. M., Morse, J. Q., et al.

(2001). Efficacy of dialectical behavior therapy in women veterans with borderline personality disorder. *Behavior Therapy, 32,* 371–390.

Levins, R., & Lewontin, R. (1985). *The dialectical biologist.* Cambridge, MA: Harvard University Press.

Lieb, K., Zanarini, M., Linehan, M., & Bohus, M. (in press). Seminar section: Borderline personality disorder. *Lancet.*

Linehan, M. M. (1987). Dialectical behavioral therapy: A cognitive behavioral approach to parasuicide. *Journal of Personality Disorders, 1,* 328–333.

Linehan, M. M. (1989). Cognitive and behavior therapy for borderline personality disorder. In A. Tasman, R. E. Hales, & A. J. Frances (Eds.), *Review of psychiatry* (Vol. 8, pp. 84–102). Washington, DC: American Psychiatric Press.

Linehan, M. M., Armstrong, H. E., Suarez, A., Allmon, D., & Heard, H. L. (1991). Cognitive-behavioral treatment of chronically parasuicidal borderline patients. *Archives of General Psychiatry, 48,* 1060–1064.

Linehan, M. M., Cochran, B. N., & Kehrer, C. A. (2001). Dialectical behavior therapy for borderline personality disorder. In D. H. Barlow (Ed.), *Clinical handbook of psychological disorders* (3rd ed., pp. 470–522). New York: Guilford Press.

Linehan, M. M., Dimeff, L. A., Reynolds, S. K., Comtois, K., Shaw-Welch, S., Heagerty, P., et al. (2002). Dialectical behavior therapy versus comprehensive validation plus 12 steps for the treatment of opioid dependent women meeting criteria for borderline personality disorder. *Drug and Alcohol Dependence, 67,* 13–26.

Linehan, M. M., & Schmidt, H. (1995). The dialectics of effective treatment of borderline personality disorder. In W. O. O'Donohue & L. Krasner (Eds.), *Theories in behavior therapy: Exploring behavior change* (pp. 553–584). Washington, DC: American Psychological Association.

Linehan, M. M., Schmidt, H., III, Dimeff, L. A., Craft, J. C., Kanter, J., & Comtois, K. A. (1999). Dialectical behavior therapy for patients with borderline personality disorder and drug-dependence. *American Journal of Addictions, 8,* 279–292.

Lynch, T. R., Morse, J. Q., Mendelson, T., & Robins, C. J. (2003). Dialectical behavior therapy for depressed older adults: A randomized pilot study. *American Journal of Geriatric Psychiatry, 11,* 33–45.

O'Leary, K. D., & Wilson, G. T. (1987). *Behavior therapy: Application and outcome.* Englewood Cliffs, NJ: Prentice-Hall.

Pennington, B. (1980). *Centering prayer.* Garden City, NY: Doubleday.

Rathus, J. H., & Miller, A. L. (2002). Dialectical behavior therapy adapted for suicidal adolescents. *Suicide and Life-Threatening Behavior, 32,* 146–157.

Reese, H. W. (1993). Contextualism and dialectical materialism. In S. C. Hayes, L. J. Hayes, H. W. Reese, & T. R. Sarbin (Eds.), *Varieties of scientific contextualism* (pp. 71–105). Reno, NV: Context Press.

Riegel, K. F. (1975). Toward a dialectical theory of development. *Human Development, 18,* 50–64.

Robins, C. J., & Chapman, A. L. (in press). Dialectical behavior therapy: Current status, recent developments, and future directions. *Journal of Personality Disorders.*

Robins, C. J., & Koons, C. R. (2004). Dialectical behavior therapy for severe personality disorders. In J. J. Magnavita (Ed.), *Handbook of personality disorders: Theory and practice* (pp. 221–253). New York: Wiley.

Robins, C. J., Ivanoff, A. M., & Linehan, M. M. (2001). Dialectical behavior therapy. In W. J. Livesley (Ed.), *Handbook of personality disorders: Theory, research, and treatment* (pp. 437–459). New York: Guilford Press.

Safer, D. L., Telch, C. F., & Agras, W. S. (2001). Dialectical behavior therapy for bulimia nervosa. *American Journal of Psychiatry, 158,* 632–634.

Sanderson, C., & Linehan, M. M. (1999). Acceptance and forgiveness. In W. R. Miller

(Ed.), *Integrating spirituality into treatment: Resources for practitioners* (pp. 199–216). Washington, DC: American Psychological Association.

Skinner, B. F. (1974). *About behaviorism.* New York: Knopf.

Staats, A. W. (1975). *Social behaviorism.* Homewood, IL: Dorsey Press.

Staats, A. W., & Staats, C. K. (1963). *Complex human behavior.* New York: Holt, Rinehart & Winston.

Swann, W. B., Jr., Stein-Seroussi, A., & Giesler, R. B. (1992). Why people self-verify. *Journal of Personality and Social Psychology, 62,* 392–401.

Telch, C. F., Agras, W. S., & Linehan, M. M. (2001). Dialectical behavior therapy for binge eating disorder. *Journal of Consulting Clinical Psychology, 69,* 1061–1065.

Turner, R. M. (2000). Naturalistic evaluation of dialectical behavioral Therapy-oriented treatment for borderline personality disorder. *Cognitive and Behavioral Practice, 7,* 413–419.

Verheul, R., van den Bosch, L. M., Koeter, M. W., de Ridder, M. A., Stijnen, T., & van den Brink, W. (2003). Dialectical behaviour therapy for women with borderline personality disorder: 12-month, randomised clinical trial in The Netherlands. *British Journal of Psychiatry, 182,* 135–140.

Weiss, F. G. (1974). *Hegel: The essential writings.* New York: Harper & Row.

Wells, H. K. (1972). Alienation and dialectical logic. *Kansas Journal of Sociology, 3,* 7–32.

Wilber, K. (1977). *The spectrum of consciousness.* Wheaton, IL: Theosophical Publishing.

3

Mindfulness-Based Cognitive Therapy

Theoretical Rationale and Empirical Status

Zindel V. Segal, John D. Teasdale, *and* J. Mark G. Williams

According to Hayes (2002), the evolution of behaviorally informed therapies has occurred over two formative epochs and is currently on the cusp of a third. In the early 1960s, the systematic application of learning theory and principles to the modification of emotional disorders suggested enough in the way of positive outcomes and reliable clinical procedures to enable its codification as a distinct therapy. The emphasis on empirical accountability and evaluation of treatment outcomes also helped to distinguish behavior therapies from more traditional psychotherapies, where concern for these issues was less central. The second phase was signaled by the arrival of cognitive therapy and the eclipsing of purely behavioral models of psychopathology in favor of accounts featuring the role of attention, memory, and mental representation. The third phase is still in its infancy. It features treatments that retain the structure associated with the two earlier phases but incorporate elements, such as dialectical philosophy, mindfulness, acceptance, relationship, and spirituality, that are outside the ken of what most would consider behavior therapy.

In this chapter, we outline the theoretical background and empirical status of one such "third-phase" treatment: mindfulness-based cognitive therapy (MBCT). MBCT is a novel, theory-driven, psychological intervention designed to reduce relapse in recurrent major depression. It incorporates as a central component mindfulness training as developed by Jon Kabat-Zinn and his colleagues at the University of Massachusetts Medical Center (Kabat-Zinn, 1990).

We begin by describing the public health significance of relapse prevention in depression and then present the thinking behind our decision to integrate mindfulness training and aspects of cognitive therapy as a potential prophylactic intervention. The empirical support for MBCT is then reviewed. We conclude by identifying possible mechanisms of change that might be operative in MBCT, along with suggestions for how this integrative approach might be extended to the treatment of other clinical disorders.

PUBLIC HEALTH BURDEN OF DEPRESSION

Major depressive disorder (MDD) remains a daunting mental health challenge, with lifetime prevalence rates estimated between 2.9 and 12.6 per 100 and lifetime risk estimated at 17–19% (Kessler et al., 1994). According to the World Health Organization (WHO), when the burden of ill health imposed by all diseases worldwide was considered, unipolar major depression imposed the fourth greatest burden (Murray & Lopez, 1998). These investigators projected that, by the year 2020, this burden will increase both absolutely and relatively, so that at that time depression will impose the second greatest burden of ill health, very close behind the top cause, ischemic heart disease.

A major reason for the scale of the burden caused by MDD is that, as well as being a condition with a high rate of incidence, it is also characterized by relapse, recurrence, and chronicity. Recent estimates project that patients will experience an average of four lifetime major depressive episodes of 20 weeks' duration each (Judd, 1997). Such data point to effective prevention of relapse and recurrence as a central challenge in the overall management of MDD. Currently, maintenance pharmacotherapy is the best validated and most widely used approach to prophylaxis in depression (e.g., Kupfer et al., 1992). In this approach, patients who have recovered following treatment of the acute episode by antidepressant medication continue to take their medication as a way to reduce risk of further episodes.

The protection from maintenance pharmacotherapy lasts only as long as patients continue to take their antidepressant medication. By contrast, it appears that a psychological treatment, cognitive-behavioral therapy (CBT) for depression (Beck, Rush, Shaw, & Emery, 1979), administered during depressive episodes, is effective in reducing subsequent rates of relapse and recurrence after treatment has been completed. Studies comparing the long-term outcome of patients who recovered following treatment of acute depression by CBT with the outcome of patients who recovered following treatment with antidepressant medication and were then withdrawn from medication, consistently find less relapse or need for further treatment in the CBT group (Blackburn, Eunson, & Bishop, 1986; Evans et al., 1992; Hollon & Shelton, 2002; Shea et al., 1992; Simons, Murphy, Levine, & Wetzel, 1986). Such findings suggest that CBT may be a treatment for acute depression that has long-term effects in reducing risk of future relapse and recurrence, presumably through patients acquiring skills that confer some degree of protection against future onsets.

RELIEVING DEPRESSION AND SUSTAINING RECOVERY

The efficacy of maintenance pharmacotherapy and psychotherapy as ways to reduce relapse in depression is welcome news for both patients and practitioners. However, each approach has its drawbacks. An operative assumption behind the use of maintenance pharmacotherapy is that patients are required to take their medication for extended periods. However, in practice, this plan is compromised by patient noncompliance in the 40% range (Basco & Rush, 1995). Providing acute-phase, structured psychotherapies, such as CBT and interpersonal psychotherapy (IPT), on a large scale may also prove to be difficult and less feasible (Olfson et al., 2002). Treatment delivery depends on scarce, expensive, professionally trained personnel. It may not be possible to administer these interventions, in their traditional formats, to make much of an impact on an illness as prevalent as depression.

In this situation, an attractive alternative strategy would be to combine pharmacotherapy for the acute episode with psychological prevention strategies administered following recovery. Doing so would allow us to take advantage of the cost-efficiency of antidepressant medication to reduce acute symptomatology, but would avoid keeping patients indefinitely on maintenance medication to reduce future relapse and recurrence.

At the time we approached this problem, there were few exemplars of a cost-efficient psychological intervention to administer to pharmacologically treated and recovered depressed patients that would reduce their subsequent risk for relapse or recurrence of depression. As a result, we decided to go back to basics for a rethink of what was actually required of such a program rather than to explore variants on the theme of standard CBT for depression. Our efforts at treatment development were guided by the need to find answers to two central questions: (1) What is the nature of cognitive vulnerability to relapse in formerly depressed patients? and (2) how does cognitive therapy reduce this vulnerability?

Cognitive Vulnerability to Relapse and Recurrence

How are we to best understand the increased relapse risk faced by formerly depressed patients (Judd, 1997)? Beck's original cognitive model suggested that vulnerability to depression was related to certain underlying dysfunctional attitudes or assumptions (Kovacs & Beck, 1978). Weissman and Beck (1978) developed a self-report questionnaire, the Dysfunctional Attitudes Scale (DAS), as a way to measure this aspect of cognitive vulnerability. From the perspective of the clinical cognitive model, DAS scores were predicted to remain elevated in patients who had previously been depressed (and who were thus known to be vulnerable) compared to never depressed controls, reflecting the presence of the hypothesized persistent dysfunctional attitudes and assumptions in the former group. Studies that have examined this prediction have generally found that although DAS scores are elevated in patients while they are in an episode of depression, DAS scores of recovered patients, tested in normal mood, are not distinguishable from those of never depressed controls (Haaga, Dyck, & Ernst, 1991). Such findings are inconsistent with the hypothesis that those vulnerable to depression manifest dysfunctional underlying assumptions or attitudes as a relatively enduring trait.

A different perspective on cognitive vulnerability to depression emerged from studies demonstrating negative biases in memory and other cognitive functions in experimentally induced depressed moods (Teasdale, 1983, 1988; see also Persons & Miranda, 1992). This work suggested that vulnerability to relapse and recurrence of depression arises from repeated associations between depressed mood and patterns of negative, self-critical, hopeless thinking during episodes of major depression, leading to changes at both cognitive and neuronal levels. As a result, individuals who have recovered from major depression differ from individuals who have never experienced major depression in the patterns of thinking that are activated by future sad moods.

Specifically, in recovered depressed patients, the thinking activated by dysphoria should be similar to the negative thinking patterns previously present in the episode. These patterns of thought typically involving views of the self as worthless and inadequate, and of the future as hopeless, are assumed to contribute to the maintenance of depressive symptoms. Reactivation of these patterns in recovered patients by dysphoria would act to maintain and intensify the dysphoric state through escalating and self-perpetuating cycles of ruminative cognitive–affective processing (Teasdale, 1988; 1997). In this way, in those with a history of major depression, states of mild dysphoria will be more likely to progress to more intense and persistent states, thus increasing risk of further onsets of episodes of major depression.

Studies that have compared the patterns of thinking activated by mild dysphoria in those with and without a history of major depression support this account; those with a history of depression typically show greater activation of globally negative views of the self and of dependence of perceived self-worth on the approval of others or the outcome of tasks (Ingram, Miranda, & Segal, 1998; Segal, Gemar, & Williams, 1999). This analysis provides a parallel explanation, at the cognitive level, to more biological accounts of episode sensitization and kindling in recurrent affective disorder (Post, 1992). Accounts at both biological and cognitive levels are consistent with the finding that less environmental stress is required to provoke relapse/recurrence with repeated experiences of episodes of major depression (Post, 1992); that is, the processes mediating relapse/recurrence appear to become progressively more autonomous with increased depressive experience (Segal, Williams, Teasdale, & Gemar, 1996). Figure 3.1 summarizes this model of depressive relapse and indicates where the effects of preventive interventions are likely to operate.

fundamental helpfulness.

What Is Reactivated?

Based on the analysis presented in Figure 3.1, a central focus of relapse prevention is to preempt the establishment of self-perpetuating and self-escalating patterns of negative thinking in states of dysphoria or at other times of potential relapse. The design of treatments capable of achieving this aim would be helped if we had a clearer understanding of the negative thinking that, according to this analysis, is reactivated.

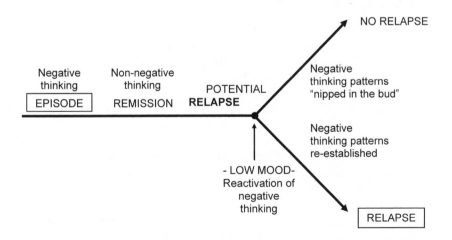

FIGURE 3.1. The conceptual model underlying the development of mindfulness-based cognitive therapy for prevention in recurrent major depression. From Segal, Williams, and Teasdale (2002). Copyright 2002 by The Guilford Press. Reprinted by permission.

Content + process

Our best hypothesis is that it is actually a whole, integrated configuration of information processing, or "mode of mind" (Teasdale, 1997) that gets "wheeled in" in states of dysphoria in depression-prone individuals. This mode involves both negative cognitive *content* and a maladaptive cognitive *process* (ruminative thought patterns). Such ruminations revolve around a globally negative view of self and are reinforced by feedback loops involving the effects of depression on other cognitive systems (e.g., attentional and memory processes) and on the body (e.g., sensations of sluggishness and fatigue) (Teasdale, Segal, & Williams, 1995). As far as depressed patients are concerned, their goal is to reduce depression. They believe that repeatedly "thinking about" negative aspects of the self or the situation will yield insights that will allow them to resolve the situation and escape the state of depression. In fact, in this mode of mind, continually dwelling on negative self-related information serves to perpetuate, rather than resolve, depression. Effectively, old, overlearned habitual patterns of cognitive processing get switched in relatively automatically, and thinking runs repeatedly around fairly well-worn "mental grooves," without finding an effective way forward out of depression.

Data supporting this view come from the work of Nolen-Hoeksema and colleagues, who have consistently demonstrated the depression-perpetuating effect of a ruminative style of responding to depression (Nolen-Hoeksema, 1991), and that a negative self-focus is characteristic of depression (Pyszczynski & Greenberg, 1987).

Protection against Depressive Relapse/Recurrence through Cognitive Therapy

Before considering the implications of this analysis for the design of novel preventive interventions in depression, it is important to understand how, according to this account, cognitive therapy achieves its effects. As previously described, the original cognitive model underlying CBT for depression suggested that vulnerability to depression stemmed from certain underlying dysfunctional attitudes or assumptions. The reduced risk of relapse faced by patients following CBT was the result of specific effects of CBT modifying those dysfunctional attitudes. To date, the specificity of this claim has not been broadly supported (Barber & DeRubeis, 1989); in studies where CBT has produced significantly better long-term outcomes than pharmacotherapy, the two treatments often have not differed on posttreatment measures of DAS (e.g., Simons, Garfield, & Murphy, 1984).

The generally held view at the time that we were trying to understand these cognitive mechanisms was that CBT, developed to change the degree of belief in depressive thoughts and dysfunctional attitudes, had its effects through changes in the *content* of depressive thinking. However, both our experience of using CBT and our theoretical analysis suggested an alternative possibility. We recognized that although the explicit emphasis in CBT is on changing thought content, CBT also leads implicitly to changes in patients' *relationships* to their negative thoughts and feelings. Specifically, as a result of repeatedly identifying negative thoughts as they arise and standing back from them to evaluate the accuracy or adaptiveness of their content, patients often make a general shift in their *perspective* on negative thoughts and feelings. Instead of viewing thoughts as absolutely true or as as descriptive of important self-attributes, patients are able to see negative thoughts and feelings as passing events in the mind that are not necessarily valid reflections of reality or central aspects of the self. While the importance of such "distancing" or "decentering" had previously been recognized in discussions of cognitive therapy (e.g., Beck et al., 1979), it was usually as a method for changing thought content rather than as an end in itself. Other investigators, such as Ingram and Hollon (1986), had, however, suggested a role for decentering that was similar to our view: "Cognitive therapy relies heavily on helping individuals switch to a controlled mode of processing that is metacognitive in nature and focuses on depression-related cognition . . . typically referred to as 'distancing'. . . . The long-term effectiveness of cognitive therapy may lie in teaching patients to initiate this process in the face of future stress" (p. 272). Our advantage in building on this alternative perspective of the way that cognitive therapy might have its effects was that it gave us the freedom to consider other approaches that while enabling a shift in relationship to negative thoughts and feelings, might, unlike cognitive therapy, have no elements explicitly directed at changing thought content. Mindfulness training was one such approach.

Prevention of Relapse and Recurrence in Depression with Mindfulness Training

While it might seem that the distance between our models of cognitive relapse vulnerability, cognitive therapy's prophylactic effects, and mindfulness training is vast, a number of sources suggested a possible link between them. We were aware, for example, that Marsha Linehan had successfully used mindfulness training as a component of her approach to borderline personality disorder (Linehan, 1993), and that Jon Kabat-Zinn and his colleagues at the University of Massachusetts Medical Center (UMASS) had developed a mindfulness-based stress reduction program (MBSR; Kabat-Zinn, 1990) relevant to a wide range of clinical conditions, including anxiety disorders. Although less familiar to us but featuring a rationale that was compatible with our account, the approach taken by Hayes (1987; Hayes, Wilson, Gifford, Follette, & Strosahl, 1996) in acceptance and commitment therapy (ACT) was also noted. As we saw it, patients in ACT learned skills in cognitive defusion and decentering aimed at reducing their experiential avoidance and allowing them to turn toward and accept distressing thoughts and feelings, as a point of departure for working with them, in effect developing a different relationship to them. With these leads in mind, we proceeded to develop an integrative theoretical model (discussed more fully in Teasdale, 1999; Teasdale et al., 1995) that outlined how mindfulness training might also be highly relevant to the prevention of relapse in depression.

Detailed analyses of the patterns of negative thinking reactivated in dysphoric mood in recovered depressed patients (Teasdale & Barnard, 1993; Teasdale et al., 1995) suggested that the critical processing modes, while "automatic" in the sense that they involved well-practiced, habitual cognitive routines, were highly dependent on central, controlled processing attentional resources. Since these resources are limited, there is competition for them between different tasks that are dependent on them and, hence, mutual interference between those tasks. Therefore, an important requirement of a relapse prevention intervention is that it should make demands on limited controlled processing resources in such a way that fewer of those resources are available for the establishment and maintenance of the depression-related processing configurations reactivated in dysphoria. "Starved" of necessary resources in this way, such configurations are less likely to be established. It is widely assumed (e.g., Norman & Shallice, 1986) that conscious awareness of task stimuli is a marker indicating that controlled processing attentional resources are being deployed to the processing of those stimuli, and that intentional action is also dependent on such limited resources. It follows that the intentional deployment of conscious awareness, which is a defining characteristic of mindfulness, will require limited attentional resources and reduce their availability for the processing configurations that might otherwise support the relapse process.

We believed that cognitive therapy achieved at least some of its relapse prevention effects through changing patients' relationship to their depressive thoughts and feelings, in particular, through fostering a "decentered" relationship to such mental contents. Such a shift is a key outcome of mindfulness training, as indicated by the following quotation from Jon Kabat-Zinn's description of the UMASS MBSR program: "It is remarkable how liberating it feels to be able to see that your thoughts are just thoughts and that they are not 'you' or 'reality.' . . . The simple act of recognizing your thoughts *as thoughts* can free you from the distorted reality they often create and allow for more clear-sightedness and a greater sense of manageability in your life" (emphasis added, Kabat-Zinn, 1990, pp. 69–70). Such observations suggested that mindfulness training might be an alternative route to achieve the decentering effect that we considered to be such an important aspect of the relapse prevention effects of cognitive therapy.

Relapse-related ruminative processing routines involve a particular "cognitive mode" of processing depression-related material, characterized by a focus at a relatively conceptual level ("thinking about") on the topic of discrepancies between present and desired states of self and world, with a view toward identifying actions to achieve the goal of reducing those discrepancies (Pyszczynski & Greenberg, 1987; Teasdale, 1999; Teasdale & Barnard, 1993). This mode might be described as "doing."

The suggestion here is that the relapse-engendering process is not simply dependent on the processing of particular types of depression-related material; rather, it is the processing of that material within a particular cognitive mode. In other words, it is not just *what* is processed that determines whether relapse ensues, but *how* that material is processed. From this perspective, an attractive strategy to preempt the establishment of relapse-related processing would be to establish a cognitive mode different from that of the relapse-engendering processing configuration, and to process depression-related and other material within that alternative cognitive mode.

Mindfulness can be seen as just such an alternative cognitive mode (Teasdale, 1999), in which the focus of processing is at a level of representation that is not conceptual, and in which specific discrepancies are not the prime topic of processing. Traditionally, this aspect of mindfulness is described as "being" rather than "doing" (Kabat-Zinn, 1990). Conceptualizing mindfulness as an alternative cognitive mode, incompatible with that characteristic of the relapse-engendering processing configuration, suggested a further attraction of mindfulness training as a route to relapse prevention.

Finally, the emphasis within mindfulness training on being fully present and attentive to the content of moment-by-moment experience, whether it is pleasant, unpleasant, or neither pleasant nor unpleasant, is of obvious relevance to the experiential avoidance that often predates relapse. In light of the how distressing the experience of depression is to patients, it is understandable that recovered patients might redirect their attention away from the early signs and symptoms of incipient relapse. Unfortunately, this leaves them less able to take adaptive action to deal skillfully with the possibility of relapse at a very early stage when relatively simple strategies may be quite helpful. Instead, by delaying action until the relapse process has gained momentum and forces itself into attention, patients end up presenting themselves with a much more difficult coping situation. Training in mindful awareness of bodily sensations, feelings, and thoughts, in particular emphasizing the importance of deliberately turning toward the unpleasant with an attitude of openness and acceptance, would clearly increase the chance of detecting difficulties early and responding more skillfully and effectively.

In summary, the analysis summarized in Figure 3.1 suggested that risk of relapse and recurrence would be reduced if patients who have recovered from episodes of major depression could learn, first, to be more aware of negative thoughts and feelings at times of potential relapse/recurrence, and, second, to respond to those thoughts and feelings in ways that allow them to disengage from ruminative depressive processing (Nolen-Hoeksema, 1991). It appeared that mindfulness training had much to offer with respect to both of these goals.

MINDFULNESS-BASED COGNITIVE THERAPY

The preventive intervention that we eventually developed, MBCT (Segal, Williams, & Teasdale, 2002), is based on an integration of elements of CBT for depression (Beck et al., 1979), with components of MBSR developed by Kabat-Zinn (1990) and colleagues. Unlike CBT, there is little emphasis in MBCT on changing the *content* of thoughts; rather, the emphasis is on changing *awareness of* and *relationship to* thoughts, feelings, and bodily sensations. Aspects of CBT included in MBCT are primarily those designed to facilitate "decentered" views such as "Thoughts are not facts" and "I am not my thoughts." Unlike MBSR, which is a generic program applicable to a wide range of problems, MBCT is specifically designed for patients who are in remission from unipolar major depression. This degree of specificity allows MBCT, like CBT, to customize sections of the program with tasks and materials that are directly tagged relative to the details of a particular clinical problem. For example, decentering can be facilitated specifically for depressive thinking by providing participants, as a group, with a list of the most frequently observed negative automatic thoughts and allowing them to recognize that their own personal "top 10" negative thoughts are actually very similar to those of other group members and to the findings reported by systematic research.

MBCT is designed to teach patients in remission from recurrent major depression to become more aware of, and to relate differently to, their thoughts, feelings, and bodily sensations (e.g., relating to thoughts and feelings as passing events in the mind rather than identifying with them or treating them as necessarily accurate readouts on reality). The program teaches skills that allow individuals to disengage from habitual ("automatic") dysfunctional cognitive routines, in particular depression-related ruminative thought patterns, as a way to reduce future risk of relapse and recurrence of depression.

Because, unlike CBT, there is little explicit emphasis in MBCT on changing the content or specific meanings of negative automatic thoughts, training in MBCT can occur in the remitted state, using everyday experience as the object of training.

MBCT and Other "Third-Wave" Behavior Therapies

While the application of mindfulness training is central to MBCT, it also features, if less prominently, in other interventions designated by Hayes

(2002) as part of the "third wave" of behavior therapies, such as dialectical behavior therapy (DBT; Linehan, 1993) and ACT (Hayes, Strosahl, & Wilson, 1999). Both DBT and ACT aim to increase patients' awareness of their inner experience (thoughts, emotions, or body sensations) through training in skills that involve observation and acknowledgment. This facilitates a decentering from the content of whatever thoughts or emotions a patient might have and suggests the possibility of new way of relating to these experiences. Training in distress tolerance in DBT incorporates mindfulness skills to help patients develop a stance of curiosity and nonjudgment to whatever comes up, rather than avoidance or control.

Another point of convergence between MBCT, DBT, and ACT is the deliberate balancing of strategies directed toward acceptance or change. While all three utilize methods derived from cognitive therapy that are intended to get patients to question the validity of prevailing automatic thoughts or beliefs, the implementation of these techniques is secondary to acceptance-based procedures. In fact, therapists/instructors in these approaches encourage patients to let go of the idea that all problems might, with enough effort, be "fixed or changed." These treatments are explicit about the risk that endless attempts at fixing or controlling one's experience might have. Chief among these is the possibility that such efforts merely reinforce the attitude that their problems are the "enemy," and that once they are eliminated, everything will be fine. The problem is that this only encourages further attempts to solve problems by ruminating on them, and these attempts often keep persons trapped in the state from which they are trying to escape. This is something that family therapists have emphasized for years (Watzlawick, Weakland, & Fisch, 1974); it is central to the concept of self-invalidation in DBT (Linehan, 1993), and there is good experimental support for the notion (Wegner, 1994).

The alternative, that of letting go of the attempts at problem solving and, instead, purposely standing back to see what it feels like to see the problem through the lens of nonreactivity, and to bring a kindly awareness to the difficulty, is common to MBCT, DBT, and ACT. The awareness practices employed in these treatments allows patients to see how fighting against their unwanted thoughts, feelings, and bodily sensations sometimes creates more tension and inner turmoil. Instead of continuously feeding the tension by participating in what their thoughts or feelings demand, patients can learn to stay close to this mental struggle by finding a calm place from which it can be observed (Kabat-Zinn, 1994).

The 8-Week MBCT Program

Participants' first exposure to the MBCT program comes during an initial interview and orientation session with the instructor. This is as much a chance for the rationale behind MBCT to be conveyed as it is for the instructor to let the participant know about the practice demands that come with attending the classes. MBCT is delivered over eight weekly, 2-hour group sessions with up to 12 recovered recurrently depressed patients. During that period, the program includes daily homework exercises. Homework invariably includes some form of guided (taped) or unguided awareness exercises directed at increasing moment-by-moment nonjudgmental awareness of bodily sensations, thoughts, and feelings, together with exercises designed to integrate application of awareness skills into daily life. A key theme of the program is a focus on awareness of experience in the moment. Participants are helped to cultivate an open and acceptant mode of response, in which they intentionally face and move into difficulties and discomfort, and to develop a "decentered" perspective on thoughts and feelings, in which these are viewed as passing events in the mind.

A core feature of the program involves facilitation of an aware mode of being, characterized by freedom and choice, in contrast to a mode dominated by habitual, overlearned "automatic" patterns of cognitive–affective processing. For patients, this distinction is often illustrated by reference to the common experience, when driving on a familiar route, of suddenly realizing that one has been driving for miles "on automatic pilot," unaware of the road or other vehicles, preoccupied with planning future activities or ruminating on a current concern. By contrast, "mindful" driving is associated with being fully present in each moment, consciously aware of sights, sounds, thoughts, and body sensations as they arise. When mindful, the mind responds afresh to the unique pattern of experience in each moment rather than reacting "mindlessly" to fragments of a total experience with old, relatively stereotyped, habitual patterns of mind. Increased mindfulness allows early detection of relapse-related patterns of negative thinking, feelings, and body sensations, thus allowing them to be "nipped in the bud" at a stage when this may be much easier than if such warning signs were not noticed or ignored. Furthermore, entering a mindful mode of processing at such times allows disengagement from the relatively "automatic" ruminative thought patterns that would otherwise fuel the relapse process. Formulation of specific relapse/recurrence prevention strategies (such as involving family members in an "early warning" system, keeping written suggestions to engage in activities that are helpful in interrupting relapse-engendering processes, or to look out for habitual negative thoughts) are also included in the later stages of the program. Following the initial phase of eight weekly group meetings, follow-up meetings are scheduled at intervals of 1, 2, 3, and 4 months.

Clinical Efficacy of MBCT

Having developed a new cost-efficient intervention to reduce relapse and recurrence in depression, it was important to see whether, in fact, MBCT achieved the aims it was designed to achieve. To do this, we conducted a clinical trial systematically evaluating the effects of the MBCT program in preventing relapse among a group of recurrently depressed patients, currently in recovery.

The choice of an appropriate trial design for the initial evaluation of a novel intervention, such as MBCT, is influenced by a number of factors. At the time we planned the trial, there was no published evidence that any psychological intervention, sequenced with pharmacologically induced depression remission could prospectively reduce risk of future recurrence in major depression. Given this situation, the first priority was to evaluate whether MBCT was of *any* benefit in reducing relapse/recurrence. If benefits were observed, future research could evaluate MBCT relative to other psychological interventions and control for the effects of group structure, attention, expectancy, and other generic factors. Comparisons with alternative approaches to prevention, such as maintenance pharmacotherapy, would also be of interest if MBCT were found to be effective.

We employed a simple additive design in which patients who continued with treatment as usual (TAU) were compared with patients who, additionally, received training in MBCT. Such a design does not aim to compare MBCT with the best available alternative preventive intervention. Nor does it allow any reduction in rates of relapse and recurrence for patients receiving MBCT to be attributed unambiguously to the specific components of MBCT rather than to the nonspecific factors that come from participating in a structured treatment program. However, this design would allow us to answer a question of primary interest: Does MBCT, when offered in addition to TAU, reduce rates of relapse and recurrence compared to TAU alone?

Teasdale, Segal, Williams, Ridgeway, Soulsby, and Lau (2000)

The first empirical evaluation of MBCT was a three-center study of 145 patients, currently in remission or recovery from major depression, who were randomized to continue with TAU or, additionally, to receive MBCT (Teasdale et al., 2000). To enter the trial, patients had to have experienced at least two previous episodes of major depression (in fact, 77% had experienced three or more). All patients had previously been treated with antidepressant medication but had been symptom-free and off medication for at least 3 months before entering the trial.

After baseline assessments and randomization to treatment condition, patients entered an initial 7-week treatment phase, after which they were followed up for a year. The primary outcome variable in which we were interested was whether and when patients experienced relapse or recurrence meeting DSM-III-R criteria for major depressive episode (American Psychiatric Association, 1987), as assessed by the Structured Clinical Interview for Diagnosis (SCID; Spitzer, Williams, Gibbon, & First, 1992) administered at bimonthly assessments throughout the trial.

In clinical trials such as those we conducted, it is conventional, prior to randomization, to stratify the sample on baseline variables that might be predictive of the primary clinical outcome of interest. In our case, we stratified on how recently the last episode of depression had occurred, and how many previous episodes of major depression patients had experienced (two vs. three or more). It is also conventional, before conducting the main statistical analyses of such a trial, to check that the effects of the treatments being compared were the same in patients in the different strata.

When we did this, we found that the pattern of results for patients with three or more previous episodes of depression was significantly different from the pattern of results for those with only two previous episodes before entering the trial. In patients with three or more episodes (who comprised 77% of the total sample), there was a statistically significant difference between the relapse rates of MBCT and TAU patients; in patients with only two episodes (who comprised 23% of the total sample), there was no difference in relapse rates between patients receiving MBCT and TAU; that is, beneficial effects of treatment were restricted to the patients with more extensive histories of depression. We consider possible explanations for this interesting finding below. For now, let us focus on the patients with three or more episodes, who were considerably in the majority in the sample we studied.

Of these patients, those who simply continued with the treatment that they would normally receive showed a 66% relapse rate over the total 60-week study period, whereas those who received a "minimum effective dose" of MBCT (at least four of the eight weekly MBCT sessions) showed a relapse rate of 37% (see Figure 3.2). The difference in relapse rates between TAU and MBCT patients remained statistically significant when all those allocated to the MBCT condition were considered (irrespective of whether they received a "minimally adequate dose" of MBCT—this is called the intention to treat sample, or ITT). For this sample, the relapse rate was 40%. The benefits of MBCT could not be accounted for by greater use of antidepressants by patients in the MBCT group; the proportion of patients using antidepressants at any time during the study period was actually less in MBCT than in TAU.

In TAU patients, risk of relapse and recurrence over the study period increased in a statistically significant linear relationship with number of previous episodes of depression: 2 episodes, 31% relapse/recurrence; 3 episodes, 56% relapse/recurrence; and 4 or more episodes, 72% relapse/recurrence. In the group receiving a minimally adequate dose of MBCT, there was no significant relationship between number of previous episodes and risk of relapse/recurrence: 54% relapsed in the group with two episodes; 37% relapsed in the group with more than two episodes; that is, MBCT ap-

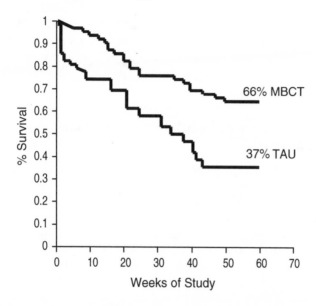

FIGURE 3.2. Survival curves comparing relapse/recurrence to DSM-III-R major depression for treatment as usual and mindfulness-based cognitive therapy, in patients with three or more previous episodes of major depression. From Teasdale et al. (2000). Copyright 2000 by the American Psychological Association. Reprinted by permission.

peared to eliminate the increased risk of relapse in those with three or more previous episodes of depression.

Ma and Teasdale (2003)

In a recently completed single-site replication study (N = 75) conducted in Cambridge, Ma and Teasdale (2003) report very similar findings. First, they found that the effects of treatment interacted with the number of previous episodes of depression experienced. Relapse rates, based on ITT analyses, for patients with three or more previous episodes of depression (who comprised 73% of their total sample) were 36% for MBCT versus 78% for TAU. They also found no protective advantage for MBCT in patients with two previous episodes of depression (27% of sample); ITT relapse rates: MBCT—50%, TAU—20%.

Taken together, the two clinical trials show that for patients with recurrent major depression, an "adequate dose" of MBCT halved relapse/recurrence rates over the follow-up period compared to TAU. Because the patients were seen in groups, this benefit was achieved for an average investment of less than 5 hours of health professional time per patient, making MBCT, as intended, a cost-efficient approach to prevention of depression. It is also important to note that MBCT was specifically designed for remitted patients and is unlikely to be effective in the treatment of acute depression, where factors such as difficulties in concentration and the intensity of negative thinking may preclude acquisition of the attentional control skills central to the program.

Greater Protection for Patients Whose Depressions Are More Recurrent?

The finding that MBCT prevented relapse and recurrence in patients with a history of three or more episodes of depression, but not in patients with only two previous episodes, is of particular interest with respect to the theoretical background to MBCT (Segal et al., 1996; Teasdale et al., 1995). This program was specifically designed to reduce the contribution of patterns of depressive thinking reactivated by dysphoria to the processes mediating relapse and recurrence. Such dysphoria-linked thinking, it was assumed, resulted from repeated associations between the depressed state and characteristic negative thinking patterns within each depressive episode. The strengthening of these associations with repeated episodes was assumed to contribute to the increased risk of subsequent episodes following each episode experienced. In particular, it was assumed that negative thinking reactivated by dysphoria contributed to the increasingly autonomous nature of the relapse/recurrence process with multiple episodes, reflected in the observation that environmental provoking events appear to play a progressively less important role in onset with increasing number of episodes (Kendler, Thornton, & Gardner, 2000; Post, 1992).

This account suggests the possibility that in this study, (1) the greater risk of relapse/recurrence in those with three or more episodes than in those with only two episodes (apparent in the TAU group) was to a large extent attributable to autonomous relapse/recurrence processes involving reactivation of depressogenic thinking patterns by dysphoria, and (2) the prophylactic effects of MBCT arose, specifically, from redirection of those processes at times of potential relapse/recurrence. Consistent with this analysis, MBCT appeared to have no prophylactic effects in those with only two previous episodes.

IMPLICATIONS FOR THE BEHAVIORAL AND COGNITIVE THERAPIES

In our work, the generic MBSR program developed by Kabat-Zinn (1990) and colleagues was modified to increase its relevance to the particular target of preventing relapse and recurrence in major depression. Taken with the results from smaller, or less controlled, evaluations suggesting the effectiveness of the generic MBSR program in treating chronic pain, generalized anxiety, and panic (Kabat-Zinn, Lipworth, Burney, & Sellers, 1986; Kabat-Zinn et al., 1992), and the effectiveness of a cognitive-behavioral program incorporating a substantial mindfulness component in reducing self-harm in borderline personality disorder (Linehan, Armstrong, Suarez, Allmon, & Heard, 1991), these findings suggest that mindfulness-based clinical interventions may hold considerable therapeutic promise either alone or in combination with other forms of intervention.

In fact, MBCT is but one example of a broader trend in treatment development within the behavioral and cognitive traditions. This trend has the potential to redefine the methods of care generated by the standard behavioral and cognitive models. As was true with the first- and second-wave behavior therapies, ACT, DBT, and MBCT all draw on empirical findings from experimental psychology, learning theory, or cognitive science to guide their problem formulation. What seems to distinguish third-wave therapies is their utilization/preference for non-language-based strategies. Clinical interventions are intended to reorient patients' understanding of their difficulties in a way that undermines the value of conceptual thought and representation as being important to their solution. They also reduce an identification with the problem in its literal form (Hayes et al., 1999). For example, whereas a panic patient's thoughts and appraisals about his or her racing heart may be taken at face value and disputed or challenged on evidentiary bases, an alternative would be to watch and acknowledge those thoughts as being in awareness while staying curious about them on a moment-by-moment basis. Thoughts are not judged as good, bad, scary, or useful. They are seen as passing events in the mind, and the challenge presented to patients is to develop this type of relationship to them. Cognitive defusion, as used in ACT and wise mind practices in DBT, offers similar ways of helping patients to sidestep the content of their thoughts and focus instead on the process.

One or two possible impacts from this shift within therapeutic practice might be predicted. If the role of language and conceptual thought is lessened, where else can attention be profitably allocated in the service of emotional regulation? One answer is in the body. If behavioral and cognitive models are influenced by these developments, we may find that they begin to include a greater emphasis on the body as a place to focus attention, especially as an alternative to ruminative or worry-driven problem solving. Staying within the cognitive tradition, it is conceivable that the next generation of thought records may well contain a separate column that asks patients to list the bodily sensations they notice in conjunction with whatever automatic thoughts are present. Behavioral and cognitive therapies might also incorporate practices that generate physical sensations by placing the body in motion, such as yoga or mindful stretching and walking. These interventions would be adjunctive to the larger treatment agenda of helping patients to learn how awareness of events in the body provides a helpful starting point when responding to powerful emotions. Note that it is not just the attentional focus that is different, but the intention to bring a kindly curiosity to what one notices is equally important. Views such as this could lead to changes in the way in which we think about and conduct exposure-based therapies.

Other impacts may range more widely than the traditions themselves and require a radical retooling of methods. For example, the fact that patients may report less disturbance and a greater sense of well-being in the presence of the very thoughts that are normally seen as defining characteristics of the disorder presents a significant challenge to the psychometrics of behavior change. Similarly, measures of mindfulness will need to be developed that capture both its state- and trait-like capacities—something for which personality theory offers few templates. These are but some of the many avenues for continued engagement with the impact of mindfulness/acceptance/radical acceptance-based clinical care on the traditional base of behavioral and cognitive therapies. With time, the newer treatments may no longer be seen as such, but might become part of the dominant tradition itself. The shift within this new wave of therapies might be seen as one of emphasis. Yet pitching interventions at levels that do not engage cognition in its propositional form challenges all those approaches that assert that changing such propositions are essential. In a similar way, the valuation of acceptance and inquiry as sufficient interventions, rather than as halfway measures in the service of change, is an important new development. Perhaps most radical within MBCT, and to some extent within DBT, is the demand placed upon therapists to acquaint themselves personally with mindfulness practice. Our experience of instructing in this mode is that it feels very different from a "therapist" mode, but we acknowledge that it will take a great deal of careful empirical work to amplify and investigate this suggestion, and to see how much it carries weight in terms of patient outcomes.

ACKNOWLEDGMENTS

The work described in this chapter was supported in part by Grant No. MH53457 from the National Institute of Mental Health (to Zindel V. Segal) and by Grant No. RA 013 from the Wales Office of Research and Development for Health and Social Care (to J. Mark G. Williams and John D. Teasdale).

REFERENCES

American Psychiatric Association. (1987). *Diagnostic and statistical manual of mental disorders* (3rd ed., rev.). Washington, DC: Author.

Barber, J. P., & DeRubeis, R. J. (1989). On second thought: Where the action is in cognitive therapy for depression. *Cognitive Therapy and Research, 13,* 441–457.

Basco, M. R., & Rush, A. J. (1995). Compliance with pharmacology in mood disorders. *Psychiatric Annals, 25*, 269–275.

Beck, A. T., Epstein, N., & Harrison, R. (1983). Cognitions, attitudes and personality dimensions in depression. *British Journal of Cognitive Psychotherapy, 1*, 1–16.

Beck, A. T., Rush, A. J. Shaw, B. F., & Emery, G. (1979). *Cognitive therapy of depression.* New York: Guilford Press.

Blackburn, I. M., Eunson, K. M., & Bishop, S. (1986). A two-year naturalistic follow-up of depressed patients treated with cognitive therapy, pharmacotherapy, and a combination of both. *Journal of Affective Disorders, 10*, 67–75.

Evans, M. D., Hollon, S. D., DeRubeis, R. J., Piasecki, J. M., Grove, W. M., Garvey, M. J., et al. (1992). Differential relapse following cognitive therapy and pharmacotherapy for depression. *Archives of General Psychiatry, 49*, 802–808.

Haaga, D. A. F., Dyck, M. J., & Ernst, D. (1991). Empirical status of cognitive theory of depression. *Psychological Bulletin, 110*, 215–236.

Hayes, S. C. (2002). Acceptance, mindfulness and science. *Clinical Psychology: Science and Practice, 9*, 101–106.

Hayes, S. C. (1987). A contextual approach to therapeutic change. In N. S. Jacobson (Ed.), *Psychotherapists in clinical practice: Cognitive and behavioral perspectives* (pp. 327–387). New York: Guilford Press.

Hayes, S. C., Strosahl, K., & Wilson, K. G. (1999). *Acceptance and commitment therapy: An experiential approach to behavior change.* New York: Guilford Press.

Hayes, S. C., Wilson, K. G., Gifford, E. V., Follette, V., & Strosahl, K. (1996). Emotional avoidance and behavioral disorders: A functional dimensional approach to diagnosis and treatment. *Journal of Consulting and Clinical Psychology, 64*, 1152–1168.

Hollon, S., & Shelton, R. (2002, June). *Cognitive therapy and the prevention of relapse in severely depressed outpatients.* Paper presented at the Society for Psychotherapy Research, Santa Barbara, CA.

Ingram, R. E., & Hollon, S. D. (1986). Cognitive therapy for depression from an information processing perspective. In R. E. Ingram (Ed.), *Information processing approaches to clinical psychology* (pp. 261–280). Orlando, FL: Academic Press.

Ingram, R. E., Miranda, J., & Segal, Z. V. (1998). *Cognitive vulnerability to depression.* New York: Guilford Press.

Judd, L. J. (1997). The clinical course of unipolar major depressive disorders. *Archives of General Psychiatry, 54*, 989–991.

Kabat-Zinn, J. (1990). *Full Catastrophe Living: The program of the Stress Reduction Clinic at the University of Massachusetts Medical Center.* New York: Delta.

Kabat-Zinn, J. (1994). *Wherever you go there you are: Mindfulness meditation in everyday life.* New York: Hyperion.

Kabat-Zinn, J., Lipworth, L., Burney, R., & Sellers, W. (1986). Four-year follow-up of a meditation-based program for the self-regulation of chronic pain: Treatment outcomes and compliance. *Clinical Journal of Pain, 2*, 159–173.

Kabat-Zinn, J., Massion, A. O., Kristeller, J., Peterson, L. G., Fletcher, K. E., Pbert, L., et al. (1992). Effectiveness of a meditation-based stress reduction program in the treatment of anxiety disorders. *American Journal of Psychiatry, 149*, 936–943.

Kendler, K. S., Thornton, L. M., & Gardner, C. O. (2000). Stressful life events and previous episodes in the etiology of major depression in women: An evaluation of the "kindling" hypothesis. *American Journal of Psychiatry, 157*, 1243–1251.

Kessler, R. C., McGonagle, K. A., Zhao, S., Nelson, C. B., Hughes, M., Eshlerman, S., et al. (1994). Lifetime and twelve-month prevalence of DSM-III-R psychiatric disorders in the United States: Results from the National Comorbidity Study. *Archives of General Psychiatry, 51*, 8–19.

Kovacs, M. B., & Beck, A. T. (1978). Maladaptive cognitive structures in depression. *American Journal of Psychiatry, 135*, 525–533.

Kupfer, D. J., Frank, E., Perel, J. M., Cornes, C., Mallinger, A. G., Thase, M. E., et al. (1992). Five-year outcomes for maintenance therapies in recurrent depression. *Archives of General Psychiatry, 49,* 769–763.

Linehan, M. M. (1993). *Cognitive-behavioral treatment of borderline personality disorder.* New York: Guilford Press.

Linehan, M. M., Armstrong, H. E., Suarez, A., Allmon, D., & Heard H. H. (1991). Cognitive-behavioural treatment of chronically parasuicidal borderline patients. *Archives of General Psychiatry, 48,* 1060–1064.

Ma, S. H., & Teasdale, J. D. (2004). Mindfulness-based cognitive therapy for depression: Replication and exploration of differential relapse prevention effects. *Journal of Consulting and Clinical Psychology, 72,* 31–40.

Murray, C. J. L., & Lopez, A. D. (1998). *The global burden of disease: A comprehensive assessment of mortality, injuries and risk factors in 1990 and projected to 2000.* Cambridge, MA: Harvard School of Public Health and the World Health Organization.

Nolen-Hoeksema, S. (1991). Responses to depression and their effects on the duration of depressive episodes. *Journal of Abnormal Psychology, 100,* 569–582.

Norman, D. A., & Shallice, T. (1986). Attention to action: Willed and automatic control of behavior. In G. E. Schwartz & D. Shapiro (Eds.), *Consciousness and self-regulation: Advances in research and theory* (Vol. 4, pp. 1–18). New York: Plenum Press.

Olfson, M., Marcus, S., Druss, B., Elinson, L., Tanielian, T., & Pincus, H. (2002). National trends in the outpatient treatment of depression. *Journal of the American Medical Association, 287,* 203–209.

Persons, J. B., & Miranda, J. (1992). Cognitive theories of vulnerability to depression: Reconciling negative evidence. *Cognitive Therapy and Research, 16,* 485–502.

Post, R. M. (1992). Transduction of psychosocial stress into the neurobiology of recurrent affective disorder. *American Journal of Psychiatry, 149,* 999–1010.

Pyszczynski, T., & Greenberg, J. (1987). Self-regulatory perseveration and the depressive self-focusing style: A self-awareness theory of reactive depression. *Psychological Bulletin, 102,* 122–138.

Segal, Z. V., Gemar, M. C., & Williams, S. (1999). Differential cognitive response to a mood challenge following successful cognitive therapy or pharmacotherapy for unipolar depression. *Journal of Abnormal Psychology, 108,* 3–10.

Segal, Z. V., Williams, J. M. G., & Teasdale, J. D. (2001). *Mindfulness-based cognitive therapy for depression.* New York: Guilford Press.

Segal, Z. V., Williams, J. M., Teasdale, J. D., & Gemar, M. (1996). A cognitive science perspective on kindling and episode sensitisation in recurrent affective disorder. *Psychological Medicine, 26,* 371–380.

Shea, M. T., Elkin, I., Imber, S. D., Sotsky, F. M., Watkins, J. T., Collins, J. F., et al. (1992). Course of depressive symptoms over follow-up: Findings from the NIMH Treatment of Depression Collaborative Research Program. *Archives of General Psychiatry, 49,* 782–787.

Simons, A. D., Garfield, S. L., & Murphy, G. E. (1984). The process of change in cognitive therapy and pharmacotherapy for depression: Changes in mood and cognition. *Archives of General Psychiatry, 41,* 45–51.

Simons, A. D., Murphy, G. E., Levine, J. L., & Wetzel, R. D. (1986). Cognitive therapy and pharmacotherapy for depression: Sustained improvement over one year. *Archives of General Psychiatry, 43,* 43–50.

Spitzer, R. L., Williams, J. B. W., Gibbon, M., & First, M. B. (1992). The Structured Clinical Interview for DSM-III-R (SCID): I. History, rationale, and description. *Archives of General Psychiatry, 49,* 624–629.

Teasdale, J. D. (1983). Negative thinking in depression: Cause, effect or reciprocal relationship? *Advances in Behaviour Research and Therapy, 5,* 3–25.

Teasdale, J. D. (1988). Cognitive vulnerability to persistent depression. *Cognition and Emotion, 2,* 247–274.

Teasdale, J. D. (1997). The relationship between cognition and emotion: The mind-in-place in mood disorders. In D. M. Clark & C. G. Fairburn (Eds.), *Science and practice of cognitive behaviour therapy* (pp. 67–93). Oxford, UK: Oxford University Press.

Teasdale, J. D. (1999). Emotional processing, three modes of mind and the prevention of relapse in depression. *Behaviour Research and Therapy, 37,* S53–S78.

Teasdale, J. D., & Barnard, P. J. (1993). *Affect, cognition and change: Re-modelling depressive thought.* Hove, UK: Erlbaum.

Teasdale, J. D., Segal, Z. V., & Williams, J. M. G. (1995). How does cognitive therapy prevent depressive relapse and why should attentional control (mindfulness) training help? *Behaviour Research and Therapy, 33,* 25–39.

Teasdale, J. D., Segal, Z. V., Williams, J. M. G., Ridgeway, V. A., Soulsby, J. M., & Lau, M. A. (2000). Prevention of relapse/recurrence in major depression by mindfulness-based cognitive therapy. *Journal of Consulting and Clinical Psychology, 68,* 615–623.

Watzlawick, P., Weakland, J., & Fisch, R. (1974). *Change: Principles of problem formation and problem resolution.* New York: Norton.

Wegner, D. (1994). Ironic processes of mental control. *Psychological Review, 101,* 34–52.

Weissman, A., & Beck, A. T. (1978, November). *The Dysfunctional Attitudes Scale.* Paper presented at the annual meeting of the Association for Advancement of Behavior Therapy, Chicago.

4

Acceptance, Mindfulness, and Cognitive-Behavioral Therapy

Comparisons, Contrasts, and Application to Anxiety

Susan M. Orsillo, Lizabeth Roemer, Jennifer Block Lerner, *and* Matthew T. Tull

Psychotherapy development and research has been particularly fruitful across the anxiety disorders, with evidence emerging for the efficacy of cognitive-behavioral interventions (typically either exposure or cognitive therapy alone, or the two combined) for each anxiety disorder. Despite this success, more work is needed to (1) validate models of the development and maintenance of anxiety disorders, (2) improve treatment efficacy (particularly in those disorders with lower success rates, such as posttraumatic stress disorder and generalized anxiety disorder), (3) determine mechanisms of change and active ingredients in complex treatment packages, and (4) improve dissemination and acceptability of interventions as efficacious treatments remain underutilized in clinical practice (Goisman, Warshaw, & Keller, 1999; Goisman et al., 1993). The acceptance-based approaches highlighted in this volume and discussed below may facilitate each of these goals.

Krasner (1992) has argued that the process of continuous creation is the core of behavioral science. The advent of behavior therapy and the "cognitive revolution" each spurred significant excitement, theory development and refinement, research, and criticism. Theories of psychopathology and treatment that integrate acceptance and mindfulness into existing cognitive-behavioral approaches seem to represent another potentially noteworthy movement within behavioral science and, as such, they require careful study and critique. In many ways, these "new" approaches to treatment are consistent with "traditional" cognitive-behavioral approaches to treating anxiety disorders. However, they highlight and make explicit some elements of intervention that have traditionally been more implicit (as we discuss below), which may be particularly important in the dissemination of treatments (where such implicit emphases may be lost).

In the first half of this chapter, we provide a brief overview of the current state of cognitive-behavioral theories and treatments for the anxiety disorders, highlight theoretical and empirical problems in these extant literatures, and explore ways that acceptance-based theories and interventions are consistent with, expand on, or challenge traditional cognitive-behavioral elements.

Our own treatment development work has focused on exploring acceptance-based approaches in the treatment of the more chronic, treatment resistant anxiety disorders, specifically posttraumatic stress disorder (Orsillo & Batten, in press), social phobia (Block & Wulfert, 2002), and generalized anxiety disorder (Orsillo, Roemer, & Barlow, 2003; Roemer & Orsillo, 2002). We are currently integrating established treatments for generalized anxiety disorder (Zinbarg, Craske, & Barlow, 1993; Borkovec & Newman, 2000) with elements of acceptance-based treatments (specifically acceptance and commitment therapy [Hayes, Strosahl, & Wilson, 1999]; mindfulness-based cognitive therapy [Segal, Williams, & Teasdale, 2002]; and dialectical behavior therapy [Linehan, 1993a]) with the hope of improving the efficacy of treatment for generalized anxiety disorder (GAD), the least successfully treated of all the anxiety disorders (Brown, Barlow, & Leibowitz, 1994). In the second half of this chapter, we provide a brief rationale for the applicability of acceptance in the treatment of GAD and describe this still evolving treatment.

THE CURRENT STATUS OF COGNITIVE-BEHAVIORAL TREATMENT FOR ANXIETY DISORDERS

Given the prevalence, chronicity, and cost associated with the anxiety disorders (Barlow, 2002; Greenberg et al., 1999; Narrow, Rae, Robins, & Regier, 2002), it is not surprising that treatment development efforts in this area have been great. Fortunately, several cognitive-behavioral and behavioral treatment packages developed for each disorder have yielded significant and large effect sizes in randomized controlled trials (see Barlow, 2002, for disorder-specific, detailed reviews), although treatments for some disorders (e.g., panic disorder and specific phobia) have yielded higher proportions of treatment responders than others (e.g., GAD and posttraumatic stress disorder [PTSD]).

Given these findings, one might question the necessity of exploring new treatment options for those with anxiety disorders. However, meta-analyses and effect sizes do not tell the whole story regarding the potential effectiveness of these treatments in clinical practice. There are a number of methodological limitations to many randomized control trials that may lead to overestimates of the effectiveness and generalizability of these treatments. For instance, the few studies for panic disorder that have included participants with more severe agoraphobic avoidance show more attrition and lower rates of clinical improvement than studies with stricter exclusion criteria (Barlow, 2002). Additionally, clinical trials often rely on narrow measures of symptom reduction as the primary indicator of treatment success rather than attending to high-end state functioning or quality of life. Few longitudinal studies are available to confirm the long-term maintenance of gains made in treatment and many studies do not measure or report on the number of participants who seek additional treatment following the termination of a clinical trial (Barlow, 2002).

The vast majority of individuals seeking psychotherapy in the community do not receive empirically supported treatments (Goisman et al., 1993, 1999), confirming that more work is required to meet the needs of individuals who are suffering with their anxiety. It may be that more vigorous dissemination efforts are needed to bridge the scientist–practitioner gap. However, the underutilization of empirically supported treatments by practitioners may also be driven in part by some limits in their effectiveness or acceptability to consumers that may not be apparent from a review of the extant treatment outcome literature. Given the importance of acceptability and ease of dissemination in determining the effectiveness of a treatment (Kazdin, 1998), these factors should be directly addressed in further treatment development efforts. For instance, methods explicitly designed to reduce fear and avoidance of internal experiences may be useful in bolstering the effectiveness of treatment for clients who may otherwise refuse exposure therapy or drop out of treatment. Acceptance-based approaches will represent a "new wave" of behavioral science only to the extent that they address these specific areas in need of improvement.

Before we explore how acceptance-based approaches may improve on existing cognitive-behavioral treatments for anxiety disorders, we provide a brief overview of both these "new" and "traditional" approaches, including the theories that underlie them and the techniques that define them.

COGNITIVE-BEHAVIORAL TREATMENTS FOR ANXIETY
AND THEIR UNDERLYING MECHANISMS

The foundation of cognitive-behavioral treatments for anxiety is based in learning theory derived from a rich history of experimental animal and human research. However, contemporary treatment packages vary widely in their connection to classical and operant learning principles. Cognitive-behavioral treatments for the anxiety disorders often consist of various techniques bundled together that, as a package, have been shown to be efficacious in reducing fear. Techniques typically include behavioral approaches such as imaginal and *in vivo* exposure, as well as some form of cognitive therapy, typically cognitive restructuring. Self-monitoring (SM) of potentially relevant stimuli and responses is often included as an assessment procedure, although it has been argued that SM serves as a cue for environmental consequences (Nelson & Hayes, 1981) and thus may be seen as an active ingredient of treatment (Korotitsch & Nelson-Gray, 1999). Other adjunctive methods included in many treatment packages for anxiety include psychoeducation, some form of relaxation training and applied relaxation, and skills training. While cognitive-behavioral treatment packages including these methods have for the most part been shown to be efficacious, dismantling and process research has failed to provide an adequate understanding as to how these multifaceted treatments actually work (Rachman, 1991; Steketee & Barlow, 2002).

Early theories on the development and treatment of anxiety disorders generally suggested that fear develops through traumatic conditioning (e.g., Marks, 1969; Wolpe, 1958), is maintained operantly through avoidance learning (Mowrer, 1947), and is reduced through extinction, or the decrease in a learned response due to repeated, nonreinforced exposure to a conditioned stimulus. However, by the late 1960s, a number of criticisms were levied at this seemingly limited viewpoint of learning and its inability to account for the selectivity of phobias (Marks, 1969) or the reduction in fear when avoidant responses are not prevented (Rachman, Craske, Tallman, & Solyom, 1986), ultimately contributing to the development of learning models (e.g., Rescorla & Wagner, 1972) that included cognitive mechanisms (Barlow, 2002).

For instance, Foa and Kozak (1986) argued that informational models of learning were needed that attended not only to stimulus–response associations but also to their meanings. Based on Lang's (1979, 1985) bioinformational model of fear, they proposed an emotional processing model by which fearful associations are altered when the associative fear network (including stimulus, response, and meaning elements of the fear) is fully accessed and new nonthreatening information is incorporated. Foa and Kozak review research that supports the proposed importance of initial activation of the fear structure (indicated by physiological responding to the feared stimulus), as well as habituation (or extinction) within and across sessions for efficacious exposure therapy.

Mineka and Thomas (1999) expanded on the emotional processing theory by proposing that the critical "meaning" information that changes through exposure is the individual's belief regarding his or her ability to control potentially threatening or aversive situations. Control, or the contingent relationship between a response and the consequent outcome (Seligman, 1975), has been shown to reduce both conditioned and unconditioned anxiety in animals exposed to aversive events (Mineka & Thomas, 1999), and perceived control is correlationally associated with lower levels of anxiety among humans (Barlow, 2002). This construct is similar to self-efficacy in Bandura's model (1977, 1986), which states that a reduction in anxiety through exposure is mediated by an individual's beliefs about the ability to cope effectively with the anxiety-provoking situation.

While the emotional processing model has had an impact on treatment development and delivery, it has also been the target of criticism. For instance, there is mounting evidence that extinction does not reflect a destruction in the stimulus–response relationship. Instead, new learning is proposed to occur in which the stimulus becomes an ambiguous signal that may elicit different reactions depending on the context (Bouton, 2002). Furthermore, some studies have failed to find an association between within-session habituation and long-term fear reduction, and other studies have found that distraction (which should minimize activation of the fear network) does not always interfere with the efficacy of exposure (see Craske, 1999, for a detailed review). Finally, because cognitive representations and schemas (as well as associative fear networks) cannot be reliably assessed, it is difficult to test the cognitive model.

Nonetheless, the interest in cognitive processes as potential mechanisms of change in the treatment of anxiety disorders has led to a vigorous effort to develop cognitive alternatives to previously established behavioral principles, particularly as a way to extend the explanatory power of behavioral theories (James, 1993). Generally, cognitive models of psychopathology assume that an individual's schemas, which include belief systems, expectancies, and assumptions, assert a strong influence on both mood and behavior by influencing how information is perceived, coded, and recalled (Beck, 1993). Anxiety disorders specifically are thought to be caused and maintained in part by a disturbance in information processing that leads to an overestimation of danger or perceived threat and an associated underestimation of personal ability to cope (Beck, Emery, & Greenberg, 1985). For instance, Clark (1986, 1988, 1996) proposed that catastrophic misinterpretations of somatic sensations are primary in the development and maintenance of panic disorder.

Although cognitive theory has become increasingly popular over the last two decades, producing a plethora of research, it is marked by a number of shortcomings. One of the main inadequacies of the model is that the constructs at its foundation remain vague and difficult to operationalize and measure. Cognitive researchers have yet to demonstrate how irrational cognitions are acquired, who acquires them, and how they can be measured independent of anxiety or panic (Bouton, Mineka, & Barlow, 2001).

Furthermore, despite an abundance of research, the basic premise of the theory, that cognition predicts behavior, has yet to be supported. Longitudinal studies have confirmed that "dysfunctional attitudes" wax and wane over time with symptoms (Persons & Miranda, 1992); the association between cognitions and emotions is bidirectional (e.g., Nolen-Hoeksema, Girgus, & Seligman, 1986; Wells & Matthews, 1994); and responses (such as panic attacks) occur without the precedence of detectable cognitions (e.g., Kenardy & Taylor, 1999).

Cognitive theories have also been criticized for ignoring situational or contextual factors that have a significant impact on emotional and behavioral responses. While cognitive theorists would posit internal mediational processes, such as attributional style or schema, if two individuals responded differently to the same event (e.g., divorce), an analysis of the contextual features of the event may result in a different explanation. When more detailed information about a life event is available, research suggests that the link between the event and the subsequent emotional reaction can be reliably established without relying on idiosyncratic, dysfunctional internal mechanisms (Coyne, 1989).

The development of cognitive therapy for anxiety disorders has also drawn criticism. One significant problem is that cognitive therapy has become a general label for a variety of techniques, any of which may actually be the active ingredient of treatment. Cognitive therapy typically includes three components: (1) self-monitoring, or the identification and labeling of thoughts; (2) logical analysis, which involves restructuring or changing the content of a dysfunctional cognition through verbal examination; and (3) hypothesis testing, or the evaluation of the validity of dysfunctional cognition through the design and implementation of behavioral experiments (Jarrett & Nelson, 1987). This mixture of cognitive and behavioral techniques makes it difficult to examine the underlying mechanism of change. Even logical analysis, the cornerstone of the theory, comprises techniques that differ significantly in form and function. For instance, some approaches emphasize content change. In other words, a seemingly irrational thought, such as "Because she will not go on a date with me, I am a loser," would be labeled as a cognitive distortion, disputed and replaced with a more rational thought, such as "There are a number of reasons as to why she might not want to go out with me," or "I am an attractive interesting man and I will eventually get a date." However, other techniques also described as logical analysis represent more of a contextual change. For instance, thoughts and feelings are viewed as independent from behavior in the following cognitive restructuring exercise when "I can't give a speech when I am anxious" is replaced with "I am still able to talk while experiencing anxious thoughts and feelings."

The most critical shortcoming of cognitive therapy is that it has failed to achieve its intended impact: Cognitive therapy is not uniquely associated with changes in cognition (Arntz, 2002; McManus, Clark, & Hackmann, 2000; Westling & Öst, 1995); there is little evidence for long-lasting overall superiority of cognitive treatments (Booth & Rachman, 1992; Craske, Glover, & DeCola, 1995; Fava et al., 1994; Foa et al., 1999; Gould, Buckminster, Pollack, Otto, & Yap, 1997; Lovell, Marks, Noshirvani, Thrasher, & Livanou, 2001; Marks, Lovell, Noshirvani, Livanou, & Thrasher, 1998; Tarrier et al., 1999); and changes in dysfunctional attitudes do not appear to mediate changes in depression and anxiety in cognitive-behavioral treatment (Burns & Spangler, 2001).

RECENT INNOVATIONS IN COGNITIVE-BEHAVIORAL THEORY AND TREATMENT FOR ANXIETY

In response to many of the shortcomings of traditional *content*-focused cognitive-behavioral approaches to psychotherapy, a number of theories and techniques focused on cognitive *processes*, particularly allocation of attention, have recently been proposed. For instance, Wells and Matthews (1994) developed the self-regulatory executive function (S-REF) model of psychological disorders that causally links psychological disturbances to a syndrome of cognitive-attentional responses characterized by self-focused attention or "online" processing of negative self-beliefs, worry/rumination, threat monitoring, resource limitation, and maladaptive coping. From this model, a key component of cognitive-behavioral treatment is presumed to be the direct modification of cognitive processes, particularly attention. The attention training technique (ATT) has been developed as an attempt to modify perseverative self-relevant processing associated with emotional disorders (Wells, 2000) and has been preliminarily applied to the treatment of panic disorder (Wells, 1990) and social phobia (Wells, White, & Carter, 1997). Situational attention refocusing (SAR), another attentional technique derived from S-REF aimed at overriding biased attention and/or facilitating the development of disconfirmatory processing routines during stressful situations, has been applied to the treatment of social phobia (Wells & Papageorgiou, 1998). A somewhat similar approach, task concentration training, was developed and evaluated for the treatment of fear of blushing (Bögels, Mulkens, & de Jong, 1997; Mulkens, Bögels, de Jong, & Louwers, 2001). While these approaches may represent improvements to existing content-based theories and therapies, their development is still in the preliminary stages and empirical support is limited.

Bouton and colleagues (2001) provided a compelling review of the basic research supporting the application of modern learning theory to the development and maintenance of anxiety (specifically panic disorder) and attempted to address the criticisms that have led to discontent with the behavioral model. They particularly underscore how cognitive and other internal experiences can be involved in learning. For instance, while interoceptive conditioning, a process by which low-level somatic sensations of anxiety or arousal may become conditioned stimuli associated with higher levels of anxiety or arousal, has been proposed to be critically important in the development of panic disorder (Bouton et al., 2001; Goldstein & Chambless, 1978; Razran, 1961), critics have argued that this theory is conceptually confusing and circular, in that anxiety or panic seem to serve arbitrarily as conditioned and unconditioned stimuli and responses (McNally, 1990, 1994; Reiss, 1987). Bouton and colleagues review a number of animal and human studies that demonstrate the viability of this model and relate it to Dworkin's (1993) description of homoreflex conditioning. This recognition that internal experiences can serve as conditioned stimuli helps set the stage for conceptualizing experiential avoidance (described more fully below), which is a key concept in several of the new behavior therapies. While Bouton and colleagues posit that cognitions, seen as a component of anxiety and panic, may also become causal through a similar process of associative learning, current evidence suggests that they are not necessary and not yet shown to be sufficient, causal stimuli.

Modern learning theory has also expanded to provide an explanation for how the "meaning" of a stimulus develops. Bouton and colleagues (2001) review a body of research examining the role of the context during extinction trials in the reemergence of fear following extinction. Contextual stimuli are thought to include both external cues in the environment and internal cues, such as drug and mood states, and even the passage of time. The cumulative research suggests that extinction does not generalize well between contexts, which has significant implications for improving the efficacy of exposure therapy as a treatment for anxiety disorders.

Modern learning theory also addresses controllability and predictability, which, as discussed earlier, have been highlighted as potentially important "meaning" variables in the development and treatment of anxiety disorders. Drawing on a growing body of animal and human research, Bouton and colleagues (2001) suggest that unpredictability and uncontrollability of aversive stimuli are factors that may affect the potency of the anxiety response and as such may strengthen fear conditioning.

While modern learning theory provides one of the best prevailing empirically based explanations for the development and treatment of anxiety, this theory is also not without its shortcomings. Although modern learning theory offers a relatively nice account for the development of panic disorder, the application to other anxiety disorders, particularly those with complex cognitive rather than somatic involvement, such as GAD, remain unstudied. Furthermore, critical gaps remain in the translation from animal research to clinical application. For instance, in the typical conditioning paradigm, animals have no learning history with the stimulus that is conditioned to elicit fear. Once the extinction process is engaged, the conditioned stimulus becomes an ambiguous stimulus, its fear eliciting properties dependent on the context. This new ambiguity may explain why the initial fear conditioning is mostly resistant to context, whereas extinction is more context-specific (Bouton, 2002). However, humans rarely develop anxiety disorders to a conditioned stimulus to which they have never been exposed. Thus, the conditioned stimulus is likely ambiguous from the initial fear acquiring experience, which may have implications for its endurance and treatment, deserving further study. Finally, and most critically, learning models based on nonhumans may be less useful in areas in which language and cognition dominate (Hayes, Barnes-Holmes, & Roche, 2001).

In summary, while it is clear that cognitive-behavioral treatments have been shown to be efficacious in reducing symptoms of anxiety disorders, efforts are still needed to improve the effectiveness and acceptability of these approaches, dismantle complex packages, and more clearly delineate the mechanism of change.

Conceptualizing Anxiety Disorders from an Acceptance-Based Behavioral Perspective

There is compelling evidence that experiential avoidance, or attempts to change the form or frequency of internal events such as thoughts, feelings, bodily sensations, or memories, contributes to the development and maintenance of many forms of psychopathology (Hayes, Wilson, Gifford, Follette, & Strosahl, 1996). From this perspective, anxiety disorders are thought to develop when individuals are unwilling to experience the anxiety (including associated thoughts, images, and possibly other accompanying distressing emotions as well) with which they are struggling. A number of internal and external control strategies may be attempted, depending on the client and his or her symptoms, in the service of alleviating these experiences. Most obviously, significant behavioral avoidance develops as the client attempts to avoid objects and situations that elicit unwanted internal events. As this avoidance or escape behavior increases and generalizes, the client may begin to make changes that have a significant impact on his or her quality of life. Similarly, individuals with anxiety disorders often engage in a variety of experiential avoidance strategies, such as distraction or suppression, aimed at decreasing or eliminating anxiety-related cognitions and sensations. A core assumption of this model is that these attempts at avoidance only serve to perpetuate distress.

One learning account of experiential avoidance (relational frame theory [RFT]; Hayes et al., 2001) focuses on the role of language and cognition.[1] Humans are able to bidirectionally associate stimuli whose relationship has been trained in only one direction. This unique form of learning means that internal experiences such as thoughts, images, and emotions can come to serve the same function as the events with which they are associated. Hayes and colleagues (2001) suggest that relational responding, or learning to respond to one event in terms of another, is initially reinforced by one's verbal community (e.g., humans reinforce one another for verbally describing the learning process of relating two stimuli). The process is thought to be maintained in part by the instrumental value of understanding stimulus relations, in that this level of understanding is often associated with an increased ability to control events.

Unfortunately, this unique ability to understand internal events is not supplemented by an ability to escape or avoid such events. Research has documented that attempts to avoid and suppress internal events such as thoughts and emotions are nonproductive (Gross & Levenson, 1993, 1997; Wegner, 1994). However, the futility of control efforts may not be readily apparent; the paradoxical effects of thought suppression often emerge after some appearance of short-term utility (Gold & Wegner, 1995). Thus, individuals often continuously attempt to apply this strategy. Furthermore, the literal and evaluative functions of human language permit humans to anxiously anticipate future, feared events, evaluate their performance in a situation as inferior to others, and label their responses as pathological and aversive (Hayes et al., 2001). These verbal products are experienced as comparable to the events they represent (including one's own construction of self), a relationship that has been described as cognitive fusion (Hayes, Strosahl, et al., 1999). Avoidance efforts are thought to be motivated by cognitive fusion, in that negatively evaluated states are viewed as more aversive and dangerous to the extent that they are perceived to have some impact and influence on one's enduring sense of self (Hayes, Strosahl, et al., 1999).

Consistent with this work, a number of behavioral psychotherapy efforts have been directed toward targeting experiential avoidance and increasing acceptance, most notably acceptance and commitment therapy (ACT; Hayes, Strosahl, et al., 1999). Similar emphases on experiential acceptance can also be seen in dialectical behavior therapy (DBT; Linehan, 1993a, 1993b), integrative behavioral couple therapy (Cordova, Jacobson,

---

[1] Of course, other psychotherapy traditions have also addressed the concepts of experiential avoidance and acceptance (e.g., Greenberg & Safran, 1987; Rogers, 1961); here, we focus only on behavioral (and cognitive-behavioral) approaches.

& Christensen, 1998), and, from the cognitive tradition, mindfulness-based cognitive therapy (MBCT; Segal et al., 2002), as well as other approaches reviewed in this volume.

In our work (described more fully below), influenced heavily by ACT, experiential acceptance is defined as a willingness to experience internal events, such as thoughts, feelings, memories, and physiological reactions, in order to participate in experiences that are deemed important and meaningful. Acceptance reflects a change in the behavior elicited by a stimulus from that which is functioning to avoid, escape, or destroy, to behavior functioning to maintain or pursue contact (Cordova, 2001). The basis of our acceptance-based behavioral therapy is first and foremost to increase actions and behaviors in the client's life that are consistent with his or her values and/or desires (e.g., being intimately connected with others, engaging in challenging and meaningful work, education, or recreational activities).

Experiential avoidance is viewed as the primary obstacle preventing individuals from engaging in valued actions. In other words, clients believe that they need to gain control over their thoughts and feelings before they can move forward with valued action, because these internal experiences are seen as pathological, painful, and behaviorally limiting. Thus, the proposed mechanism of change is the enhancement of a stance from which internal events are viewed as natural, universal, transient responses that arise from our cumulative interactions with the environment that need not direct behavior, as well as an increased contact with naturally reinforcing contingencies for valued behavior.

This working definition is important, because it addresses many of the misconceptions associated with acceptance. For instance, acceptance is often misunderstood to be resignation, or accepting the fact that one will live with chronic anxiety or some psychological disability forever. However, an acceptance approach assumes that the most distressing component of anxiety will lessen once anxiety is no longer habitually evaluated and suppressed (although acceptance is not seen as a control strategy, as discussed more fully below). Chronic anxiety is thought to be maintained by efforts at escape and avoidance. Furthermore, inherent in acceptance is behavioral change aimed at eliminating the notion of anxiety as a disability. Our therapy is directed at opening up behavioral possibilities where behavioral restriction had been the norm, thus helping client develop more flexible behavioral repertoires (Goldiamond, 1974).

Another misconception is that acceptance implies that experiencing negative thoughts and feelings is a noble goal, and that one "should" choose to live this way rather than "choosing" to control internal experiences. We do not see the option of controlling internal events as a choice. Although there are some techniques that can be used for the short-term control of internal events, such as distraction, relaxation, or substance use, there is widespread evidence from experimental research (e.g., Purdon,

1999; Wegner, 1994), epidemiological data, and our clients' lives that internally directed control efforts are not associated with long-term, maintained success.

A variety of clinical methods are used to enhance experiential acceptance (more fully described as used in our current treatment efforts below). Generally, we use psychoeducational methods designed to introduce key concepts such as the limits and cost of experiential avoidance and control. In-session experiential exercises and between-session assignments are seen as the primary methods of increasing experiential acceptance and concurrent value-driven behavior.

One set of techniques that we have found to be useful in facilitating an acceptance stance is mindfulness practice. Mindfulness is a construct that has recently gained considerable attention as a potentially powerful clinical method. While it is similar in some ways to experiential acceptance, mindfulness arises from a spiritual rather than a scientific tradition. Mindfulness is a process that involves moving toward a state in which one is fully observant of external and internal stimuli in the present moment, and open to accepting (rather than attempting to change or judge) the current situation (e.g., Kabat-Zinn, 1994; Segal et al., 2002).

Given the current adoption of mindfulness into psychotherapy, several existing theories have been applied to explain the potential efficacy of mindfulness skills. In a review of the literature, Baer (2003) suggests that mindfulness may promote exposure to previously avoided internal experiences, lead to cognitive change or a change in attitude about one's thoughts, increase self-observation and management, produce a state of relaxation, or increase acceptance. Teasdale and colleagues (2002) suggest that mindfulness practice may be efficacious through increasing metacognitive awareness, a cognitive set associated with "decentering" or "disindentification," in which negative thoughts and feelings are experienced as mental events rather than as the self. Breslin, Zack, and McMain (2002) suggest that mindfulness may be a sensitizing process that increases an individual's awareness of the relationship between certain stimuli and responses, which may decrease the continued automatic response to the stimulus, and at the same time a desensitizing process that promotes exposure and tolerance of negative affect and cognition.

While there is mounting evidence that mindfulness practice is associated with improved physical and psychological functioning (Baer, 2003), at present, there is no clear evidence as to how mindfulness works and no single theory of psychopathology serving as the foundation for its use in psychotherapy (Hayes & Wilson, 2003). We (Roemer & Orsillo, 2003) and others (e.g., Baer, 2003; Hayes & Wilson, 2003; Teasdale, Segal, & Williams, 2003) have begun to theoretically explore how this spiritual tradition fits into current theories of psychopathology, but more work is needed to investigate empirically the mechanism through which mindfulness operates and to integrate this technique into a theoretical context (Hayes, 2002; Teasdale et al., 2003). Considerably more research is also needed to support current theories of experiential avoidance and acceptance, and their role in psychopathology and psychotherapy. However, the initial promise of acceptance-based approaches suggests that further inquiry into their relationship with traditional approaches is indicated.

Similarities and Differences between Cognitive-Behavioral and Acceptance-Based Behavioral Approaches to Anxiety

Approach and Avoidance

Acceptance-based behavioral models of psychopathology are consistent with existing cognitive-behavioral formulations of and treatments for anxiety, in that both include internal avoidance as a causal and/or maintaining factor. For instance, "interoceptive avoidance" or the avoidance of behaviors that produce somatic symptoms (e.g., drinking caffeinated beverages, exercise, sexual relations), has been shown to be characteristic of panic disorder (Rapee, Craske, & Barlow, 1995), and interoceptive exposure is a cornerstone of cognitive-behavioral treatment for this disorder (Barlow, 2002). Similarly, fear of emotional responding (specifically fear, Goldstein & Chambless, 1978; but also other emotions, Williams, Chambless, & Ahrens, 1997) has been identified as a precipitating or maintaining factor in panic and other anxiety disorders. Thought–action fusion, or the belief that thoughts can directly influence external events (e.g., "If I imagine my son being hit by a car, it will happen") and that having negatively evaluated intrusive thoughts (e.g., "I want to stab my children") is morally equivalent to carrying out a prohibited action, which is consistent with the concept of cognitive fusion in ACT (Hayes, Strosahl, et al., 1999), has been implicated in the development and maintenance of obsessive–compulsive disorder (OCD; Shafran, Thordarson, & Rachman, 1996). Avoidance of trauma-related emotions seems to predict the emergence of more distress and severity of symptoms among those who experience a traumatic event (Gilboa-Schechtman & Foa, 2001).

Drawing from this shared conceptualization of the role of avoidance in the persistence of fear and avoidance, both traditional and acceptance-based behavioral therapies advocate approach behavior as an integral part of treatment. Traditional approaches typically develop a fear and avoidance hierarchy of anxiety-eliciting situations and prescribe a systematic and progressive program of exposure to those situations, with the primary goal being the eventual extinction of fear. As described earlier, traditional approaches typically involve exposure to objects and situations, as well as internal events such as somatic sensations, as in the case of panic disorder, and thoughts and images, as in the treatment of OCD and PTSD. Although behavioral models have begun to identify emotions themselves as potential conditioned stimuli (e.g., Goldstein & Chambless, 1978; Williams et al., 1997), it has been less common to include such emotional responses as specific targets of exposure in manualized treatments.

While approach is advocated in acceptance-based behavioral therapies and the methods used are topographically similar to those used in traditional exposure therapy, the rationale and goal are different. Acceptance-based therapies explicitly connect approach behavior to increasing quality of life. Clients are encouraged to identify valued directions in their lives and to commit to actions that are consistent with these values. It is acknowledged that this action will inevitably bring up painful thoughts, feelings, images, and sensations and urges to avoid. Engaging in behavioral or "exposure" assignments is directed at reducing avoidance but not extinguishing internal responses (although it is acknowledged that extinction may occur). Engagement in the actions themselves is seen as inherently valuable.

While this approach is not inconsistent with traditional behavior therapy, it makes explicit a component of therapy that has become implicit in many manualized treatments. This emphasis on clinically significant change may address a major shortcoming of the extant treatment literature, in that the operationalization of clinical significance, if done at all, is often done a priori using outcome measures that may or may not represent the client's ability to function better in some palpable way (Kazdin, 1998). It is also likely that explicitly connecting approach or exposure with values may increase the willingness of a previously reluctant client to experience private events, since the purpose and benefit of doing so may be more obvious and salient than in traditional behavioral approaches.

Acceptance is also intended to increase "decentering," "defusion," or "deliteralization" of language or "metacognitive awareness"; all processes propose to demonstrate to clients that internal events are transient responses rather than personally threatening stimuli that need to be avoided. This altered relationship to one's internal experience may increase clients' willingness to engage in exposure and experience the accompanying distress.

Preliminary support for the potential utility of an acceptance rationale for enhancing traditional exposure therapy comes from an experimental study with panic disorder. Levitt, Brown, Orsillo, and Barlow (in press) compared the physiological arousal, self-reported anxiety, and willingness of participants diagnosed with panic disorder who were randomly assigned to a suppression, acceptance, or control instruction condition before engaging in a CO_2 inhalation challenge. Although the groups did not differ in their physiological response to the challenge, clients in the acceptance group reported less anxiety and a greater willingness to participate in a second challenge than did the other two groups. While the generalizability of these experimental findings to clinical practice is unknown, the results of the study do provide some support for continued examination of the potential integration of acceptance into the interoceptive treatment for panic disorder.

Finally, while modern learning theory has made significant gains in including interoceptive conditioning and exposure in its model, the impact of complex human phenomena on fear acquisition and resistance to change remains underaddressed in this model. Both traditional and acceptance-based behavioral theories underscore the role of learning in the development of anxiety disorders, but newer learning theories (e.g., Hayes et al., 2001) expand on this conceptualization by including potential pathways by which language, cognition, and access to private events affect emotional learning. More basic and applied research is needed from both traditions to develop treatment models more fully.

Cognitive Factors

Acceptance-based and cognitive approaches are similar in that they both acknowledge the role of life experiences (learning or programming) in contributing to the content of thoughts and experiences commonly associated with anxiety disorders. However, they differ radically in the presumed role of cognitions in the development and treatment of the disorders. As discussed earlier, the basis of the cognitive model is that cognitions (or schemas) are at least partially causal in the development of anxiety disorders. In contrast, acceptance-based (and more traditional) behavioral approaches view cognitions as responses.

Based on the cognitive model, cognitive therapy is aimed at directly modifying cognitive content and processes, most traditionally through the Socratic method of questioning the rationality of presumably dysfunctional thoughts. Acceptance-based approaches focus on changing one's *relationship to* one's thoughts and feelings, viewing thoughts as thoughts rather than as reality (Hayes, Strosahl, et al., 1999; Segal et al., 2002; Teasdale et al., 2002). Thus, cognitive approaches are aimed at changing thought content, whereas acceptance-based approaches include methods such as mindfulness practice and deliteralization exercises aimed at changing one's relationship with his or her internal responses.

However, as discussed earlier, cognitive therapy involves a number of techniques, some of which are consistent with acceptance-based approaches. Interestingly, there is some evidence that MBCT (an acceptance-based approach) and traditional cognitive therapy both may work through a similar mechanism. Teasdale and colleagues (2002) demonstrated that the success of both MBCT and cognitive therapy in decreasing depressive relapse was associated with increases in metacognitive awareness (the ability to view thoughts and feelings from a decentered perspective). Although similar studies have yet to be conducted exploring the role of metacognitive awareness in the treatment of anxiety, it may also be an important underlying mechanism in cognitive therapy for anxiety disorders.

Attention

Traditional, contemporary, and acceptance-based cognitive-behavioral models all acknowledge the role of attention in the development and treatment of anxiety, although the theories differ in the importance and function that they ascribe to this construct. Early behavioral models identified attention as a response that could be brought under operant control (Ullman & Krasner, 1975). As mentioned earlier, self-monitoring has been conceptualized as an active ingredient through its modification of attentional focus.

Cognitive-behavioral models posit that attention is narrowed and biased toward threat cues among clients with anxiety disorders, and that worry disrupts one's contact with the full range of internal and external stimuli. Thus, in addition to extinguishing conditioned stimuli and preventing avoidance, cognitive-behavioral approaches attempt to increase clients' attention to naturally occurring contingencies in order to reinforce and support more flexible behavioral responding.

Several techniques are used to engage this process. As discussed earlier, self-monitoring increases attention to environmental cues. Cognitive therapy teaches clients to notice maladaptive thoughts and consider more rational aspects of a given situation or circumstance. Contemporary models include specific attentional training aimed at modifying maladaptive processes, and shifts in attention aimed at providing information that may be inconsistent with irrational beliefs.

It is quite likely that similar mechanisms at least partially explain the efficacy of acceptance-based therapies. Acceptance differs from experiential avoidance in that internal and external experiences that may be unpleasant are acknowledged rather than avoided. This expanded attention increases contact with present-moment contingencies, which may facilitate adaptive, flexible responding to environmental contingencies, as opposed to more rigid, rule-governed (e.g., Hayes, Strosahl, et al., 1999) patterns of responding that are not based in current circumstances (Borkovec, 2002; Kabat-Zinn, 1994). Baer (2003) has also suggested that the present-moment awareness associated with mindfulness may facilitate self-management in that individuals may be more likely to use a range of coping skills as a result of being more self-aware.

However, traditional cognitive-behavioral and acceptance-based approaches differ in at least two potentially important ways. In traditional cognitive-behavioral treatment, attention is typically altered by directing the client to attend to specific types of stimuli and responses (e.g., notice anxious cues, physiological responses), while acceptance encourages a broader attentional focus. Also, the quality of attention in acceptance-based approaches is proposed to be quite different. Specifically, efforts are made to encourage an "observer" point of view that brings compassionate, nonjudgmental attention to experiences in order to reinforce a sense of self that is separate from momentary, transient responses, which should ultimately decrease efforts to avoid negatively valenced internal events.

Control

Traditional theories propose that a fundamental component of anxiety-provoking situations is that individuals perceive them as being out of their control (Mineka & Thomas, 1999). It has been suggested that the basic motivational drive to reduce anxiety is likely directed in part toward reestablishing a perception of control (Craske & Hazlett-Stevens, 2002; Mineka & Thomas, 1999). Disconfirming a low sense of perceived control by decreasing avoidance and increasing effective coping has been described as one of the critical cognitive changes that occurs as a function of exposure therapy (Barlow, 2002; Mineka & Kelly, 1989). Traditional cognitive approaches assert that one may increase control over his or her emotional experiences (and behavior) by actively changing the content of thoughts from irrational to rational.

Control is also critical in conceptualization and treatment from an acceptance perspective. Consistent with the basic tenets of behavioral therapy, acceptance-based approaches encourage behavioral control by encouraging clients to identify actions that they value and by developing new, more adaptive rules that may support behavioral action that is consistent with those values even in the absence of immediate reinforcement (e.g., the rule "I want to be intimately connect with others" may support disclosure in an interaction even when emotional responses and sometimes the other person's reaction may be immediately punishing). However, acceptance-based approaches differ significantly from traditional approaches in their philosophy regarding attempts to control internal responses. As discussed, acceptance-based therapies underscore the role of efforts to control internal experiences as key in the development and maintenance of psychological problems.

Acceptance-based treatment of anxiety has come under some criticism, because acceptance of threat-related thoughts and feelings is seen as inconsistent with the primary, adaptive function of fear and anxiety (Craske & Hazlett-Stevens, 2002). However, we contend that this approach may actually be more consistent with evolutionary theories of emotion than cognitive approaches aimed at changing the nature and content of cognitive and emotional reactions. In our treatment, we acknowledge the function of emotion and the cost of attempting to automatically ignore or alter responses. We encourage clients to explore the function of an emotional response in a given situation and to consider whether a behavioral reaction is indicated (e.g., "I am sad because this work is not fulfilling to me"), or whether the emotion is an indicator that the client is taking risks and pursuing something that is consistent with values (e.g., "I am feeling anxious because I am allowing myself to be vulnerable with someone else").

Acceptance approaches have also been described as forms of control (e.g., "When I feel out of control, I can do something—accept my feelings" or "I will accept my feelings so that they will dissipate") (Craske & Hazlett-Stevens, 2002). However, acceptance-based approaches predict that attempts to use acceptance as a control strategy will backfire and result in increased negative thoughts and feelings given that acceptance often will not result in an immediate reduction in anxious feelings (leading to increased distress among individuals who were attempting to control their anxiety). Thus, although a response of acceptance is likely to lead to longer term reductions in general levels of anxiety (presumably through reductions in avoidance efforts that paradoxically increase anxiety, and through behavioral changes that improve the client's quality of life), engaging in acceptance strategies in order to reduce or control anxiety immediately is not expected to be beneficial. While our clinical experience is consistent with this prediction, more research is needed to determine whether this distinction is a valid one.

Having raised some general points about the ways in which traditional and acceptance-based approaches compare and contrast in theory and technique, we now present an overview of our work in the area of GAD to demonstrate how acceptance-based approaches may advance the field. We provide an empirical and conceptual basis for the development of this work and briefly describe our approach to treatment.

INTEGRATIVE ACCEPTANCE-BASED CONCEPTUALIZATION AND TREATMENT OF GENERALIZED ANXIETY DISORDER

Cognitive-behavioral interventions have demonstrated efficacy for GAD (Borkovec & Ruscio, 2001). Although the most common treatment packages include applied relaxation, cognitive therapy, and some form of exposure/desensitization, there is evidence for the efficacy of both cognitive therapy and applied relaxation/coping desensitization alone (with all treatments including psychoeducation and self-monitoring; Borkovec, Newman, Pincus, & Lytle, 2002). Nonetheless, GAD remains one of the least successfully treated of the anxiety disorders, with fewer than 60% of participants meeting criteria for high-end state functioning at 12-month follow-up in even the most successful trials (e.g., Borkovec & Costello, 1993; Ladouceur et al., 2000). This suggests a need for future treatment development, capitalizing on the efficacy of established treatments, but increasing their impact. Several recent conceptual and empirical developments in understanding worry and GAD suggest connections to similar developments in the application of acceptance-based approaches to other areas of psychopathology, prompting us to explore the utility of these approaches in our treatment of GAD. We briefly review the conceptual and empirical basis for this integration below (see Roemer & Orsillo, 2002, for a full review).

Worry Is Future Focused

As Borkovec and Sharpless note in Chapter 10, this volume, worry, the central defining feature of GAD, is inherently future-focused. Chronic worriers repeatedly engage in verbal–linguistic activity (thought) that posits numerous potential future catastrophes. In addition to generating further anxiety and increasing attentional bias toward threat, worry precludes adaptive responding to present-moment contingencies by diverting attention from what is happening currently. The demonstrated efficacy of both applied relaxation and cognitive therapy in treating GAD is likely due in part to the present-moment attentional focus inherent in both approaches (and also from the self-monitoring that is included in all cognitive-behavioral treatments). Borkovec and Sharpless highlight the ways that their cognitive-behavioral approach increases present-moment focus by intervening across multiple domains (physiological, cognitive, etc.). However, as noted earlier, acceptance-based approaches that incorporate mindfulness practice provide explicit strategies for increasing (nonjudgmental) awareness of the present moment that may enhance cognitive-behavioral treatment for GAD. Preliminary support for this approach comes from an effective open trial of mindfulness-based stress reduction (MBSR) for a mixed group of individuals with anxiety disorders, including those with GAD (Kabat-Zinn et al., 1992).

Worry and GAD Are Characterized by Rigid, Habitual Responses

A wealth of information-processing research highlights the habitual nature of anxious responding and attentional biases for threat among anxious individuals (Barlow, 2002). Cognitive-behavioral therapy targets this rigidity by teaching new ways of responding at cognitive, behavioral, and somatic levels. However, Borkovec (e.g., Borkovec & Newman, 2000) stresses the importance of presenting clients with multiple response options, so that one rigid pattern is not replaced with another but instead flexible responding is encouraged. Acceptance-based therapies encourage a broadened awareness of internal and external cues aimed at enhancing flexible, adaptive responding. The mindfulness stance of "beginner's mind" explicitly counters the tendency to see things in the way they have always been seen and allows for new, flexible responding to current stimuli. While some cognitive therapy strategies (such as replacing negative beliefs with positive beliefs) might in fact lead to rigid responding (although this is not the intent of cognitive therapy and is unlikely when it is skillfully applied), an emphasis on noticing, acknowledging, and accepting whatever is present rather than habitually trying to alter it may increase flexibility and choice.

Flexible, intentional behavior can also be facilitated and strengthened through an emphasis on identifying and clarifying what matters to the client (values; Hayes, Strosahl, et al., 1999; Wilson & Murrell, Chapter 6, this volume). This approach may enhance adaptive rule-governed behavior that is resistant to contingencies that would otherwise elicit avoidance. For instance, individuals with GAD may habitually avoid intimate relationships because they can elicit anxiety. Identifying the development of intimate relationships as a valued direction (and a rule) may lead to increased approach behavior toward potential partners even in the presence of threat cues that discourage this behavior. Acceptance may facilitate the identification and salience of values, further increasing intentional responding in the moment.

Worry Serves an Experientially Avoidant Function

We (Roemer & Orsillo, 2002) have recently noted the apparent overlap between Borkovec's avoidance model of GAD (Borkovec, Alaine, & Behar, 2004) and Hayes and colleagues' (Hayes et al., 1996; Hayes, Strosahl, et al., 1999) experiential avoidance model of psychopathology. Basic research has found that worry is associated with reduced physiological reactivity to a fearful image (Borkovec & Hu, 1990) and reduced self-reported anxiety following a distressing film (Wells & Papageorgiou, 1995), suggesting that worry may function to reduce distress in the short term. In self-report studies, the use of worry to distract from more distressing topics has reliably distinguished those with GAD from those with subthreshold GAD symptoms (Borkovec & Roemer, 1995; Freeston, Rhéaume, Letarte, Dugas, & Ladouceur, 1994). These findings suggest that worry may be negatively reinforced by reducing emotional distress; in other words, worry may serve an experientially avoidant function (see Roemer & Orsillo, 2002, for a more extensive review of the evidence). Consistent with this, we found that both worry and self-reported impairment associated with GAD were significantly correlated with reports of experiential avoidance, as well as fear of emotional responding (Roemer, Salters, Raffa, & Orsillo, in press). Relatedly, Mennin, Heimberg, Turk, and Fresco (2002) have found that GAD is associated with nonacceptance of emotional responses.

As both Borkovec (1994) and Hayes, Strosahl, and colleagues (1999) note, experiential avoidance may initially seem advantageous but can eventually have long-term deleterious consequences. In the case of worry as a form of experiential avoidance, despite findings of initial reductions in distress and arousal (reviewed earlier), studies find that worry may interfere with physiological habituation to feared stimuli (Borkovec & Hu, 1990) and lead to intrusions (Wells & Papageorgio, 1995). Borkovec suggests that by reducing arousal, worry interferes with functional exposure to feared stimuli, thereby maintaining threatening meanings and interfering with new learning.

If, in fact, as many researchers have proposed (e.g., Borkovec et al., 2004; Mennin et al., 2002; Roemer & Orsillo, 2002), worry functions to reduce emotional distress that individuals with GAD find aversive but has long-term negative consequences, it may be beneficial to target directly experiential avoidance in treating GAD. Psychoeducation and experiential exercises that increase emotional awareness and understanding of the function of emotion (such as those used in DBT; Linehan, 1993b) may facilitate awareness, understanding, and acceptance of emotional experience. Elements of ACT (Hayes, Strosahl, et al., 1999), such as an emphasis on the problems associated with experiential control and introduction of the concept of willingness as an alternative to control efforts, may also reduce experiential avoidance. Also, mindfulness practice, along with cognitive defusion exercises, may help facilitate acceptance and willingness to experience rather than avoidance of emotional responses. Experiencing one's emotions and distressing thoughts as just thoughts or feelings (as opposed to stable, enduring features of oneself) can reduce the threat associated with certain emotions and thoughts, thereby minimizing the desire to avoid them. Finally, in-session reinforcement of behavior that maintains, and extinction of behavior that avoids, contact with feared internal experiences can promote and enhance willingness (Cordova, 2001).

Worry May Inhibit Action in Valued Directions

Unlike other anxiety disorders, GAD is not characterized by focal behavioral avoidance. However, one study found that 64% of individuals with GAD did report avoidance of certain situations (Butler, Gelder, Hibbert, Cullington, & Klimes, 1987). It is likely that GAD is also associated with more subtle forms of avoidance, because a continual focus on potential future catastrophes likely interferes with action in the present moment. Our clients often report feeling "frozen." Fears of potential negative outcomes following action in any direction immobilize them to the extent that they take no purposeful action at all. Rather than engaging in actions in valued directions (e.g., meeting new people, opening themselves up to an intimate partner, pursuing a new career direction), they often report engaging in protective actions aimed at preventing potential threat. This is not to say that individuals with GAD are inactive; in fact, they often seem almost hyperactive, although these actions tend not to be in valued directions. In addition, their chronic attentional focus on future potential catastrophes can distract them from valued aspects of their current behavior.

As we discussed earlier, drawing from Hayes and colleagues (1999), we advocate an expansion of traditional exposure models, so that emphasis is placed on helping clients move toward what matters to them rather than solely toward what they fear. In addition to providing a stronger rationale for exposure, this also allows clients to approach areas that elicit other unwanted emotions (beyond fear), such as sadness or shame. This can be accomplished through imaginal and in vivo exposure exercises that proceed from values identification exercises (Wilson & Murrell, Chapter 6, this volume). We have also found that some of our clients are already living the lives they want to be living in many ways, but their constant anxious future-focus interferes with their ability to experience the lives they are living. In these cases, values work often takes the form of increasing awareness within valued contexts (e.g., relationships, work), typically using informal mindfulness techniques.

Current Form of Treatment

At the time of this writing we are 1 year into our treatment development grant, so our treatment is in a much earlier stage than most others in this volume, and it continues to evolve. Nonetheless, we provide a brief overview of our current protocol below, highlighting its relationship to other approaches described in this volume.

Psychoeducation

Consistent with traditional cognitive-behavioral approaches, our introduction to treatment includes psychoeducation. In addition to reviewing the model of worry and anxiety described earlier, we present the concept of mindfulness and mindfulness skills (Linehan, 1993b; Segal et al., 2002), the function of emotions (e.g., emotions provide important information to ourselves and others; Linehan, 1993b), and the problems associated with efforts at experiential control, along with the potential solution of willingness to have one's internal experience (Hayes, Strosahl, et al., 1999). We also present the concept of values, discussed more fully below. Although these concepts are initially presented somewhat didactically (in conjunction with handouts), we also use metaphors, in-session exercises, and homework assignments throughout treatment to help the clients experience rather than simply understand them.

Acceptance

Methods aimed at increasing awareness and acceptance are at the foundation of our treatment. We assume that awareness increases contact with natural contingencies and the probability that valued behavior will be maintained, and that mindfulness skills facilitate willingness to engage in behavior that might bring up negatively evaluated internal experiences. We increase awareness in part through self-monitoring (first of worry, then of emotions, efforts to control, willingness, and valued action, as each concept is introduced). We introduce the concept of mindfulness early in treatment, highlighting that it is a process and a habit that can be developed. We emphasize multiple aspects of mindfulness (e.g., awareness, nonjudgmental observation, beginner's mind, staying in the moment, acceptance/letting go) and cultivate these aspects through numerous forms of practice. Mindfulness exercises are done at the beginning of each session, and clients practice mindfulness between sessions both formally (setting aside time to practice mindfulness through meditation, progressive muscle relaxation, or imagery) and informally (bringing mindful awareness to whatever they are engaged in, such as walking, doing dishes, driving; Hanh, 1992). Although progressive muscle relaxation is often used as a way of altering one's experience, we emphasize attention to physical sensations during both tense and release cycles, and encourage clients to practice acceptance in response to any sensations that emerge (including anxious thoughts and feelings while "relaxing"). Clients also engage in mindful emotion exercises in which they imagine recent emotional events and are encouraged to take a mindful stance in response to the thoughts, feelings, and sensations that arise. These exercises are designed to increase awareness of emotional experience, to provide experiential evidence that acceptance can be tolerated, and to allow for reinforcement of acceptance behaviors. Clients learn that they can allow their emotional experience, and that their emotional experience is multifaceted and evolving. They are also able to experience their emotional reactions, providing them with important information that is often lost through experiential avoidance.

We also introduce clients to the concept of clear versus muddy emotions (similar to clean and dirty emotions in ACT; Hayes, Strosahl, et al., 1999). We explore with clients the ways that our emotional responses can become clouded (e.g., due to lack of sleep, chronic worry, unresolved emotional responses to a previous event, or efforts to control that paradoxically increase the intensity of responses). Clients practice bringing mindfulness and awareness to their emotional reactions in order to clarify them, allowing them to serve as more effective guides for behavior when appropriate.

We also use numerous acceptance strategies to increase clients' experience of their thoughts and feelings as constantly in flux and distinct from what they represent (e.g., *milk* is a word, not a white creamy substance). These include cognitive defusion exercises used in ACT (Hayes, Strosahl, et al., 1999) such as referring to thoughts as thoughts (e.g., "I'm having the thought that I'm going to fail") and replacing *but's* with *and's* (e.g., "I want to go to the party *and* I feel anxious" rather than "I want to go to the party *but* I feel anxious"). We also use several meditation practices, such as putting thoughts on leaves on a stream (Hayes, Strosahl, et al., 1999) or onto clouds in the sky (Linehan, 1993b), as well as the mountain and lake metaphors (Kabat-Zinn, 1994), in which clients imagine they are these natural forms and notice how their surface is constantly changing, while their core remains the same. These strategies are used to help clients become aware of and separate from their thoughts, thus defusing or distancing them from those thoughts and allowing them to act independently of those thoughts.

Valued (Mindful) Action

We introduce the concept of values, or living a life worth living, during the assessment phase immediately preceding treatment by having clients complete a questionnaire that assesses the importance of a number of life domains (family relations, social relations, physical well-being, etc.) and the degree to which they feel their living is consistent with their values in these domains (Wilson & Murrell, Chapter 6, this volume). We address values in each session, first by defining values (as a process, a choice, a direction in life rather than an outcome), then through a series of writing exercises to help clients clarify their values (as distinct from what they feel they "should" value or what others would like them to value). Common themes that emerge among our clients are opening up to other people (particularly in intimate relationships), finding work options that are challenging and fulfilling, and engaging in self-care activities (e.g., spiritual practice, physical exercise, creativity). Clients then monitor their actions in identified valued domains (we typically choose two or three in which importance and consistency ratings are particularly discrepant). Finally, clients and therapists work together to choose actions for the coming week, identify potential obstacles, and subsequently review actions and obstacles while planning for the next week.

As mentioned earlier, in some cases, a significant alteration in behavior is what is needed to bring valued action into our client's life. However, it is also often the case in our work with GAD that clients are actually behaving in accordance with their values, but their subtle distraction and avoidance is preventing them from truly being in contact or participating in those actions (e.g., the mother who spends a lot of "quality time" with her children that is filled with activities during which she is distracted by worry). Also, although we often begin values work by focusing on one or two specific domains, we encourage a broader emphasis in the spirit of making choices and living in accordance with values, allowing for more flexible action between sessions. Clients initially monitor actions and obstacles to action in specific domains, but then move to daily monitoring of more general valued living (i.e., acting intentionally in a way that is consistent with what matters to the individual).

CONCLUSIONS

While the literature on the efficacy and underlying mechanisms of cognitive-behavioral treatments for anxiety is expansive, more work is needed to improve our ability to understand and treat these disorders. Acceptance-based theories and therapies offer some promise in their ability to extend and refine the work that has been completed to date. Research on the theories supporting acceptance-based approaches and the efficacy of preliminary treatment efforts is in its infancy. However, we contend that these approaches may significantly improve our ability to provide some relief to those suffering with anxiety.

Acceptance-based approaches improve on existing treatments in that clinically significant change is an explicit, primary goal of treatment. Efforts are made to intervene directly on fear and avoidance of internal experiences, the variables that have been shown to interfere with traditional exposure (e.g., Jaycox, Foa, & Morral, 1998), which may increase the acceptability and potency of more established approaches. Time and continued research will tell if acceptance-based behavioral approaches will be able to build on the strengths and address the limitations of earlier behavioral and cognitive-behavioral theories and interventions. Creative, scientifically sound studies that explore explicitly operationalized intervention strategies, mechanisms of change, and broad definitions of clinically relevant outcomes, coupled with an open, skeptical stance are needed as we work to advance science and help our clients lead meaningful, valued lives.

REFERENCES

Arntz, A. (2002). Cognitive therapy versus interoceptive exposure as treatment of panic disorder without agoraphobia. *Behaviour Research and Therapy, 40*, 325–341.

Baer, R. A. (2003). Mindfulness training as a clinical intervention: A conceptual and empirical review. *Clinical Psychology: Science and Practice, 10*, 125–143.

Bandura, A. (1977). Self-efficacy: Towards a unifying theory of behavior change. *Psychological Review, 84*, 191–215.

Bandura, A. (1986). *Social foundations of thought and action: A social cognitive theory.* Englewood Cliffs, NJ: Prentice-Hall.

Barlow, D. H. (2002). *Anxiety and its disorders: The nature and treatment of anxiety and panic*(2nd ed.). New York: Guilford Press.

Beck, A. T. (1993). Cognitive therapy: Nature and relation to behavior therapy. *Journal of Psychotherapy Practice and Research, 2*, 345–356.

Beck, A. T., Emery, G., & Greenberg, R. L. (1985). *Anxiety disorders and phobias.*New York: Basic Books.

Block, J. A., & Wulfert, E. (2002, May). Acceptance or change of private experiences: A comparative analysis in college students with a fear of public speaking. In R. D. Zettle (Chair), *Recent outcome research on acceptance and commitment therapy (ACT) with anxiety disorders.* Symposium conducted at the 28th annual meeting of the Association for Behavior Analysis, Toronto, Canada.

Bögels, S. M., Mulkens, S., & de Jong, P. J. (1997). Task concentration and fear of blushing. *Clinical Psychology and Psychotherapy, 4*, 251–258.

Booth, R., & Rachman, S. (1992). The reduction of claustrophobia: I. *Behaviour Research and Therapy, 30*, 207–221.

Borkovec, T. D. (1994). The nature, functions, and origins of worry. In G. Davey & F. Tallis

(Eds.), *Worrying: Perspectives on theory, assessment, and treatment*(pp. 5–35). Sussex, UK: Wiley.

Borkovec, T. D. (2002). Life in the future versus life in the present. *Clinical Psychology: Science and Practice, 9*, 76–80.

Borkovec, T. D., Alcaine, O. M., & Behar, E. (2004). Avoidance theory of worry and generalized anxiety disorder. In R. G. Heimberg, C. L. Turk, & D. S. Mennin (Eds.), *Generalized anxiety disorder: Advances in research and practice* (pp. 77–108). New York: Guilford Press.

Borkovec, T. D., & Costello, E. (1993). Efficacy of applied relaxation and cognitive-behavioral therapy in the treatment of generalized anxiety disorder. *Journal of Consulting and Clinical Psychology, 61*, 611–619.

Borkovec, T. D., & Hu, S. (1990). The effect of worry on cardiovascular response to phobic imagery. *Behaviour Research and Therapy, 28*, 69–73.

Borkovec, T. D., & Newman, M. G. (2000). Worry and generalized anxiety disorder. In P. Salkovskis (Ed.), *Comprehensive clinical psychology* (Vol. 6, pp. 439–460). Oxford, UK: Elsevier.

Borkovec, T. D., Newman, M. G., Pincus, A. L., & Lytle, R. (2002). A component analysis of cognitive-behavioral therapy for generalized anxiety disorder and the role of interpersonal problems. *Journal of Consulting and Clinical Psychology, 70*, 288–298.

Borkovec, T. D., & Roemer, L. (1995). Perceived functions of worry among generalized anxiety disorder subjects: Distraction from more emotionally distressing topics? *Journal of Behavior Therapy and Experimental Psychiatry, 26*, 25–30.

Borkovec, T. D., & Ruscio, A. M. (2001). Psychotherapy for generalized anxiety disorder. *Journal of Clinical Psychiatry, 62*(Suppl. 11), 37–42.

Bouton, M. E. (2002). Context, ambiguity, and unlearning: Sources of relapse after behavioral extinction. *Biological Psychiatry, 52*, 976–986.

Bouton, M. E., Mineka, S., & Barlow, D. H. (2001). A modern learning theory perspective on the etiology of panic disorder. *Psychological Review, 108*, 2–32.

Breslin, F. C., Zack, M., & McMain, S. (2002). An information-processing analysis of mindfulness: Implications for relapse prevention in the treatment of substance abuse. *Clinical Psychology: Science and Practice, 9*, 275–299.

Brown, T. A, Barlow, D. H., & Leibowitz, M. R. (1994). The empirical basis of generalized anxiety disorder. *American Journal of Psychiatry, 151*, 1272–1280.

Burns, D. D., & Spangler, D. L. (2001). Do changes in dysfunctional attitudes mediate changes in depression and anxiety in cognitive behavioral therapy? *Behavior Therapy, 32*, 337–369.

Butler, G., Gelder, M., Hibbert, G., Cullington, A., & Klimes, I. (1987). Anxiety management: Developing effective strategies. *Behaviour Research and Therapy, 25*, 517–522.

Clark, D. M. (1986). A cognitive approach to panic. *Behaviour Research and Therapy, 24*, 461–470.

Clark, D. M. (1988). A cognitive model of panic attacks. In S. Rachman & J. D. Maser (Eds.), *Panic: Psychological perspectives* (pp. 71–89). Hilldale, NJ: Erlbaum.

Clark, D. M. (1996). Panic disorder: From theory to therapy. In P. M. Salkovskis (Ed.), *Frontiers of cognitive therapy: The state of the art and beyond* (pp. 318–344). New York: Guilford Press.

Cordova, J. V. (2001). Acceptance in behavior therapy: Understanding the process of change. *Behavior Therapist, 24*, 213–226.

Cordova, J. V., Jacobson, N. S., & Christensen, A. (1998). Acceptance versus change interventions in behavioral couple therapy: Impact on couples' in-session communication. *Journal of Marital and Family Therapy, 24*, 437–455.

Coyne, J. C. (1989). Thinking postcognitively about depression. In A. Freeman, K. M. Simon, L. E. Beutler, & H. Arkowitz (Eds.), *Comprehensive handbook of cognitive therapy* (pp. 227–244). New York: Plenum Press.

Craske, M. G. (1999). *Anxiety disorders: Psychological approaches to theory and treatment.* Boulder, CO: Westview Press.

Craske, M. G., & Hazlett-Stevens, H. (2002). Facilitating symptom reduction and behavior change in GAD: The issue of control. *Clinical Psychology: Science and Practice, 9,* 69–75.

Craske, M. G., Glover, D., & DeCola, J. (1995). Predicted versus unpredicted panic attacks: Acute versus general distress. *Journal of Abnormal Psychology, 104,* 214–223.

Dworkin, B. R. (1993). *Learning and physiological regulation.* Chicago: University of Chicago Press.

Fava, M., Bless, E., Otto, M.W., Pava, J. A., & Rosenbaum, J. F. (1994). Dysfunctional attitudes in major depression: Changes with pharmacotherapy. *Journal of Nervous and Mental Disease, 182,* 45–49.

Foa, E. B., Dancu, C. V., Hembree, E. A., Jaycox, L. H., Meadows, E. A., & Street, G. P. (1999). A comparison of exposure therapy, stress inoculation training, and their combination for reducing posttraumatic stress disorder in female assault victims. *Journal of Consulting and Clinical Psychology, 67,* 194–200.

Foa, E. B., & Kozak, M. J. (1986). Emotional processing of fear: Exposure to corrective information. *Psychological Bulletin, 99,* 20–35.

Freeston, M. H., Rhéaume, J., Letarte, H., Dugas, M. J., & Ladouceur, R. (1994). Why do people worry? *Personality and Individual Differences, 17,* 791–802.

Gilboa-Schechtman, E., & Foa, E. B. (2001). Patterns of recovery from trauma: The use of intraindividual analysis. *Journal of Abnormal Psychology, 110,* 392–400.

Goisman, R. M., Rogers, M. P., Steketee, G. S., Warshaw, M. G., Cuneo, P., & Keller, M. B. (1993). Utilization of behavioral methods in a multicenter anxiety disorders study. *Journal of Clinical Psychiatry, 54,* 213–218.

Goisman, R. M., Warshaw, M. G., & Keller, M. B. (1999). Psychosocial treatment prescriptions for generalized anxiety disorder, panic disorder, and social phobia, 1991–1996. *American Journal of Psychiatry, 156,* 1819–1821.

Gold, D. B., & Wegner, D. M. (1995). Origins of ruminative thought: Trauma, incompleteness, nondisclosure, and suppression. *Journal of Applied Social Psychology, 25,* 1245–1261.

Goldiamond, I. (1974). Toward a constructional approach to social problems. *Behaviorism, 2,* 1–84.

Goldstein, A. J., & Chambless, D. L. (1978). A reanalysis of agoraphobia. *Behavior Therapy, 9,* 47–59.

Gould, R. A., Buckminster, S., Pollack, M. H., Otto, M. W., & Yap, L. (1997). Cognitive behavioral and pharmacological treatment for social phobia: A meta-analysis. *Clinical Psychology: Science and Practice, 4,* 291–306.

Greenberg, L. S., & Safran, J. D. (1987). *Emotion in psychotherapy.* New York: Guilford Press.

Greenberg, P. E., Sisitsky, T., Kessler, R. C., Finkelstein, S. N., Berndt, E. R., Davidson, J. R. T., et al. (1999). The economic burden of the anxiety disorders in the 1990s. *Journal of Clinical Psychiatry, 60,* 427–435.

Gross, J. J., & Levenson, R. W. (1993). Emotional suppression: Physiology, self-report, and expressive behavior. *Journal of Personality and Social Psychology, 64,* 970–986.

Hanh, T. N. (1992). *Peace is every step: The path of mindfulness in everyday life.* New York: Bantam.

Hayes, S. C. (2002). Acceptance, mindfulness, and science. *Clinical Psychology: Science and Practice, 9,* 101–106.

Hayes, S. C., Barnes-Holmes, D., & Roche, B. (Eds.). (2001). *Relational frame theory: A post-Skinnerian account of human language and cognition.* New York: Plenum Press.

Hayes, S. C., Bissett, R. T., Korn, Z., Zettle, R. D., Rosenfarb, I. S., Cooper, L. D., et al.

(1999). The impact of acceptance versus control rationales on pain tolerance. *Psychological Record, 49*, 33–47.

Hayes, S. C., Strosahl, K. D., & Wilson, K. G. (1999). *Acceptance and commitment therapy: An experiential approach to behavior change.* New York: Guilford Press.

Hayes, S. C., & Wilson, K. G. (2003). Mindfulness: Method and process. *Clinical Psychology: Science and Practice, 10*, 161–165.

Hayes, S. C., Wilson, K. G., Gifford, E. V., Follette, V. M., & Strosahl, K. (1996). Experiential avoidance and behavioral disorders: A functional dimensional approach to diagnosis and treatment. *Journal of Consulting and Clinical Psychology, 64*, 1152–1168.

James, J. E. (1993). Cognitive-behavioural theory: An alternative conception. *Australian Psychologist, 28*, 151–155.

Jarrett, R. B., & Nelson, R. O. (1987). Mechanisms of change in cognitive therapy of depression. *Behavior Therapy, 18*, 227–241.

Jaycox, L. H., Foa, E. B., & Morral, A. R. (1998). Influence of emotional engagement and habituation on exposure therapy for PTSD. *Journal of Consulting and Clinical Psychology, 66*, 185–192.

Kabat-Zinn, J. (1994). *Wherever you go there you are.* New York: Hyperion.

Kabat-Zinn, J., Massion, A. O., Kristeller, J., Peterson, L. G., Fletcher, K. E., Pbert, L., et al. (1992). Effectiveness of a meditation-based stress reduction program in the treatment of anxiety disorders. *American Journal of Psychiatry, 149*, 936–943.

Kazdin, A. E. (1998). *Research design in clinical psychology.* Boston: Allyn & Bacon.

Kenardy, J., & Taylor, C. B. (1999). Expected versus unexpected panic attacks: A naturalistic prospective study. *Journal of Anxiety Disorders, 13*, 435–445.

Korotitsch, W. J., & Nelson-Gray, R. O. (1999). An overview of self-monitoring research in assessment and treatment. *Psychological Assessment, 11*, 415–425.

Krasner, L. (1992). The concepts of syndrome and functional analysis: Compatible or incompatible? *Behavioral Assessment, 14*, 307–321.

Ladouceur, R., Dugas, M. J., Freeston, M. H., Léger, E., Gagnon, F., & Thibodeau, N. (2000). Efficacy of a new cognitive-behavioral treatment for generalized anxiety disorder: Evaluation in a controlled clinical trial. *Journal of Consulting and Clinical Psychology, 68*, 957–964.

Lang, P. J. (1979). A bio-informational theory of emotional imagery. *Psychophysiology, 16*, 495–512.

Lang, P. J. (1985). The cognitive psychophysiology of emotion: Fear and anxiety. In A. H. Tuma & J. D. Maser (Eds.), *Anxiety and the anxiety disorders* (pp. 131–170). Hillsdale, NJ: Erlbaum.

Levitt, J. T., Brown, T. A., Orsillo, S. M., & Barlow, D. H. (in press). The effects of acceptance versus suppression of emotion on subjective and psychophysiological response to carbon dioxide challenge in patients with panic disorder. *Behavior Therapy.*

Linehan, M. M. (1993a). *Cognitive-behavioral treatment of borderline personality disorder.* New York: Guilford Press.

Linehan, M. M. (1993b). *Skills training manual for treating borderline personality disorder.* New York: Guilford Press.

Lovell, K., Marks, I. M., Noshirvani, H., Thrasher, S., & Livanou, M. (2001). Do cognitive and exposure treatments improve various PTSD symptoms differently?: A randomized controlled trial. *Behavioural and Cognitive Psychotherapy, 29*, 107–112.

Marks, I. (1969). *Fears and phobias.* London: Heinmann Medical Books.

Marks, I., Lovell, K., Noshirvani, H., Livanou, M., & Thrasher, S. (1998). Treatment of posttraumatic stress disorder by exposure and/or cognitive restructuring: A controlled study. *Archives of General Psychiatry, 55*, 317–325.

McManus, F., Clark, D. M., & Hackmann, A. (2000). Specificity of cognitive biases in social phobia and their role in recovery. *Behavioural and Cognitive Psychotherapy, 28*, 201–209.

McNally, R. J. (1990). Psychological approaches to panic disorder: A review. *Psychological Bulletin, 108*, 403–419.

McNally, R. J. (1994). *Panic disorder: A critical analysis*. New York: Guilford Press.

Mennin, D. S., Heimberg, R. G., Turk, C. L., & Fresco, D. M. (2002). Applying an emotion regulation framework to integrative approaches to generalized anxiety disorder. *Clinical Psychology: Science and Practice, 9*, 85–90.

Mineka, S., & Kelly, K. A. (1989). The relationship between anxiety, lack of control and loss of control. In A. Steptoe & A. Appels (Eds.), *Stress, personal control and health* (pp. 163–191). Oxford, UK: Wiley.

Mineka, S., & Thomas, C. (1999). Mechanisms of change in exposure therapy for anxiety disorders. In T. Dalgleish & M. Power (Eds.), *Handbook of cognition and emotion* (pp. 747–764). New York: Wiley.

Mowrer, O. H. (1947). On the dual nature of learning—a re-interpretation of "conditioning" and "problem-solving." *Harvard Educational Review, 17*, 102–148.

Mulkens, S., Bögels, S. M., de Jong, P. J., & Louwers, J. (2001). Fear of blushing: Effects of task concentration training versus exposure *in vivo* on fear and physiology. *Journal of Anxiety Disorders, 15*, 413–432.

Narrow, W. E., Rae, D. S., Robins, L. N., & Regier, D. A. (2002). Revised prevalence based estimates of mental disorders in the United States: Using a clinical significance criterion to reconcile 2 surveys' estimates. *Archives of General Psychiatry, 59*(2), 115–123.

Nelson, R. O., & Hayes, S. C. (1981). Theoretical explanations for reactivity in self-monitoring. *Behavior Modification, 5*, 3–14.

Nolen-Hoeksema, S., Girgus, J. S., & Seligman, M. E. P. (1986). Learned helplessness in children: A longitudinal study of depression, achievement, and attributional style. *Journal of Personality and Social Psychology, 51*, 435–442.

Orsillo, S. M., & Batten, S. V. (in press). ACT in the treatment of PTSD. *Behavior Modification*.

Orsillo, S. M., Roemer, L., & Barlow, D. H. (2003). Integrating acceptance and mindfulness into existing cognitive-behavioral treatment for GAD: A case study. *Cognitive and Behavioral Practice, 10*, 223–230.

Persons, J. B., & Miranda, J. (1992). Cognitive theories of vulnerability to depression: Reconciling negative evidence. *Cognitive Therapy and Research, 16*, 485–502.

Purdon, C. (1999). Thought suppression and psychopathology. *Behaviour Research and Therapy, 37*, 1029–1054.

Rachman, S. J. (1991). Neo-conditioning and the classical theory of fear acquisition. *Clinical Psychology Review, 11*, 155–173.

Rachman, S. J., Craske, M. G., Tallman, K., & Solyom, C. (1986). Does escape behavior strengthen agoraphobic avoidance?: A replication. *Behavior Therapy, 17*, 366–384.

Rapee, R. M., Craske, M. G., & Barlow, D. H. (1995). Assessment instrument for panic disorder that includes fear of sensation-producing activities: The Albany Panic and Phobia Questionnaire. *Anxiety, 1*, 114–122.

Razran, G. (1961). The observable unconscious and the inferable conscious in current Soviet psychophysiology: Interoceptive conditioning, semantic conditioning, and the orienting reflex. *Psychological Review, 68*, 81–147.

Reiss, S. (1987). Theoretical perspectives on the fear of anxiety. *Clinical Psychology Review, 7*, 585–596.

Rescorla, R. A., & Wagner, A. R. (1972). A theory of Pavlovian conditioning: Variations in the effectiveness of reinforcement and nonreinforcement. In A. H. Black & W. F. Prokasy (Eds.), *Classical conditioning: II. Current research and theory* (pp. 64–99). New York: Appleton–Century–Crofts.

Roemer, L., & Orsillo, S. M. (2002). Expanding our conceptualization of and treatment for generalized anxiety disorder: Integrating mindfulness/acceptance-based approaches with existing cognitive-behavioral models [Featured article]. *Clinical Psychology: Science and Practice, 9, 54–68.*

Roemer, L., & Orsillo, S. M. (2003). Mindfulness: A promising intervention strategy in need of further study. *Clinical Psychology: Science and Practice, 10, 172–178.*

Roemer, L., Salters, K., Raffa, S., & Orsillo, S. M. (in press). Fear and avoidance of internal experiences in GAD: Preliminary tests of a conceptual model. *Cognitive Therapy and Research.*

Rogers, C. R. (1961). *On becoming a person: A therapist's view of psychotherapy.* Boston: Houghton Mifflin.

Segal, Z. V., Williams, J. M., & Teasdale, J. D. (2002). *Mindfulness-based cognitive therapy for depression: A new approach to preventing relapse.* New York: Guilford Press.

Seligman, M. E. P. (1975). *Helplessness: On depression, development, and death.* San Francisco: Freeman.

Shafran, R., Thordarson, D., & Rachman, S. (1996). Thought action fusion in obsessive compulsive disorder. *Journal of Anxiety Disorders, 5, 379–391.*

Steketee, G. S., & Barlow, D. H. (2002). Obsessive–compulsive disorder. In D. H. Barlow, *Anxiety and its disorders: The nature and treatment of anxiety and panic* (2nd ed., pp. 516–551). New York: Guilford Press.

Tarrier, N., Pilgrim, H., Sommerfield, C., Faragher, B., Reynolds, M., Graham, E., et al. (1999). A randomized trial of cognitive therapy and imaginal exposure in the treatment of chronic posttraumatic stress disorder. *Journal of Consulting and Clinical Psychology, 67, 13–18.*

Teasdale, J. D., Moore, R. G., Hayhurst, H., Pope, M., Williams, S., & Segal, Z. V. (2002). Metacognitive awareness and prevention of relapse in depression: Empirical evidence. *Journal of Consulting and Clinical Psychology, 70, 275–287.*

Teasdale, J. D., Segal, Z. V., & Williams, J. M. G. (2003). Mindfulness training and problem formulation. *Clinical Psychology: Science and Practice, 10, 157–160.*

Ullman, L. P., & Krasner, L. (1975). *A psychological approach to abnormal behavior* (2nd ed.). Upper Saddle River, NJ: Prentice-Hall.

Wegner, D. M. (1994). Ironic processes of mental control. *Psychological Review, 101, 34–52.*

Wells, A. (1990). Panic disorder in association with relaxation-induced anxiety: An attentional training approach to treatment. *Behavior Therapy, 21, 273–280.*

Wells, A. (2000). *Emotional disorders and metacognition: Innovative cognitive therapy.* New York: Wiley.

Wells, A., & Matthews, G. (1994). *Attention and emotion: A clinical perspective.* Hillsdale, NJ: Erlbaum.

Wells, A., & Papageorgiou, C. (1995). Worry and the incubation of intrusive images following stress. *Behaviour Research and Therapy, 33, 579–583.*

Wells, A., & Papageorgiou, C. (1998). Social phobia: Effects of external attention on anxiety, negative beliefs, and perspective taking. *Behavior Therapy, 29, 357–370.*

Wells, A., White, J., & Carter, K. (1997). Attention training: Effects on anxiety and beliefs in panic and social phobia. *Clinical Psychology and Psychotherapy, 4, 226–232.*

Westling, B. E., & Öst, L. (1995). Cognitive bias in panic disorder patients and changes after cognitive-behavioral treatments. *Behaviour Research and Therapy, 33, 585–588.*

Williams, K. E., Chambless, D. L., & Ahrens, A. (1997). Are emotions frightening?: An extension of the fear of fear construct. *Behaviour Research and Therapy, 35, 239–248.*

Wolpe, J. (1958). *Psychotherapy by reciprocal inhibition.* Stanford, CA: Stanford University Press.

Zinbarg, R. E., Craske, M. G., & Barlow, D. H. (1993). *Therapist guide for the Master of your Anxiety and Worry (MAW) program.* Albany, NY: Graywind.

5

Functional Analytic Psychotherapy, Cognitive Therapy, and Acceptance

Robert J. Kohlenberg, Jonathan W. Kanter, Madelon Bolling, Reo Wexner, Chauncey Parker, *and* Mavis Tsai

While treating clients with cognitive-behavioral therapy (CBT), Kohlenberg and Tsai (1991) noticed a curious and clinically significant phenomenon. Some of their CBT clients were transformed in their ability to be intimate and caring in their relationships with others. This occurred in addition to notable improvements in the specific goals of the CBT (e.g., reduced anxiety, obsessions, compulsions, or depression). In their search for answers as to why this occurred with some clients but not with others, Kohlenberg and Tsai noticed that these cases involved a naturally occurring, intense, and close therapist–client relationship—with features beyond those of the usual collaborative relationship required to conduct CBT effectively (Callaghan, Naugle, & Follette, 1996). Functional analytic psychotherapy (FAP; Kohlenberg & Tsai, 1991) is the behavioral treatment that evolved from these early observations. It purposely produces an unusually curative therapist–client relationship, while remaining true to the theory and practice that underlie CBT.

In this chapter, we describe the guiding principles of FAP, show specific techniques for using these principles, and specify how they integrate with acceptance techniques to enhance cognitive therapy for depression (Beck, Rush, Shaw, & Emery, 1979).

FUNCTIONAL ANALYTIC PSYCHOTHERAPY: GUIDING PRINCIPLES

FAP is guided by the notion that much behavior is shaped and maintained by a process of reinforcement that is ubiquitous and occurs naturally during the therapy session. This principle suggests that all therapists and clients inevitably and naturally shape each other's behavior, whether the therapy being conducted is categorized as behavioral, cognitive, or psychodynamic. This often occurs outside of the awareness of either the therapist or the client. Examples include a client who stops asking for extra sessions in response to the therapist's continued unavailability, a client who becomes aware of a previously "repressed" memory after an overeager therapist presses for abuse details, a therapist who tends to end the session 10 minutes late with a seductive and attractive client or 5 minutes early with a depressed client. More subtle examples of influence on what a client says, thinks, or feels in session include changes in body posture, eye contact, smiling, or affirmative nods (Kanter, Kohlenberg, & Loftus, 2002).

A well-known property of reinforcement is that the closer in time and place a behavior is to its consequences, the greater will be the effect of those consequences. Thus, treatment effects will be stronger if clients' problems and improvements occur during the therapy session, because they then are closest in time and place to potential natural reinforcement from the therapist. In this view, the client–therapist relationship is a social environment with the potential to evoke and change actual instances of the client's problematic behavior in the here and now. (For detailed discussion of the client–therapist relationship in behavioral terms, see Follette, Naugle, & Callaghan, 1996; Kohlenberg & Tsai, 1991.)

Consider a male client, Mr. G., who wants more intimacy and close relationships. The therapist observes that the client becomes distant and somewhat threatening or ominous when the therapist expresses caring for him. Other examples include a client whose problem is that she has no friends, who avoids eye contact with the therapist, talks at length in-session in an unfocused and tangential manner, and frequently gets angry at the therapist for not having all the answers. Still another is a woman with a pattern of getting into relationships with unattainable men, who develops a crush on her therapist. And finally, a man who is recently divorced because his wife found him distant and avoidant of intimacy cancels the next session after making an important self-disclosure. These situations offer therapists extraordinary opportunities to identify and change pervasive and significant interpersonal problems in the here and now. We refer to these opportunities as therapist–client relationship learning opportunities (TCRLOs), and they are the foundation of any FAP-based treatment approach. We describe their use in more detail below.

USING FUNCTIONAL ANALYTIC PSYCHOTHERAPY TO ENHANCE EXISTING TREATMENTS

In this chapter, we describe the use of these therapy learning opportunities to enhance cognitive therapy for depression. We note that in addition to our approach, several recent cognitive therapy variants—including Safran and Segal (1990), Young (1990), and the cognitive behavioral analysis system of psychotherapy (CBASP; McCullough, 2000)—emphasize the therapist–client relationship as an important treatment component. CBASP, in particular, has provided compelling data showing that a greater emphasis on the therapist–client relationship is associated with better client outcomes. In addition, two newer behavior therapies—acceptance and commitment therapy (ACT; Hayes, Strosahl, & Wilson, 1999) and dialectical behavior therapy (DBT; Linehan, 1993)—also highlight the key role of the therapist–client relationship and the in-session interaction. However, most cognitive-behavioral therapies, other than noting the importance of building a strong therapeutic alliance and collaborative working relationship, do not explicitly highlight the utility of TCRLOs (Follette et al., 1996; Jacobson, 1989).

This positions FAP, which provides a framework and technology that explicates and optimizes these in-session learning opporunties, as a potential enhancement that can supercharge existing psychotherapeutic treatments. Alternatively, FAP can function as a stand-alone treatment. As such, it may be most appropriate for clients whose behaviors are not targeted by, or who have not improved with standard cognitive-behavioral treatments, and clients with long-standing interpersonal difficulties typically characterized as personality disorders (Follette et al., 1996). FAP-enhanced treatment rather than stand-alone FAP is the focus of this chapter.

When FAP is used to enhance existing treatments, an additional consideration becomes important—the treatment rationale. The rationale underlies the treatment and guides the choice of therapeutic interventions. Most modern treatments for depression have a specific rationale that suggests specific interventions. For example, cognitive therapy (Beck et al., 1979) focuses on cognitive interventions, interpersonal therapy (Klerman, Weissman, Rounsaville, & Chevron, 1984) focuses on interpersonal interventions, and behavioral activation (Jacobson, Martell, & Dimidjian, 2001) focuses on behavioral interventions. FAP instead is guided by functional analysis (Kohlenberg & Tsai, 1991; Kohlenberg, Tsai, & Kohlenberg, 1996). This imbues FAP with a flexibility and adaptability unmatched by treatments with more specific rationales.

USING FUNCTIONAL ANALYTIC PSYCHOTHERAPY
TO ENHANCE COGNITIVE THERAPY FOR DEPRESSION

We used FAP to enhance Beck and colleagues' (1979) cognitive therapy for depression in a National Institute of Mental Health (NIMH)–sponsored treatment development study (Kohlenberg, Kanter, Bolling, Parker, & Tsai, 2002). The enhanced treatment is referred to as FECT (FAP-enhanced cognitive therapy). The two major FECT enhancements to standard cognitive therapy are (1) the use of an expanded rationale for the causes and treatment of depression, and (2) a greater use of the therapist–client relationship as an in-the-moment learning opportunity.

Our treatment development study (Kohlenberg et al., 2002) employed most of the standard features of depression treatment outcome studies, including structured assessment for major depressive disorder, typical inclusion and exclusion criteria, and outcome assessment with the Beck Depression Inventory (Beck, Ward, Mendelson, Mock, & Erbaugh, 1961), the Hamilton Rating Scale for Depression (Hamilton, 1967), and other measures of specific areas of functioning. However, because it was a treatment development study in which we were interested in our ability to train cognitive therapists to conduct FECT, the same four research therapists first conducted cognitive therapy (18 clients) and then FECT (28 clients), and random assignment was not employed. Results suggested that FECT achieved incremental efficacy over cognitive therapy, even though cognitive therapy performed well (79% of FECT clients and 60% of cognitive therapy clients responded to treatment). In addition, compared to standard cognitive therapy, FECT clients showed large improvements on measures of interpersonal functioning—a result predicted by FECT's increased use of TCRLO. Additional analyses from this study are presented below, as we describe the two major FECT enhancements.

Enhancement 1: Use of an Expanded Rationale

The process of providing a treatment rationale to clients is considered to be a common characteristic of the beginning of nearly all cognitive-behavioral psychotherapies. A treatment rationale generally comprises a description of a specific model of the etiology and treatment for a specific psychological problem (Addis & Carpenter, 2000). In general, treatment rationales have become more specific over time, perhaps due to the increasing influence of specific treatment manuals on the field. While this specificity may benefit researchers and research therapists whose priorities include differentiating and explicating treatment components to ensure that research protocols are delivered with integrity (Moncher & Prinz, 1991), this specificity may negatively impact the practicing clinician who wishes to conduct empirically supported treatments but retain sufficient flexibility to respond to diverse clients whose problems may not match a particular treatment rationale, or who do not agree with or accept a particular treatment rationale.

For example, the treatment rationale for cognitive therapy (Beck et al., 1979) describes the relationship between cognition and affect, then links this model to treatment techniques specifically aimed at correcting maladaptive cognitions. The cognitive theory is represented as an ABC sequence in which A represents an event or stimulus, B represents cognition in response to A, and C represents the resulting behavior or emotional response (Beck, 1967, p. 322). By the conclusion of this explanation, the client has been presented an overview of the cognitive theory of depression and the corresponding treatment that will ensue. As presented in Beck's treatment manual, the cognitive rationale is limited to the cognitive theory of depression, and alternative views are not presented (Kanter et al., 2002). Most of the time, this is not a problem. However, cognitive therapists sometimes have difficulty when clients do not respond favorably to the rationale, and treatment outcomes suffer. For example, Castonguay, Goldfried, Wiser, Raue, and Hayes (1996) reported descriptive analyses of nine cognitive therapy sessions in which therapeutic alliance ruptures were noted. In all but one of these sessions, the clients disagreed with the relevance of dysfunctional thoughts to their problems, or showed reluctance to engage in cognitive restructuring, but the therapist persisted in trying to fit the client's experience into the cognitive rationale. All of these clients had poor outcomes at the end of treatment.

It is well accepted that clients who respond favorably to the treatment rationale in cognitive therapy for depression are more likely to improve following treatment (Addis & Jacobson, 2000; Fennell & Teasdale, 1987; Ilardi & Craighead, 1994). Addis and Carpenter (2000) hypothesized that the match between the client and the treatment rationale promotes a more favorable outcome due to such factors as increased rapport, therapeutic alliance, and willingness to do homework. Several researchers have shown that a poor reaction to the treatment rationale negatively affects the therapeutic alliance, which in itself is a strong predictor of treatment outcome (Greenberg & Pinsof, 1986).

An alternative approach that avoids this pitfall is suggested by the behavioral underpinnings of FAP. The FAP view is that cognition, although covert, is simply behavior. Thinking, planning, believing, and categorizing (generally referred to as verbal or cognitive behavior) are things people do or behaviors in which people engage, and are subject to the same historical shaping processes (e.g., reinforcement) as are other behaviors. The degree of control exerted by cognition over subsequent behavior is on a continuum and varies depending on a particular client's history. In addition, modern behavior analysis is now focused on new shaping processes that may be unique to verbal behavior (Hayes, Barnes-Holmes, & Roche, 2001). This research provides behaviorally oriented clinicians a new conceptualization and technology for working with human language and cognition that heretofore has lacked richness, depth, and sophistication, and has often led to criticisms that behavioral approaches are overly simplistic and superficial.

Likewise, in FAP, the guiding principle that cognition is behavior leads to an expanded rationale for FECT that not only includes the traditional cognitive account but also provides alternatives to those clients for whom this is a mismatch. This results in a larger, more diverse set of intervention options. When presenting the rationale, FECT therapists do the same thing that is done by cognitive therapists; that is, they present the standard ABC cognitive model and tell clients that their beliefs, attitudes, and thoughts about external events can lead to problematic feelings and maladaptive behavior. This is illustrated in Figure 5.1a. For clients whose experience matches ABC, FECT proposes that the methods of cognitive therapy are usually effective and probably maximize the therapy–client match and outcome. FECT therapists differ from cognitive therapists, however, in that an acceptance intervention aimed at distancing the client from the cognitive content rather than changing the content may be used if cognitive therapy interventions are not effective in a particular case (we discuss FECT and acceptance below).

Departing from the cognitive therapy rationale, FECT therapists also tell clients that other possibilities might also exist in addition to the ABC paradigm. For clients whose experience corresponds to one of these other paradigms, standard cognitive therapy might result in a client–therapy mismatch and a less effective treatment. For example, Figure 5.1b represents a client who says, "I just reacted, I didn't have any preceding thoughts or beliefs." A cognitive therapist might respond to this with additional assignments aimed at bringing cognition into awareness. In contrast, the FECT therapist is more accepting of the idea that there is no cognition at work

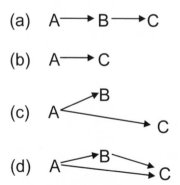

FIGURE 5.1. Some cognition–behavior relationships according to the FECT expanded rationale. A, antecedent event; B, belief/cognition; C, consequence (emotional reaction).

and may, for example, engage in an activation or exposure intervention aimed at noncognitive features of the problem.

As another example, Figure 5.1c represents a client who says, "I truly believe that I do not have to be perfect, but I still feel like I have to be." In this case, as Beck and colleagues (1979, pp. 302–303) describe, a patient is suggesting that he has already changed his thoughts to be accurate, but it has not helped him feel better. (Another typical example is, "I know I'm not worthless but I don't believe it emotionally.") While the cognitive therapist is encouraged to persist in application of the cognitive model in this situation, the FECT model accommodates the possibility that the client may have a "B" that does not play a role in causing the problematic "C" even though there is a temporal sequencing that resembles the one posited by the cognitive model; that is, the FECT view is that it is possible to have a belief that precedes the problematic emotion and/or behavior but is not causally related to the emotion.

The FECT approach is not limited to simply adding versions (b) and (c) to the cognitive hypothesis (a) in Figure 5.1; rather, these examples demonstrate the flexibility that the view affords. Other variants of the ABC model exist. For example, Figure 5.1d represents a situation in which the problematic response is influenced both by beliefs or cognitions and directly by the activating event (as in a classical conditioning paradigm). In this situation, sole reliance on cognitive restructuring may have the effect of partial or temporary, but not complete, amelioration of the problematic response. We speculate that problems with relapse may at times be due to such multiple influences.

The improved client–treatment matching of the expanded rationale is illustrated in the case of Mr. D., a participant in the FECT treatment development study. Mr. D. had a problem of getting angry too easily. During a therapy session, he brought up an example of getting angry at other drivers at a four-way stop while driving to his appointment. He explained how the driver in front of him could have moved forward a little and allowed Mr. D. to make a right-hand turn. In this example, the therapist does a brief assessment to determine whether ABC or an alternate paradigm should also be considered at this moment in Mr. D.'s treatment:

Mr. D.: I thought, "You idiot!"

Therapist: You remember during our discussion of the [FECT] brochure that thought sometimes precedes feelings but can also occur after. At the four-way stop, you thought, "You idiot!" Were you aware as to whether you had that thought first and then got angry, or did you get angry first and then have the thought?

Mr. D.: I got angry first.

Thus, the expanded rationale has led the therapist to ask a very simple question, the answer to which suggests that it may not be useful to attempt a cognitive intervention at this moment in therapy. We recognize that a well-trained cognitive therapist is equipped to handle this situation with the tools of standard cognitive therapy (e.g., by retreating from direct restructuring and using this situation as an opportunity to help the client recognize any fleeting automatic thoughts that may have occurred), and that cognitive theory (Clark, Beck, & Alford, 1999) provides an account for the client's experience of feeling before thinking that is consistent with the cognitive model. We want to underscore that outcome studies show that standard cognitive therapy is often, if not usually, effective and is an important component of FECT. FECT, however, increases the flexibility of the therapist to follow different paths when treatment is not working and, as mentioned earlier, research examining the relationship between cognitive therapy process and outcome (Castonguay et al., 1996) suggests that flexibility may be beneficial in these situations.

Data from the FECT study (Kohlenberg et al., 2002) provide additional support for the benefits of an expanded rationale. We assessed clients' reactions to their treatment rationales by training blind raters in an observational coding system based on Addis's Reaction to Rationale (unpublished) scale. Figure 5.2 shows that clients who received the expanded

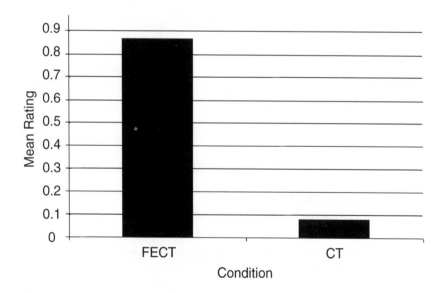

FIGURE 5.2. Overall positive reaction by clients to the rationales given in FAP-enhanced cognitive therapy (FECT) and standard cognitive therapy (CT).

rationale had a significantly greater overall positive response to the rationale than did standard cognitive therapy clients. Also, regression analyses revealed that clients with a more positive overall reaction to their rationale were more likely to achieve sustained remission (defined as a client who was not clinically depressed at the end of acute treatment, and who remained depression-free throughout the follow-up period).

The Expanded Rationale for Cognitive and Behavior-Analytic Clinicians

We suggested earlier that Mr. D.'s response might indicate that a cognitive intervention may not be useful. Of course, the choice of intervention in any FAP-based therapy should be guided by functional analysis (Follette, Naugle, & Linerooth, 1999; Kohlenberg, Tsai, & Kohlenberg, 1996) and case conceptualization (Kohlenberg & Tsai, 2000). In addition, because FECT may be attractive to both behaviorally oriented clinicians and cognitive therapists, who enter psychotherapy with quite different histories and worldviews (Hayes, Hayes, & Reese, 1988), we recognize that the nature of the intervention conducted in FECT also has to do with the therapist's history and previous experience. For an experienced cognitive therapist trying FECT for the first time, an awareness of the possibilities suggested by the expanded rationale may foster an increased sensitivity to situations in which standard cognitive therapy interventions are not working. For this clinician, the use of the expanded rationale may function as a limited functional analysis and serve as a point of entry for learning the utility of functional analysis in more detail.

On the other hand, a clinician with a background in behavior analysis who is now trying FECT, may be less likely to use cognitive therapy techniques in the first place, placing more emphasis on explicit behavioral techniques or acceptance techniques. Paradoxically, the use of FECT—a thoroughly behavior analytic approach—may increase the sensitivity of this clinician to situations in which standard cognitive therapy interventions are appropriate. To this clinician, we emphasize that FECT therapists maintain a consistent behavioral framework, use cognitive interventions with caution, and consider that such interventions can be behaviorally reconceptualized (Kohlenberg & Tsai, 1991) using verbal behavior concepts (Skinner, 1957) and rule governance (Hayes & Gifford, 1997).

Enhancement 2: Use of Therapist–Client Relationship Learning Opportunities

The comments of client Mr. G. provide a thumbnail sketch of how the use of in-session relationship learning transforms standard cognitive therapy into FECT. Mr. G., a 44-year-old with a long-standing history of major depression and poor responses to several previous medications and psychosocial treatments, presented with a deep dissatisfaction in his interpersonal relationships. He felt that people rejected him, and he was unable to achieve closeness with others. Mr. G. was no longer depressed at the end of our treatment and reported making progress in being more intimate with his wife and children. In contrast to the other 46 subjects in our study, Mr. G. received only eight sessions of standard cognitive therapy, because his therapist had a medical emergency. Mr. G. was then transferred to another therapist who used FECT for the remaining 12 sessions. Although Mr. G. was dropped from the treatment development study because he received both treatments, he was the only client who experienced both cognitive therapy and FECT. Thus, he was in the unique position of being able to describe and compare his experience of both treatments, which he did during the final session:

> "There's a lot of stuff going on in my personal life that we've been working on here in depression and so on, and that has led to maybe the cognitive therapy way of handling things and looking at ah, you know, the daily activity log and then doing the thought records and analyzing thoughts and how they lead to things. So that's over here [with the first eight sessions of cognitive therapy]. And then this other part, which I definitely got into with you [the next 12 sessions of FECT], was in my personal relationships and how that works, on both sides, myself and the other person. And then it became how that occurred for you and me as an example of that, [my appearing to others as] ominous. It's something I learned with you so that it would not persist in unintentionally coloring my relationships."

Here is our interpretation of Mr. G.'s comments.

1. Mr. G. acknowledged the utility of standard cognitive therapy techniques. FECT recognizes that cognitive therapy is a well-established therapy with proven effectiveness, and good cognitive therapy is the foundation on which FECT builds.

2. Mr. G. stated that during FECT, he became aware, for the first time, of an interpersonal problem involving others perceiving something ominous about him that interferes with his relationships. Mr. G. identified that this interpersonal problem occurred not only in his daily life but also in the therapy session between himself and his therapist. When a daily life problem occurs in the therapy session, it becomes a TCRLO, and FECT is designed specifically to use these opportunities to maximum benefit. Mr. G.'s awareness of a daily life problem that also occurs in the therapist–client relationship captures the focus that FECT has on identifying and using the therapist–client relationship for this purpose.

3. Finally, Mr. G. suggested that learning to deal with this problem

with the therapist will help him in his future relationships with others. This statement by Mr. G. hints that the TCRLO focus was effective and highlights the FECT contention that therapeutic change is maximized when here-and-now learning occurs.

Clinically Relevant Behaviors

TCRLOs are based on the notion that the therapist–client relationship is a social environment with the potential to evoke and change actual instances of the client's problematic behavior as they occur. Thus, therapy focuses on those therapist–client interactions that are examples of the client's daily life problems. For example, Mr. G., who had interpersonal problems in his daily life in part because of his belief that "People should just say what is on their minds," might at times appear ominous or intimidating to the therapist because of a bluntness that results from that belief. As previously noted, TCRLO's occur when here-and-now, in-session behaviors that are functionally similar to the daily life behaviors that are the targets of therapy occur. These in-session behaviors are referred to as clinically relevant behavior (CRB). CRB1s are client problems that occur in session. CRB2s are client improvements that occur in session. It should be noted that CRBs are real, occur naturally during therapy, and differ from the prompted and/ or scripted within-session behaviors of role playing, behavioral rehearsal, or social skills training (Kohlenberg, Tsai, & Dougher, 1993).

CRBs may also be catalogued as either cognitive CRBs and/or interpersonal CRBs. Cognitive CRBs are in-session, actual occurrences of problematic cognition (CRB1) or improved cognition (CRB2). For example, Mr. G.'s belief that "I should just say what is on my mind," if it occurs in therapy and is related to the kind of difficult behavior that causes him interpersonal problems in his daily life, is a cognitive CRB1. Any occurrence of a problematic cognition having to do with the therapy, the therapeutic relationship, or the therapist would be considered a cognitive CRB1. The occurrence of a problematic cognitive CRB provides a special opportunity for the therapist to do *in vivo* cognitive therapy. For example, the therapist could use a thought log or empirical hypothesis-testing pertaining to the here-and-now client–therapist interaction. However, as discussed earlier, in the presence of a cognitive CRB, the therapist may elect to intervene with an alternative intervention based on the expanded rationale, the case conceptualization, and functional assessment.

The Mr. G. example involved both cognitive and interpersonal CRBs. Interpersonal CRBs are actual in-session problematic interpersonal behaviors. For example, one interpersonal CRB1 was that Mr. G. was not aware of when he was acting ominously with the therapist. The therapist could have encouraged and prompted Mr. G. to develop more awareness of this behavior instead of employing an *in vivo* cognitive intervention targeting the belief that "You should say what is on your mind," if such increased awareness was conceptualized as a CRB2 (an in-session improvement in client behavior). This points up the importance of generating a clear case conceptualization from the outset and updating it as treatment progresses.

As an aid in case conceptualization, Callaghan (2001) has developed a comprehensive system for assessing interpersonal CRBs in FAP and FAP-enhanced treatments. CRBs are classified into five functional classes: (1) assertion of needs, (2) bidirectional communication, (3) conflict, (4) disclosure and interpersonal closeness, and (5) emotional experience and expression. Mr. G.'s problem of not recognizing the impact of his behavior on others would be considered an exemplar of (2) bidirectional communication, which is defined as "behaviors that function to inhibit an interpersonal relationship between the client and therapist or the client and other people due to the client's inability to discriminate, or respond effectively to the impact he or she has on other people, or problems with providing feedback to others" (p. 18). Callaghan's model provides therapists an initial idiographic assessment of interpersonal CRBs and a template for tracking changes in specific interpersonal CRBs over the course of therapy (Callaghan, Summers, & Weidman, 2003).

Developing awareness of CRB1s and CRB2s as they occur in therapy and change over time is the cornerstone of FECT. Since CRBs occur in the here and now, therapist awareness of CRBs requires that the therapist be fully present and aware during the therapy session. Thus, the FECT therapist's awareness of CRBs has much in common with the practice of mindfulness (Linehan, 1993; Marlatt, 2002; Teasdale et al., 2000). An initial task of the FECT therapist, once a CRB has been identified, is changing the focus of the therapy session to the TCRLO as it is occurring. The following transcript segment from a session with Mr. G. illustrates how a therapist might first identify an interpersonal CRB1 to a client. In this session, the therapist and Mr. G. had been discussing Mr. G.'s daily life problem of being very strict and detail-oriented, and how Mr. G. has difficulty identifying the impact of this behavior on others. The therapist has observed these behaviors in the therapeutic relationship and sees the current situation as a potential point for intervention. In this segment, the therapist demonstrated some fundamental FECT techniques that are highlighted in this text:

MR. G.: In personal relationships . . . maybe that tendency is too strict, or too, um, unforgiving. Now it isn't like I'm unforgiving, like I hate somebody, but if, if . . . we say something or if we agree to do something, I expect us to act on that.

THERAPIST: [After more discussion of how this strictness affects his relationships.] We've been around this topic a bit, between you and I. How do you think I react to that? [The therapist is interested in this topic as a potential TCRLO, so he directs the client to focus on the therapeutic relationship.]

MR. G.: A, that's a wonder to me, and B, I project that in the beginning it may have been a little confronting or irritating, because I don't think a lot of people just say what's on their mind . . . but I don't know, really, I wonder how you take it. . . . [The client's response suggests that he is unaware of the therapist's reactions, so this could be a TCRLO. The client's unawareness of the therapist's reaction could be considered a CRB1.]

THERAPIST: I didn't really feel a sense of confrontation but I did feel, um, there's times when it feels, even, the word might be a bit much for it, but a little scary, and it is for the things that seem unsaid. . . . It seems to be this, this sort of ominous potential consequence [Mr. G.: Hmm.] . . . which feels ominous. Ominous I think is a good term for it. . . . [The therapist self-discloses his personal reactions to the client, which functions both to increase the client's awareness and to highlight a related CRB1 of being ominous. Being ominous and being aware of being ominous are conceptualized as different behaviors.]

MR. G.: That's intriguing to me. I'd like to hear more about that.

THERAPIST: What's your reaction to hearing that?

MR. G.: Immediately I think I'm missing some human interaction skills, because I'm certainly not here to cause people pain or ominous feelings . . . in fact, that takes me a little bit by surprise. The only thing I can think of in a very personal way is, um, is this "emotional blackmail." Do people feel like I won't like them if they don't interact with me the way I dictate that they should? I don't know. [Continued discussion of how he could make an interaction feel ominous.]

THERAPIST: I wonder if this [my feeling this ominous potential consequence from you], if there is any sense of this being a parallel, or having a relationship to how you might feel others' reactions are? Does it seem like it is possible that others could have a sense of this as well? [This is an important question that is expected to facilitate generalization of improvements from the therapist–client interaction to daily life. Generalization is expected to occur naturally but can be augmented by offering interpretations that compare within-session interactions to daily life.]

MR. G.: You mean other than yourself?

THERAPIST: Correct.

MR. G.: I think I see some of that. To a certain extent, people, when they interact with me, it may be a little different than when they interact with other people. . . . I like detail, I like to know what's going on . . . and that may cause some people some tension . . . [The client's identification that his behavior may cause tension in others is not technically a CRB2, because it is not related to the therapeutic relationship, but it nonetheless does demonstrate increased awareness in daily life.]

THERAPIST: I want to let you know that as I've grown to know you, I find you real likeable. I really enjoy working with you. There's a little less sense of that [being ominous over time], and it is part of the dynamic that I'm trying to unravel. [The therapist amplifies his positive feelings about the client in response to the client's statement of increased awareness. This natural reinforcement of improved behavior is a cornerstone of the treatment.] . . . Now I want to circle back around. . . . What's happening with your interaction with your wife . . . what's going on for you in all your reactions and dynamics, and so on, past and present, when, as you experience it, your wife is trying to control you? [This weaving back and forth between in-session and daily life behavior is another typical intervention, again expected to facilitate generalization.]

Do Cognitive Therapists Already Use TCRLO?

In grant reviews and informal discussions with cognitive therapists, it is often asserted that cognitive therapists use the therapeutic relationship for *in vivo* learning routinely during cognitive therapy. There is no reason why this could not be the case. To be sure, there are no prohibitions on using the therapeutic relationship during standard cognitive therapy, and several examples are included in Beck and colleagues' treatment manual (1979).

We have collected data that bear on this issue based on an adherence scale developed for the FECT study (Kohlenberg et al., 2002). The scale is called the Therapist In-Session Strategy Scale (THISS) and is based on the method, structure and some of the content of the Collaborative Study Psychotherapy Rating Scale (CSPRS; Hollon et al., 1987). The THISS includes the CSPRS Cognitive Therapy subscale, as well as two additional subscales entitled FAP and *In Vivo* Cognitive Therapy. The FAP subscale measures the frequency and extent of therapeutic attention to TCRLOs, such as the therapist commenting on some aspect of the client's in-session behavior or disclosing his or her own thoughts or feelings about the client's in-session behavior. The *In Vivo* Cognitive Therapy subscale measures the frequency and extent of cognitive interventions regarding TCRLOs. This subscale was constructed by recasting standard cognitive therapy items from the CSPRS Cognitive Therapy subscale to focus on therapist–client issues. See Table 5.1 for subscale item examples. The THISS subscales demonstrated good internal consistency, and THISS raters demonstrated good interrater and rater-criterion reliability (Kohlenberg et al., 2002). As shown in Figure 5.3, we found that our cognitive therapists did not use FAP types of interven-

TABLE 5.1. Examples of THISS Items

Cognitive Therapy subscale, item 18, Specific Examples: Therapist urges client to give concrete, specific examples of beliefs OR events from daily life. For example:

    C: I can never do anything right.
    T: Can you give me an example, like, from this last week?
    C: Oh, like stuff around the house.
    T: You never do stuff right around the house? Like what?
    C: Like cleaning.

In Vivo Cognitive Therapy subscale, item 17, Specific *In Vivo* Examples: Therapist urges client to give concrete, specific examples of beliefs or events *in vivo* OR *about therapy*. For example:

    C: I don't do anything right.
    T: Does that apply in here, too?
    C: Of course.
    T: Give me an example of something wrong you do here.
    C: Well, I answer too quickly, without considering.

FAP subscale, item 12, Comments on Client Behavior: Therapist describes, notes, acknowledges, or otherwise comments on some aspect of client's behavior (thoughts, feelings, or actions) toward or relevant to the therapist. For example:

    T: I notice that when I say positive things about you, you do a couple of different things. Sometimes you discredit or qualify what I say, sometimes you kind of close up or shut down, and other times you sort of ignore it and change the subject and start into some long-winded monologue.

---

tions while conducting standard cognitive therapy, but did use these interventions while doing FECT. This provides some evidence that standard cognitive therapy does not generally involve a focus on TCRLO. However, it may be argued that the cognitive therapists in our study were not practicing typical cognitive therapy.[1]

To address this concern, we also used the THISS to rate 52 cognitive therapy sessions from Jacobson and colleague's (1996) component analysis of cognitive therapy for depression. All therapists were qualified research cognitive therapists and had been rated as competent by expert raters using the Cognitive Therapy Scale (Dobson, Shaw, & Vallis, 1985). As shown in Figure 5.3, cognitive therapists in both the component analysis and in the FECT study rarely used TCRLO interventions, while FECT therapists consistently did. These differences were statistically reliable. In the FECT study, we also found that the use of the particular TCRLO interventions assessed by the *In Vivo* Cognitive Therapy subscale predicted positive treatment outcomes.

---

[1] However, they were rated as competent by Keith Dobson on the Cognitive Therapy Scale (Dobson, Shaw, & Vallis, 1985), and ratings were comparable to those found in the NIMH Treatment for Depression Collaborative Research Program (Shaw et al., 1999).

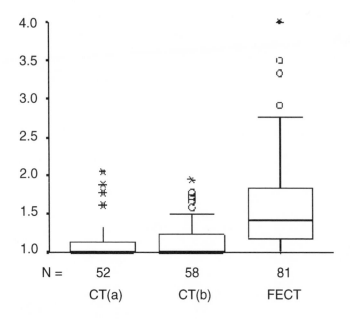

FIGURE 5.3. Box plots showing TCRLO interventions during cognitive therapy (CT) in (a) the Jacobson (Jacobson et al., 1996) study, and (b) the FECT (Kohlenberg et al., 2002) study and during FECT in the FECT study.

Putting It Together: FECT in Practice

Kohlenberg and colleagues (2002) outline seven specific techniques for practicing FECT (Table 5.2). First, FECT therapists conduct Beck and colleagues' (1979) cognitive therapy for depression and maintain its 20-session length and individual session structure (setting and following an agenda; working on targeted problems with CBT techniques and homework assignments; eliciting feedback from the client at the end of the session). However, at the beginning of therapy, the FECT therapist presents an expanded rationale rather than the standard cognitive therapy rationale. This presentation includes *Coping with Depression* (Beck & Greenberg, 1995), the FECT brochure (Kohlenberg & Tsai, 1997), and a verbal presentation. For example, the therapist might say:

> "The focus of our therapy will depend on the causes of your problems. It is often the case that when people become depressed, how they think about and perceive the world changes, and then their negative thinking keeps them depressed. So we'll look at your thoughts and see if they are keeping you depressed, and there are strategies to help you change your thinking. In addition, depressed people often have stopped doing the

TABLE 5.2. Seven FECT Techniques

Technique	Description	Purpose
1. Set the scene early	Assign autobiographical statement homework.	• Emphasizes historical factors. • Aids case conceptualization. • Possible TCRLO.
2. Present expanded rationale	• Present *Coping with Depression*. • Present FECT brochure. • Present rationales verbally. • Assess client response to rationales.	• Increases therapist flexibility. • Aids case conceptualization. • Possible TCRLO.

3. Use FECT case conceptualization	• Describe:
	  1. Relevant history
	  2. Daily life problems
	  3. Corresponding cognitive CRB1s
	  4. Corresponding interpersonal CRB1s
	  5. In-session goals (CRB2s)
	  6. Daily life goals
		• Emphasizes historical factors.
		
		• Identifies potentially important cognitive phenomena.
		• Identifies possible TCRLOs and CRBs.

4. Notice CRBs	• Ongoing observation of possible CRBs.	
5. Evoke CRBs	• Ask questions to focus on therapist–client relationship.	
6. Increase therapist self-awareness	• Focus on therapist reactions to clients in supervision. • Use self-disclosure appropriately in session.	• Aids detection and appropriate response to CRBs. • Evoke CRB1s or naturally reinforce CRB2s.

7. Use Daily Record	• Same columns as Beck's Thought Record
	• Client also considers:
	  1. Causal sequence of thoughts and feelings
	  2. In-session versions of daily life problematic responses
	  3. Alternative actions, as well as alternative thoughts
		• Consistent with cognitive rationale.
		
		• Consistent with expanded rationale.
		• Aids focus on TCRLOs.
		
		• Consistent with expanded rationale; increases likelihood of activation or acceptance interventions.

things in their life that used to be important to them; if this has happened for you, we will help you get moving again. We might do lots of other things, such as grieving your losses, contacting your feelings—especially those that are difficult for you to experience, and developing relationship skills. The important thing is that there are many different ways to treat depression, and we'll do what works for you."

This expansion requires the flexibility to change the approach if it does not match the client's experience and/or if the client is not progressing.

When presenting the expanded rationale, FECT therapists also prepare the client for the focus on TCRLOs. For example, the therapist might say:

"One other thing will be important in our work; that is, sometimes the things you are depressed about, and your depression itself, will show up in our sessions. For example, I know you feel hopeless about your relationship with your wife, and in turn there may be times when you feel hopeless in here, with me, about our work. That is OK if that happens. When things like that happen, when your depression shows up in here, it will be very important for us to take notice. That is because when things happen live between us, they are special opportunities for us to do real work and to really help you understand and change what is happening to you, as it is happening."

While using the expanded rationale and expanded set of techniques throughout the course of therapy, FECT therapists are poised to use in-session learning opportunities as they occur. They use a FECT case conceptualization that aids in the detection of TCRLOs and CRBs. They continuously observe the client–therapist interaction and look for the occurrence of the client's daily life problems and dysfunctional thoughts in the here and now, within the context of the client–therapist relationship. As one example, the client's response to the initial autobiographical homework assignment may be an early TCRLO, and even if it is not directly addressed as such, it may nonetheless help the therapist generate hypotheses about potential CRBs that might appear later in therapy. For example, does the client procrastinate, give sparse information, complete volumes of writing, or give up and feel hopeless in response to the assignment? How are these responses related to the client's presenting daily life problems?

FECT therapists use a modified Dysfunctional Thought Record (Beck et al., 1979), the Daily Record of Thinking, Feeling, and Doing, that retains the major columns of the original (including the situation; the client's actions, thoughts, and feelings in response to the situation; and alternative thinking) but adds several features. First, the instructions were modified to include the expanded rationale:

"Begin filling out this record with the problematic situation, what you did, or what you felt. If possible, denote whether the thinking, feeling, or doing came first, second, or third (which did you experience first, second, and third?)."

Asking the client to consider the sequence of behaviors provides additional information to the therapist to help determine if the ABC, AC, ACB, or other paradigms fit the client's particular experience.

Second, after the client denotes the thoughts, feelings, and actions that occurred in response to the particular event in daily life, a new column asks the client, "How might similar problematic thoughts, feelings, and/or actions come up in session, about the therapy, or between you and your therapist?" This *In Vivo* column increases the focus on TCRLOs and helps the client learn to recognize relationships between in-session and daily life behaviors, which facilitates generalization of in-session improvements to daily life.

A third new column, consistent with the expanded rationale, facilitates behavioral activation and acceptance by asking clients to come up with alternative ways of acting that would help them achieve their goals. This column is discussed more fully in the next section.

FECT AND ACCEPTANCE

Although FECT uses the structure and techniques of cognitive therapy (Beck et al., 1979), it is consistent with an acceptance rationale (Hayes et al., 1999) that some believe contraindicates the use of cognitive interventions. Briefly, the acceptance rationale is: Human suffering is at least in part due to the ubiquitous human agenda of experiential (cognitive and emotional) avoidance (Hayes, Wilson, Gifford, Follette, & Strosahl, 1996). Specifically, humans spend considerable effort trying to alter the form, frequency, or situational sensitivity of thoughts and emotions in order to avoid their aversive features. Paradoxically, this avoidance, rather than alleviating suffering, produces and maintains it. Research and theorizing on relational frame theory, a modern, behavior-analytic account of human language and cognition (Hayes et al., 2001), and other research suggests that this agenda is a natural by-product of human language and is ultimately ineffective and detrimental. In addition, the avoidance agenda is supported by cultural processes, such as modeling, and behavioral processes, such as negative reinforcement. Cognitive restructuring strategies, as deliberate attempts to control and avoid aversive emotional experiences, are thus seen as part of the problem of experiential avoidance rather than a solution to it. Alternatively, the interventions of ACT (Hayes et al., 1999) aimed at relinquishing pseudocontrol over thoughts and feelings, psychological acceptance of aversive thoughts and feelings, and commitment to valued action in the presence of aversive thoughts and feelings are recommended.

A key feature of any clinical behavior-analytic therapy (Dougher, 1999) is that the choice of treatment interventions should be based on functional analysis rather than topographical features of the problem. Simply put, one should do what works, and the determination of what works should not be based on preformed rules, as in "If depressed, do behavioral activation." Therefore, the FECT view is that cognitive interventions may be appropriate in several circumstances, and the choice of intervention should be based on case conceptualization and functional analyses of the situation at hand. Cognitive interventions may benefit the client if avoidance of aversive thoughts has been ruled out as a major factor in the client's distress, the client has experienced significant benefits from cognitive intervention in the past, or the client is new to therapy and has not been exposed to any sort of previous therapeutic intervention. As in standard cognitive therapy, FECT therapists typically start treatment with behavioral and cognitive therapy interventions. These interventions may be particularly useful if they result in the client engaging in new, improved behaviors for which natural, positive reinforcement is readily available. On the other hand, working under the expanded rationale, FECT therapists are prepared to drop the cognitive therapy if it becomes apparent that the client's primary problem is emotional avoidance rather than behavioral activation and eventual contact with positive reinforcement. In addition, FECT therapists may move into acceptance strategies if the client is not improving with standard cognitive interventions, or if the client rejects or does not respond favorably to the cognitive rationale.

FECT incorporates acceptance in several ways. First, it is important to note that TCRLOs can facilitate and create intense experiences of psychological acceptance that would be difficult to achieve otherwise. ACT itself is geared to reap the full benefits of in-session work, because ACT is a behavioral treatment that, like FAP, was developed with an appreciation for the role of the immediate environment in shaping behavior. Many ACT interventions are experiential exercises that the client and therapist do together, in the here and now, with the purpose of creating an in-session learning experience rather than making a didactic point. For example, the ACT Eye Contact exercise (Hayes et al., 1999, pp. 244–245) involves the therapist and client pulling their chairs together so they may look into each other's eyes for about 3 minutes. This exercise usually elicits a host of uncomfortable reactions in both parties and can be a powerful example of commitment to valued action in the face of aversive private experiences. The use of TCRLO to facilitate acceptance in FAP is discussed fully in Cordova and Kohlenberg (1994).

Second, behavioral activation, which is conducted at the beginning of standard cognitive therapy but generally underemphasized as treatment progresses except in cases of more severe depression, is highlighted in FECT's expanded rationale and given a more prominent role in the overall FECT approach. Although based on a simpler behavioral rationale than ACT, the interventions of behavioral activation (Martell, Addis, & Jacobson, 2001) also are consistent with the priority of commitment to and engagement in action rather than direct modification of thoughts and feelings. For example, the Activity Log emphasizes activation and accomplishment without requiring the absence of depression. Following the standard cognitive therapy structure and the expanded rationale, the FECT therapist will begin treatment with activation assignments and may elect to continue activation strategies rather than switching to cognitive content as treatment progresses, and if activation is producing results. This is consistent with research on behavioral activation by Jacobson and colleagues (1996), which suggests that activation alone produces results equivalent to the full cognitive therapy package.

Third, FECT's Daily Record, which, as in standard cognitive therapy, often structures the therapeutic work during the bulk of the treatment, contains a new column that facilitates acceptance interventions and maintains therapeutic awareness of the client's degree of experiential avoidance. The Alternative More Productive Ways of Acting column contains the question, "Committing to act more effectively: How committed are you to acting more effectively in the future even if you have negative thoughts and feelings?" The client responds on the following scale:

- 0%: None (I can't act better while I have negative thoughts and/or feelings).
- 50%: I am willing to give it a try.
- 100%: Very much—I will act effectively and have my negative thoughts and feelings at the same time.

FECT therapists use this column as a continual reminder to themselves and their clients that it is possible to improve even if one has negative thoughts and feelings.

CONCLUSIONS

This chapter has provided an overview of the basic principles of FAP, a treatment that utilizes basic behavioral principles to produce an intense and curative therapist–client relationship. In practice, due to the focus on TCRLOs, FAP may at times appear more like psychoanalysis than standard behavior therapy (Kohlenberg & Tsai, 1991, pp. 169–188). It rarely appears strictly behavioral in form, although it rests on solid behavioral foundations, and all interventions can be viewed through the lens of modern behavioral theory. FAP can be used as a stand-alone treatment or to enhance other treatments.

FECT is the use of FAP as an enhancement to standard cognitive therapy for depression in several ways. First, the standard cognitive therapy rationale and interventions are employed, but in FECT, they are part of an expanded rationale that gives the therapist more flexibility to drop cognitive therapy when it is not working or is not appropriate. Acceptance, activation, and many other interventions are used in conjunction with or instead of cognitive therapy interventions, based on a case conceptualization that emphasizes an idiographic functional analysis of client problems. Second, throughout treatment, FECT therapists are poised to capitalize on TCRLOs as they occur to maximize the potential for the client to learn new, more productive behaviors in the here and now.

In a preliminary, uncontrolled trial, FECT clients preferred the expanded rationale and evidenced incremental improvements in depression and major gains in interpersonal functioning. Notably, adherence analyses found that standard cognitive therapy did not employ a TCRLO focus, and this focus—specifically in the context of cognitive therapy interventions—enhanced outcomes. Therefore, FECT adds to a growing list of new, cognitive-behavioral treatments, including Safran and Segal (1990), Young (1990), CBASP (McCullough, 2000), ACT (Hayes et al., 1999), and DBT (Linehan, 1993) that appreciate and place special emphasis on the therapist–client relationship as a vehicle for client change. We believe there may be a much-needed movement afoot in this direction that will expand the scope, depth, sophistication, and ultimate success of cognitive-behavioral therapy.

REFERENCES

Addis, M. E., & Carpenter, K. M. (2000). The treatment rationale in cognitive behavioral therapy: Psychological mechanisms and clinical guidelines. *Cognitive and Behavioral Practice*, 7(2), 147–156.

Addis, M. E., & Jacobson, N. S. (2000). A closer look at the treatment rationale and homework compliance in cognitive-behavioral therapy for depression. *Cognitive Therapy and Research*, 24(3), 313–326.

Beck, A. T. (1967). *Depression: Clinical, experimental and theoretical aspects.* New York: Harper & Row.

Beck, A. T., & Greenberg, R. L. (1995). *Coping with depression.* Bala Cynwyd, PA: Beck Institute for Cognitive Therapy and Research.

Beck, A. T., Rush, A. J., Shaw, F. B., & Emery, G. (1979). *Cognitive therapy of depression.* New York: Guilford Press.

Beck, A. T., Ward, C. H., Mendelson, M., Mock, J., & Erbaugh, J. (1961). An inventory for measuring depression. *Archives of General Psychiatry, 4,* 561–571.

Callaghan, G. M. (2001). *Functional Idiographic Assesment Template (FIAT).* Unpublished manual, San Jose State University.

Callaghan, G. M., Summers, C. J., & Weidman, M. (2003). The treatment of histrionic and narcissistic personality disorder behaviors: A single-subject demonstration of clinical effectiveness using functional analytic psychotherapy. *Journal of Contemporary Psychotherapy*, *33*, 321–339.

Callaghan, G. M., Naugle, A. E., & Follette, W. C. (1996). Useful construction of the client–therapist relationship. *Psychotherapy: Theory, Research, Practice, Training*, *33*(3), 381–390.

Castonguay, L. G., Goldfried, M. R., Wiser, S., Raue, P. J., & Hayes, A. M. (1996). Predicting the effect of cognitive therapy for depression: A study of unique and common factors. *Journal of Consulting and Clinical Psychology*, *63*(3), 497–504.

Clark, D. A., Beck, A. T., & Alford, B. A. (1999). *Scientific foundations of cognitive theory and therapy of depression*. New York: Wiley.

Cordova, J. V., & Kohlenberg, R. J. (1994). Acceptance and the therapeutic relationship. In S. C. Hayes, N. S. Jacobson, V. M. Follette, & M. J. Dougher (Eds.), *Acceptance and change: Content and context in psychotherapy* (pp. 125–142). Reno, NV: Context Press.

Dobson, K. S., Shaw, B. F., & Vallis, T. M. (1985). Reliability of a measure of the quality of cognitive therapy. *British Journal of Clinical Psychology*, *24*(4), 295–300.

Dougher, M. J. (Ed.). (1999). *Clinical behavior analysis*. Reno, NV: Context Press.

Fennell, M. J. V., & Teasdale, J. D. (1987). Cognitive therapy for depression: Individual differences and the process of change. *Cognitive Therapy and Research*, *11*(2), 253–271.

Follette, W. C., Naugle, A. E., & Callaghan, G. M. (1996). A radical behavioral understanding of the therapeutic relationship in effecting change. *Behavior Therapy*, *27*, 623–641.

Follette, W. V., Naugle, A. E., & Linerooth, P. J. (1999). Functional alternatives to traditional assessment and diagnosis. In M. J. Dougher (Ed.), *Clinical behavior analysis* (pp. 99–125). Reno, NV: Context Press.

Greenberg, L. S., & Pinsof, W. M. (Eds.). (1986). *The psychotherapeutic process: A research handbook*. New York: Guilford Press.

Hamilton, M. (1967). Development of a rating scale for primary depressive illness. *British Journal of Social and Clinical Psychology*, *6*(4), 278–296.

Hayes, S. C., Barnes-Holmes, D., & Roche, B. (Eds.). (2001). *Relational frame theory: A post-Skinnerian account of human language and cognition*. New York: Kluwer Academic/Plenum.

Hayes, S. C., & Gifford, E. V. (1997). The trouble with language: Experiential avoidance, rules, and the nature of verbal events. *Psychological Science*, *8*(3), 170–173.

Hayes, S. C., Hayes, L. J., & Reese, H. W. (1988). Finding the philosophical core: A review of Stephen C. Pepper's "World hypotheses: A study in evidence." *Journal of the Experimental Analysis of Behavior*, *50*(1), 97–111.

Hayes, S. C., Strosahl, K. D., & Wilson, K. G. (1999). *Acceptance and commitment therapy: An experiential approach to behavior change*. New York: Guilford Press.

Hayes, S. C., Wilson, K. G., Gifford, E. V., Follette, V. M., & Strosahl, K. (1996). Experiential avoidance and behavioral disorders: A functional dimensional approach to diagnosis and treatment. *Journal of Consulting and Clinical Psychology*, *64*(6), 1152–1168.

Hollon, S. D., Evans, M. D., Auerbach, A., DeRubeis, R. J., Elkin, I., Lowery, A., et al. (1987). *Development of a system for rating therapies for depression: Differentiating cognitive therapy, interpersonal psychotherapy, and clinical management pharmacotherapy*. Unpublished manuscript.

Ilardi, S. S., & Craighead, W. E. (1994). The role of nonspecific factors in cognitive-behavior therapy for depression. *Clinical Psychology: Science and Practice*, *1*(2), 138–156.

Jacobson, N. S. (1989). The therapist–client relationship in cognitive behavior therapy: Implications for treating depression. *Journal of Cognitive Psychotherapy*, *3*(2), 85–96.

Jacobson, N. S., Dobson, K. S., Truax, P. A., Addis, M. E., Koerner, K., Gollan, J. K., et al. (1996). A component analysis of cognitive behavioral treatment for depression. *Journal of Consulting and Clinical Psychology, 64,* 295–304.

Jacobson, N. S., Martell, C. R., & Dimidjian, S. (2002). Behavioral activation treatment for depression: Returning to contextual roots. *Clinical Psychology: Science and Practice, 8*(3), 255–270.

Kanter, J. W., Kohlenberg, R. J., & Loftus, E. F. (2002). Demand characteristics, treatment rationales, and cognitive therapy for depression. *Prevention and Treatment, 5,* Article 41. Available at http://journals.apa.org/prevention/volume5/pre0050041c.html

Klerman, G. L., Weissman, M. M., Rounsaville, B. J., & Chevron, E. S. (1984). *Interpersonal psychotherapy of depression.* New York: Basic Books.

Kohlenberg, R. J., Kanter, J. W., Bolling, M. Y., Parker, C., & Tsai, M. (2002). Enhancing cognitive therapy for depression with functional analytic psychotherapy: Treatment guidelines and empirical findings. *Cognitive and Behavioral Practice, 9*(3), 213–229.

Kohlenberg, R. J., & Tsai, M. (1991). *Functional analytic psychotherapy: Creating intense and curative therapeutic relationships.* New York: Plenum Press.

Kohlenberg, R. J., & Tsai, M. (1997). *Functionally enhanced cognitive therapy.* Seattle: University of Washington, FECT Treatment Project.

Kohlenberg, R. J., & Tsai, M. (2000). Radical behavioral help for Katrina. *Cognitive and Behavioral Practice, 7*(4), 500–505.

Kohlenberg, R. J., Tsai, M., & Dougher, M. J. (1993). The dimensions of clinical behavior analysis. *Behavior Analyst, 16*(2), 271–282.

Kohlenberg, R. J., Tsai, M., & Kohlenberg, B. S. (1996). Functional analysis in behavior therapy. In M. Hersen, R. M. Eisler, & P. M. Miller (Eds.), *Progress in behavior modification* (pp. 1–24). Newbury Park, CA: Sage.

Linehan, M. M. (1993). *Cognitive-behavioral treatment of borderline personality disorder.* New York: Guilford Press.

Marlatt, G. A. (2002). Buddhist philosophy and the treatment of addictive behavior. *Cognitive and Behavioral Practice, 9*(1), 44–99.

Martell, C. R., Addis, M. E., & Jacobson, N. S. (2001). *Depression in context: Strategies for guided action.* New York: Norton.

McCullough, J. P. (2000). *Treatment for chronic depression: Cognitive behavioral analysis system of psychotherapy (CBASP).* New York: Guilford Press.

Moncher, F. J., & Prinz, R. J. (1991). Treatment fidelity in outcome studies. *Clinical Psychology Review, 11,* 247–266.

Safran, J. D., & Segal, Z. V. (1990). *Interpersonal process in cognitive therapy.* New York: Basic Books.

Shaw, B. F., Elkin, I., Yamaguchi, J., Olmsted, M., Vallis, T. M., Dobson, K. S., et al. (1999). Therapist competence ratings in relation to clinical outcome in cognitive therapy of depression. *Journal of Consulting and Clinical Psychology, 67*(6), 837–846.

Skinner, B. F. (1957). *Verbal behavior.* East Norwalk, CT: Appleton–Century–Crofts.

Teasdale, J. D., Segal, Z. V., Williams, J.M. G., Ridgeway, V. A., Soulsby, J. M., & Lau, M. A. (2000). Prevention of relapse/recurrence in major depression in mindfulness-based cognitive therapy. *Journal of Consulting and Clinical Psychology, 68,* 615–623.

Young, J. E. (1990). *Cognitive therapy for personality disorders: A schema-focused approach.* Sarasota, FL: Professional Resource Exchange.

6

Values Work in Acceptance and Commitment Therapy

Setting a Course for Behavioral Treatment

Kelly G. Wilson *and* Amy R. Murrell

What is the purpose of behavior therapy? Although skills-building components inform many behavioral treatments, goals and outcome assessments typically focus on reductions in psychological complaints of one sort or another. Behavior therapy, like medicine, has taken as its task the reduction of suffering. Embedded in our choice of outcome measures is an assumption about the relationship between psychological complaints and psychological well-being. Behavior therapy, along with most of behavior health perspectives, has adopted the position that (1) psychological suffering is anomalous, and (2) psychological health is inversely related to the number and intensity of psychological complaints.

Hayes, Strosahl, and Wilson call this the "assumption of healthy normality" (1999, p. 4). According to this assumption, psychological health is the normal state of affairs and is interrupted only when some abnormal pathological condition intervenes. The behavior therapy variant of this view differs in two significant ways from the traditional medical model. First, in terms of pathogenesis, the behavior therapist is more likely to point to learning history than to biological malfunction. Second, behavior therapy has typically understood behavior problems in terms of learning processes that are not unlike the learning processes that generate normal nonpathological behavior patterns. What it shares with the traditional medical model is that well-being is the normal state of affairs. However, rather than the intrusion of some biological malfunction, infectious agent, or toxic insult, the behavior therapist posits anomalous, pathogenic learning histories. From this perspective, such learning histories generate negative thoughts, emotions, memories, bodily states, and behavioral predispositions—the behavioral equivalents of tumors, viruses, and bacteria—that must be excised in order for good psychological health to return.

SOURCES OF SUFFERING

Learning History as Pathogen

Consider the standard behavioral approach to panic disorder, in which treatment is executed at the level of person–environment interaction. While acknowledging that genetic and/or physiological factors may predispose someone to develop panic disorder, traditional state-of-the-art behavioral treatments focus on providing an individual with a new learning history that will reduce anxiety in what have been anxiety-producing contexts. Central to this new learning history is systematic exposure to feared events. The most promising new interventions include exposure to both feared external events, such as shopping malls, and feared interoceptive events, such as accelerated heart rate (e.g., Barlow, 2002; Bouton, Mineka, & Barlow, 2001). The key marker for successful therapy is that the client be panic-free for some period following treatment.

An Alternative View

An alternative to this pathology-oriented view is described by Hayes and colleagues as the "assumption of destructive normality" (1999, pp. 4–12). From this perspective, as with the traditional behavioral view, it is *normal* psychological processes that primarily lead to suffering. The behavior therapy movement has always viewed psychological problems in terms of normal learning processes, but psychological problems were argued to be the result of an anomalous learning history (e.g., Kanfer & Phillips, 1970). The alternative view argues that nonanomalous learning processes may be the primary source of suffering, or may exacerbate the effects of abnormal learning histories or primary biological pathogenesis (e.g., see Bach & Hayes, 2002).

The critical normal processes involved in this account are the learning processes underlying human language. Recent developments in the behavioral analysis of language suggest that special properties of human language generate suffering among humans over and above the suffering of nonhuman species (Hayes, Barnes-Holmes, & Roche, 2001; Wilson & Blackledge, 1998; Wilson, Hayes, Gregg, & Zettle, 2001). This perspective does not rule out the effects of abnormal processes. It simply suggests that the possession of language alone will produce suffering, and that processes underlying language will compound the suffering that results from either anomalous biological processes or anomalous learning histories.

If this is so, we ought to see psychological problems virtually everywhere we look, and indeed, the prevalence of psychological problems is staggering. The National Comorbidity Survey, for example, found that 29% of the nationally representative sample of 8,098 adults (ages 15–54) met criteria for at least one psychiatric disorder during the previous year, and 48% in their lifetime (Kessler et al., 1994). Fully 79% of those with lifetime disorders were comorbid for another DSM-III-R disorder (Kessler et al., 1994).

Language and Suffering

We assume that language evolved as a result of its survival value. There are a few methods of ensuring survival. Some creatures reproduce by the millions. Others, with smaller reproductive capacity, develop other means to serve this central evolutionary imperative. Over and above our need to reproduce, find food, and all else, we must avoid being eaten. Humans are relatively fragile creatures. We cannot tolerate cold as well as a polar bear. We are not as strong as an elephant. We are not as swift as a cheetah. Still, humans have come to dominate the planet. We have devised means to overcome many of the physical disadvantages that we have with respect to other more robust creatures. If we cannot live in an environment, we have the capacity to alter it dramatically. This success in protecting ourselves from a hostile world has made it possible for us to live in the most inhospitable places on (or even off) the planet.

Language developed as an adaptation that fulfilled a central role in protecting humans from a hostile environment. One of the extraordinary outcomes of the basic processes underlying language is that they allow humans to compare, evaluate, and respond effectively to contingencies that are small and cumulative, temporally remote, of extremely low probability, or otherwise defective, in ways that would not support effective behavior on the part of nonhuman organisms. For example, for consequences to be effective for nonhumans, they must (1) occur relatively close in time to the behavior that produced them and (2) be relatively large in magnitude. Lacking these two qualities, behavior is not altered. Even with relatively sophisticated nonhuman organisms such as primates, the negative health consequences of smoking, which are tiny, cumulative, and years away, would never overcome the short-term positive effects of tobacco, because the basic processes underlying language in humans are absent or weak (Hayes et al., 2001).

Similarly, positive events that are much delayed or small and cumulative will not reinforce the behavior of animals lacking human language. A food pellet delivered 15 minutes after a lever press will not increase the probability that a rat will press the lever again. The same is true of classical conditioning processes. In order for classical conditioning to be effective, the unconditioned stimulus must follow the neutral stimulus very closely in time. Additionally, in both operant and respondent conditioning, the order of events must be correct. In operant conditioning, the reinforcer cannot precede the response; it must follow. In respondent conditioning, the unconditioned stimulus must follow the neutral stimulus or conditioning will not occur. Exceptions do exist. For example, some animals store food for the next winter. And, in the area of classically conditioned responses, taste aversions can be conditioned even though the illness does not follow for many hours. However, these exceptions tend to involve very fixed patterns of behavior that cannot be established outside these narrow domains. The special cases appear to be determined by millions of years of evolutionary history rather than by the organization of contingencies within the lifetime of the organism.

Humans, in the most extraordinary contrast, can respond effectively to a host of contingencies that would fail to control the behavior of nonverbal organisms. Events can be made present verbally and become psychologically present as dangerous (or desirable) even though they are not apparent in the immediate environment. The ability to respond effectively to what would otherwise be an ineffective organization of contingencies is thought to be the result of relational conditioning processes (Hayes et al., 2001). Through these processes, humans avoid the verbally established event just as they would avoid the event itself, because the actual event is psychologically present in the verbal event. Take, for example, death. If we were to ask readers to think about the death of the person who they most love in the world, many would balk. We do not merely avoid death, which has genuine survival value; we also avoid thoughts about death, which has no apparent survival value. The acceptance and commitment therapy (ACT) model, to be further discussed later, labels this tendency to avoid aversive psychological events "experiential avoidance." The creators and proponents of ACT see this avoidance as a natural outcome of relational learning processes (i.e., verbal processes), and, critical to this position, a primary obstacle to effective living (Hayes, Wilson, Gifford, Follette, & Strosahl, 1996; Hayes et al., 1999; Wilson & Luciano, 2002).

LANGUAGE, PSYCHOPATHOLOGY, AND EXPERIENTIAL AVOIDANCE

A great deal of suffering emerges from persistent and uniquely human attempts to control different aspects of experience. Here, we are not speaking of events in the world, but instead the experiential precipitants of those events. Our culture teaches us that positive thoughts and feelings are desirable; negative thoughts and feelings are bad and ought to be removed, diminished, or at least minimized. We devise strategies in our schools to raise self-esteem and confidence and to encourage cheerfulness and optimism. By contrast, we work actively to reduce negative thoughts and feelings—unless they are relatively transient.

From the time we are very young, we are taught that we can and should control negative aspects of experience. Children who cower when they have to speak in front of the class are told that they have nothing to fear. The boy who cries on the soccer field is called a baby. An adult who tells a friend that he or she will always be passed over for promotion at work is told that he or she ought not think that. The supportive friend will likely try to convince the person either that it is not true now or that it will not be true forever. It is as if feeling fearful and rejected is as much the enemy as frightening and rejecting circumstances. The underlying assumption is that one must feel courageous to be courageous, and that one must believe one can succeed in order to succeed. Thus, we learn to fight not only aversive circumstances but also our own reactions to those circumstances. Furthermore, we fight not only the present circumstances but also those that occur in our imagined futures and remembered past.

Models of psychopathology also commonly assume that negative thoughts and emotions must be supplanted by positive thoughts and emotions, so that clients can move on with their lives. In traditional cognitive therapy and in rational-emotive behavior therapy, clients are taught to dispute irrational thoughts directly (Beck, Rush, Shaw, & Emery, 1979; Ellis, 1962). Some treatments focus on elimination or reductions of problematic emotional states, such as anxiety, through exposure (e.g., Barlow, Craske, Cerny, & Klosko, 1989; Borkovec et al., 1987). In the area of substance abuse, attempts are made to reduce conditioned cravings through cue exposure (Monti, Kadden, Rohsenow, & Cooney, 2002). All of these treatments appear to share the view that certain cognitions, emotions, and bodily states cause bad behavioral outcomes, and that in order to improve the behavioral outcomes, these causes must be eliminated, or at least reduced.

Paradoxical Effects of the Control of Negative Cognition and Emotion

Although it is not wholly uniform, there is a considerable amount of evidence in the experimental literature on thought suppression (see Purdon, 1999, for recent review), in the literature on coping with depression (Bruder-Mattson, & Hovanitz, 1990; DeGenova, Patton, Jurich, & MacDermid, 1994) and surviving child sexual abuse (Leitenberg, Greenwald, & Cado, 1992; Polusny

& Follette, 1995), in the literature on alcoholism (Cooper, Russell, Skinner, Frone, & Mudar, 1992; Moser & Annis, 1996), and in work on recovery from traumatic events (Foa & Riggs, 1995), that suggests that avoidant means of coping predict poorer long-term outcomes. There is also a rapidly expanding clinical literature on treatments that emphasize a focus on acceptance and valued living as an alternative to pure change-oriented treatments. Linehan (1987) has for quite some time argued theoretically and empirically for the role of acceptance in the treatment of borderline personality disorders. Christensen, Jacobson, and Babcock (1995) have pursued the implications of acceptance in the treatment of couples. Others have developed acceptance and/or mindfulness-oriented strategies in the treatment of depression relapse (Segal, Williams, & Teasdale, 2001), anxiety (Forsyth & Eifert, 1998; Roemer & Orsillo, 2002), substance abuse (Marlatt, 2002), and eating disorders (Wilson, 1996).

Experiential Avoidance and Valued Living

Experiential avoidance is not problematic in and of itself. If the experiences avoided are relatively discrete and time-limited, few or no problems may arise. So, for example, if one's daughter is out on a date and is a little late getting home, one might distract oneself by working. This distraction might moderate one's contact with worries associated with her whereabouts, the character of her boyfriend, possible car accidents, and the like. Most probably, she arrives home safe and sound that evening and the outcome is completed work. The problem arises when the avoided experiences are more or less permanent fixtures of an individual's life. If what are avoided are thoughts, memories, and bodily states related to a sexual abuse history, that history is permanent. When the source of the troubling aspects of experience is permanent, the avoidance may also be permanent—to the extent that the individual refuses to accept psychological contact with those thoughts, memories, and bodily states. Lack of acceptance can also be detrimental when the experiences avoided are likely to occur in the pursuit of some value. So, for example, if the sexual abuse survivor is *wholly* committed to avoiding distressing thoughts, emotions, and memories connected to the abuse, he or she may act in the service of the reduction of these aversive aspects of experience at the expense of rich intimate interactions.

Management of aversive private events can become a sort of occupation. It is not a pleasant occupation, but like a lot of not-so-pleasant occupations, people may comfort themselves with the thought that once the job is done, they will be able to do what they *really* want to do in their lives. In this way, lives are put on hold in the service of managing thoughts and emotions. And, a life that is lived outside a person's most closely held values feels lousy.

PURPOSES OF TREATMENT IN ACCEPTANCE
AND COMMITMENT THERAPY

From an ACT perspective, negative cognition and emotion may, but need not, produce bad behavioral outcomes. ACT adopts a somewhat different focus than has been traditional in the behavior therapy movement. Because we believe that suffering is a natural by-product of language, we see the removal of suffering as futile. Complete removal of suffering would only be possible by the removal of language (in addition to the nonlanguage sources of suffering), and that is impossible. So instead, ACT is aimed at finding a way to accept the dark side of language processes, even while taking advantage of what language has to offer us. The core ACT goal, in the most abstract sense, is to help a client live a rich and meaningful life, while accepting the suffering that surely comes to all of us. Of course, few therapeutic schools or individual therapists would claim otherwise, but how to approach that goal might be very different depending on the specifics of the underlying theory.

From the pathology-oriented perspective just described, removal of pathology frees individuals to pursue whatever life direction they might take. From an ACT perspective, psychological suffering is not anomalous. It is normal and pervasive. The struggle to remove psychological adversity fixes, and intensifies, that adversity in an individual's experience. Even more importantly, it is a struggle that interferes with a life lived persistently in the pursuit of one's values. ACT is aimed squarely at helping clients to relinquish this struggle in order to live a life in pursuit of their most deeply held values.

VALUES-DIRECTED BEHAVIOR THERAPY

Behavior therapy has made extraordinary progress over the past 40 years. In what follows, we examine two mainstay behavior therapy interventions. We discuss underlying mechanisms of change, and finally, we describe the ways in which these interventions can be refined and directed by the addition of a strong, systematic values orientation.

Exposure Procedures in Behavior Therapy

Our largest effect sizes in behavior therapy can be found among treatments that use exposure-based interventions for anxiety disorders. These interventions are an excellent example of the translation research that defined the development of the early behavior therapy movement (Wilson, 1997). Early on in the behavior therapy movement, we asked whether our knowledge base on conditioned fear and avoidance in the laboratory could be applied to clinical cases of fear and avoidance. The answer has been an unmitigated "yes." Although some fear and avoidance has been refractory, exposure-based procedures have revolutionized the treatment of anxiety disorders. Simple phobias, for example, can be treated successfully in less than a day (Öst, 1985). We believe that the applicability of exposure-based procedures may be even broader if we expand our understanding of the nature of conditioning and extinction and the ways that respondent and operant contingencies interact.

What Occurs in Exposure-Based Treatment?

Assessment of the efficacy of exposure-based treatments has been influenced by the laboratory preparations from which these procedures were derived. Laboratory studies on classical conditioning and extinction require readily accessible dependent measures in order to know whether conditioning has occurred, or in an extinction preparation, whether the effects of conditioning have been extinguished. Heightened autonomic arousal and avoidance are readily assessed dependent measures that change reliably in aversive conditioning procedures. In the clinic, we use actual avoidance (e.g., behavioral approach tasks) and proxies for avoidance (e.g., questionnaires about avoidance), and direct or proxy measures of autonomic arousal to gauge the severity of the anxiety disorder, or alternatively, as a measure of treatment efficacy.

It is unquestionable that aversive conditioning increases avoidance and autonomic arousal, and that extinction procedures reduce them. However, these two effects do not exhaust the effects of aversive conditioning. Conditioned aversives have effects on operant behavior that go beyond avoidance and have implications for psychological problems. We know from the basic behavioral science literature that when conditioned aversives are superimposed on a free operant baseline, we will see *conditioned suppression* of operant responding. This occurs even though the operant behavior that is suppressed has no connection to the production of the conditioned aversive stimulus. For example, Geller (1960) established key pecking in a pigeon under a variable interval schedule. He then superimposed a tone that lasted 3 minutes, followed by an electric shock. Over a series of trials, the pigeon's key pecks were entirely suppressed during the period in which the tone was sounding, even though key pecking had no effect on either the tone or the subsequent shock.

In short, aversive conditioning has three primary effects on behavior that are of interest for understanding psychopathology: (1) It produces conditioned elicitation (i.e., arousal, tension); (2) it increases behaviors that terminate the aversive stimulus (i.e., avoidance and escape); and (3) it suppresses other operant responding, except those operant responses that terminate the aversive stimulus (conditioned suppression). Taken together, aversive stimuli, including *conditioned* aversives, generate a sharp narrowing of behavioral response patterns. In the presence of aversives, or events correlated with aversives, organisms become physically ready to act, and their voluntary behavior narrows to responses that terminate the threat.

Consider an example in nature that demonstrates the evolutionarily sensible advantage afforded by this response to aversive events and their correlates. If a rabbit were to see a lion on the savannah, it would not be advantageous, from a survival perspective, for the rabbit to continue foraging or to notice the flowers and other features of the landscape. The evolutionary advantage would go to the rabbit that had an immediate and narrow pattern of response—that is, the rabbit that showed high autonomic arousal, the immediate suppression of less critical behaviors (conditioned suppression), and rapid movement to its hidey-hole (avoidance). Likewise, if some sound or smell reliably preceded the appearance of the lion, the adaptive advantage would go to the rabbits that showed the same pattern of behavior with respect to the sound or smell as they showed to the actual lion. It is important to emphasize that these correlated events need to occur both close together in time and in a particular order. Events that follow the presence of the lion do not take on the threatening psychological functions of the lion. If backward conditioning were robust, the hidey-hole might take on the functions of the lion, causing the rabbit to run from the hidey-hole. To the contrary, the hidey-hole precedes the removal of threat and so takes on those safety functions.

In the world outside human language, this is a pretty neat evolutionary trick. Unfortunately, the emergence of language, which has provided many adaptive advantages, also has a dark side. The dark side of language is that through relational conditioning processes, events can come to have aversive properties even without the close temporal pairing that is necessary for all of the other creatures of the earth. As described in the earlier section on experiential avoidance, we humans avoid not only that which is dangerous but also anything that is conditioned relationally to events that are dangerous. If you were an early, language-capable hominid, for example, another hominid might say to you after an aborted attack by a lion, "That was a lion." Because of the special properties of relational conditioning (Hayes et al., 2001; Wilson & Blackledge, 1998; Wilson et al., 2001) the word *lion* would take on some of the threatening psychological functions of the lion, even though it occurred far beyond the temporal bounds necessary for good classical conditioning, and even though the word *lion* followed rather than preceded the presence of the actual lion. Now if you heard someone say the word *lion*, you might become aroused, stop what you are doing (conditioned suppression), and run to a safe place (avoidance). This is all to the good if it helps us avoid lions, but what happens when the thing we avoid is not some external event, such as a lion, but instead an aspect of experience, such as a disturbing memory, thought, or emotion?

The upshot of this relational conditioning process is that humans have the capacity to develop narrow and inflexible patterns of behavior with respect to many, many events, including many of the contents of our own conscious experience. We are quite clear, as behavior therapists, about what to do when some external event generates these narrow and inflexible patterns of behavior: We do exposure. We are somewhat less clear when the events generating these patterns are aspects of our own experience. When a thought of failure is the event that generates a narrow and inflexible pattern of behavior, we often work to refute the thought. Why? It does little good to refute fears about phobic objects. In fact, the DSM requires there to be some insight into the excessiveness of the fears in order to qualify as a phobia rather than as a delusion. When someone is fearful of an object, the best treatment is to get them interacting with the feared object in a variety of ways (except ways of interacting that involve avoidance or escape). We do not simply ask the snake phobic to peer at the snake. We ask him or her to approach the snake, to notice the colors of the snake, to observe the way it moves, and to touch the snake. In other words, we attempt to establish a broad and flexible repertoire with respect to the snake. Why would we not use exactly the same procedures with thoughts, memories, bodily states, emotions, and other aspects of experience? Bouton and colleagues (2001) have noted the inconsistency in treating personal experiences, such as thoughts, by attempting to refute them. Their view that panic disorder, for example, is the result of conditioned anxiety to both interoceptive and exteroceptive cues, allows for a broadened use of exposure. In fact, the single most significant addition of Barlow's treatment of panic has probably been the systematic application of exposure procedures to interoceptive cues (Barlow, 2002; Bouton et al., 2001).

This perspective on aversive conditioning suggests that the primary problem with conditioned aversives is not that the individual avoids or becomes aroused. The problem is that they *only* become aroused and avoid. We do not want the snake phobic to become incapable of arousal and avoidance; sometimes these are just the right responses. What we seek is a broad and flexible repertoire with respect to snakes. Using the snake phobia example, we can think of the difference between pre- and postexposure as a change in a population of potential responses. Preexposure, the individual has a very narrow, high probability set of responses (see Figure 6.1). Almost regardless of context, the snake phobic has a 100% probability of becoming alarmed and acting to minimize contact with the snake. Postexposure, the snake phobic shows a broad and flexible repertoire (Figure 6.2). With the postexposure repertoire, whether, for example, the phobic stopped to look in the window of a pet store would be controlled not *merely* by the presence or absence of snakes, but by contextual factors such as available time, whether he or she was with a friend interested in snakes, whether there were colorful examples of snakes displayed, and any of myriad contextual features of this kind.

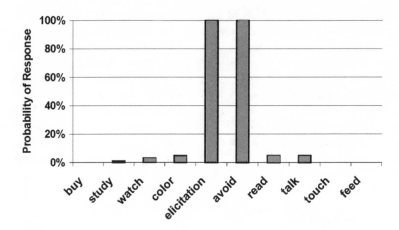

FIGURE 6.1. Preexposure, the snake phobic shows a narrow set of responses, with a near 100% probability of occurrence.

Implications for Treatment

Taking this view of exposure, we might intervene when an event, either external or internal, generates a narrow and inflexible pattern of behavior. The purpose of the intervention is not merely to lessen arousal and avoidance, but instead to build a broad and flexible repertoire with respect to the

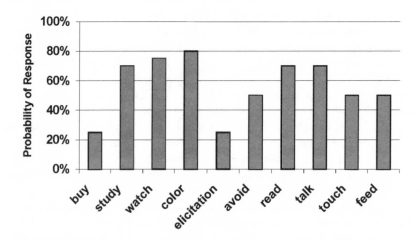

FIGURE 6.2. Postexposure, the snake phobic shows a broad and flexible set of responses. The breadth of potential responses allows for other features of context to exert control over the actual response emitted.

avoided event. Although elicitation and avoidance will generally be reduced given such treatment, these reductions are not the goal of the treatment. At a practical level, it means that anything we do with avoided events that is not avoidance behavior is good, in that it broadens the individual's repertoire. Our negative thoughts, memories, bodily states, and emotions are calls to action. When they arise, we have a characteristic pattern of response with respect to them. Whatever the pattern observed, our concern as clinicians is not so much with its form as with its fixedness. Exposure procedures are aimed at making these patterns of behavior broad and flexible.

Acceptance, Mindfulness, Cognitive Defusion, and Their Relation to Exposure

When thoughts are responded to in terms of their literal content, we term this *cognitive fusion*. Interventions that attenuate the relationally conditioned functions of thoughts can be considered defusion strategies. Cognitive defusion can be considered a special case of exposure. The language of classical conditioning and extinction, from which exposure-based treatments were derived, is adequate in the analysis of directly conditioned aversive stimuli. Cognitive defusion, by contrast, refers to procedures that broaden repertoires with respect to stimuli that have acquired their psychological functions through relational (or verbal) processes.

Exposure, or defusion in the case of relationally conditioned stimuli, means psychological exposure, not mere physical exposure. Humans have a plethora of means to avoid, even when the events are "right there in front of them." For exposure to have its optimal effect, clients must put themselves in intimate psychological contact with the event in question. Coaching an open and accepting posture with respect to aversive psychological content facilitates the process of exposure. Similarly, teaching mindfulness with respect to disturbing psychological content can bring a client into contact with disturbing material in a new way. From this perspective, acceptance and mindfulness can be seen as activities that violate the narrowness of the avoidant repertoire. Considered as a type of defusion strategy, being mindful is not part of the narrow pattern of responses that are typical with respect to thoughts and feelings, especially not aversive thoughts and feelings. Kabat-Zinn, for example, states that mindfulness involves "paying attention in a particular way: on purpose, in the present moment, non-judgmentally" (1995, p. 4). Two things occur when we can shape such a response. First, the client's repertoire has broadened. This is a new pattern of behavior with respect to his or her thoughts. Second, the client has the direct experience (not merely the insight) that broadening is possible. The latter is probably the most critical feature of the defusion experience.

BEHAVIORAL ACTIVATION

Behavioral activation is likewise an old and venerable weapon in the behavior therapy armamentarium. Like exposure-based procedures, it represents a translation from laboratory science to clinical science.

The Reinforcement Deprivation Hypothesis

We can readily generate something that looks like depression in a laboratory animal. If an organism is in an environment that is free from threat, rich in sources of food, water, and opportunities to explore and exercise, it will be quite active in the environment. If opportunities for positive reinforcement are systematically stripped from the environment, the animal will initially explore the available space, foraging for food, water, and other necessities. Perhaps it will attempt to escape, if possible. Eventually, however, the animal will greatly reduce its activities. In a manner of speaking, it waits for something in the environment to change. Again, this can be seen as an evolutionarily sensible response to a very impoverished environment. Pervasive threat has the same effects.

Consider, for example, the series of experiments carried out to produce what has been termed "learned helplessness" (Seligman & Maier, 1967; see Miller & Norman, 1979, for review). When animals are subjected to uncontrolled aversive conditions, they initially attempt to escape. However, over time, these operant responses extinguish, because they do not eliminate the aversive events. Again, this is a sensible response from an evolutionary perspective. The evolutionary imperative to survive suggests that energy be conserved for a time when action might make a difference. Until there is a change in context, activity is wasteful of resources (Ferster, 1973). As with aversive conditioning, described earlier, such conditions produce narrow and inflexible patterns of behavior. Rats in Seligman's work, for example, did not attempt to escape even when escape became possible (Seligman & Beagley, 1975). In order to change this state of affairs, something in the psychologically present environment of the organism must change. This can be brought about either by a perceptible change in the environment or by compelling the organism to produce the behavior that terminates the aversive event (e.g., Seligman, Maier, & Geer, 1968).

The necessary change in the environment is much more complex for humans. Humans may have a seemingly safe and rich environment—one that it is free from physical threat and is full of food, water, and opportunity—and still suffer. In our world, unlike that of the rat, these primary reinforcers are not enough. Verbal relations can lead to a deprivation of a different sort. For example, humans may experience an apparently rich environment as one in which they lack a sense of adequacy, or in which their suffering has no meaning. These deprivations are not eliminated when physical needs are met, or with material wealth. There are people who seem to have every-thing who can barely live through one day—and there are those who choose not to. Something very powerful must become psychologically pres-ent in order for a human to become active under these conditions.

Early Clinical Application of the Reinforcement Deprivation Hypothesis

Intervention strategies have been developed that capitalized on the relation-ship between depressive symptomatology and availability of positive rein-forcement. Lewinsohn, Sullivan, and Grosscup (1980) applied this perspec-tive by collecting a list of potentially pleasant activities. They focused treatment on increasing the frequency and variety of pleasant events in the depressed person's life. Increases in activity do appear to make a difference in depression, and some recent studies suggest that behavioral activation may be a critical, if not the most important, component in cognitive ther-apy for depression (Jacobson et al., 2000; Martell, Addis, & Jacobson, 2001).

APPLYING EXPOSURE, DEFUSION, AND BEHAVIORAL ACTIVATION

Given these behavioral technologies, we now focus on two problems that can be addressed by values-centered interventions. First, what will the tar-gets of these interventions be? What activities will we seek to increase? What events will we target with our exposure and defusion strategies? The second problem relates to issues of motivation; that is, having selected tar-gets for exposure, defusion, and activation, how will we motivate our cli-ents to expose themselves to difficult psychological material? How will we motivate them to increase their activity? Mindfulness and acceptance will be our natural allies as we pursue valued activities and, in the process, en-counter difficult psychological material.

Therapy and Its Targets

We do not apply exposure to just any conditioned aversion. For example, we have a conditioned aversion to images of swastikas (probably relational conditioning, since we have no direct conditioning history with respect to swastikas), but there is no reason to defuse this conditioned aversion. Simi-larly, with regard to behavioral activation, pleasantness alone is inadequate to direct activation, since many activities are pleasing but entirely incom-patible with what anyone would consider "the good life." Persistent drug use might, for example, be pleasant *and* incompatible with important valued activities. Although pleasant and valued activities may overlap, we are careful in ACT about the propensity to seek pleasantness and avoid pain. We pursue values and take our pleasure when it occurs along the way. Values can provide us with the targets for exposure and guide the choice of what activities to pursue in behavioral activation.

Therapy and Motivation

Having selected targets for exposure, defusion, and behavioral activation, how do we get our clients to participate? It is no surprise to clients with obsessive–compulsive disorder that they need to touch the doorknob and stop washing their hands. Likewise, it is not news to the person who is depressed that he or she needs to get out of bed and meet the world. However, why would these individuals engage in treatment that promises to provide benefits later, instead of engaging in behavior that provides some relief immediately? Exposure-based procedures are quite aversive. The client may do them so that anxiety *eventually* goes down. However, terminating treatment will make anxiety go down immediately. Likewise, for the depressive, the comfort of sleep provides immediate respite from ongoing thoughts of hopelessness and despair. Not only do we need to provide motivation for treatment but we also need this motivating factor to be more substantial than the motivation provided by ongoing participation in fixed patterns of behavior that provide a modicum of immediate relief.

VALUES-CENTERED BEHAVIOR THERAPY

Client values can provide both direction and motivation for the hard work of treatment and may thus offer solutions to the issues raised earlier. *From an ACT perspective, exposure and defusion are done when there is any event that generates narrow and inflexible patterns of behavior, and, when these inflexibilities are obstacles to our clients moving actively in the direction of a chosen value.* Values interventions direct therapy by targeting exposure and defusion events that function as barriers to valued living. Likewise, the dimension that directs behavioral activation is not pleasantness, but is instead deeply held personal values. This perspective generates what might be thought of as "valued-events scheduling," in contrast to the pleasant-events scheduling in earlier forms of behavior therapy (cf. Martell et al., 2001).

When obstacles prevent movement in a valued domain, we target those obstacles with exposure and defusion strategies aimed at building a broad and flexible repertoire with respect to them (including both external and internal psychological obstacles). If events that "must be avoided" can be transformed though exposure and defusion into events with which clients have behavioral flexibility, new options open up for clients. Consider the example of the sexual abuse survivor who has high elicitation and avoidance with respect to memories of her abuse history. If a memory arises during an intimate interaction with a partner, she becomes anxious. Her attention narrows to the memory. Other behaviors are suppressed, including her intimate interactions with her partner, and avoidant repertoires are activated. If she were to develop greater flexibility with respect to these memories, her ability to interact effectively in intimate contexts would be increased.

Thus, from this perspective, decisions about the targets for exposure, defusion, and behavioral activation are determined by a close examination of this fundamental question: "In a world where you could choose to have your life be about something, what would you choose?" In what follows, we examine the ways we have implemented asking this question in the context of psychotherapy. ACT is an evolving treatment technology (Hayes et al., 1999), and we are not sure whether this approach to values-directed treatment is "right." Data will ultimately tell the story. Although we do not know the end point of the development of values intervention technology, we offer this as one potential starting point.

VALUES ASSESSMENT

Systematic reinforcer preference procedures are often used in interventions with developmentally disabled individuals and with children who have behavior problems (Fox, Rotatori, Macklin, & Green, 1983; Northup, 2000; Tighe & Tighe, 1969), but less commonly in other populations. These efforts have largely focused on the identification of relatively discrete reinforcers for use in relatively tightly controlled environments. Although there have been some efforts to assess reinforcers for other populations, they have typically involved the development of reinforcer surveys (e.g., Houlihan, Rodriguez, & Levine, 1990). When direct reinforcement-based technologies have been used among outpatient adults, such as in the treatment of substance abuse, they have still focused on relatively discrete reinforcers that are provided for relatively discreet behaviors, such as using monetary rewards for clean urinalyses among substance abusers (e.g., Higgins, Wong, & Badger, 2000). However, for most adults, the most powerful values in our lives are not discrete reinforcers. We like $100 bills, but if we were asked about the relative value of a $100 bill as compared to, say, a rich relationship with our children, money becomes relatively unimportant. There is no good science that tells us precisely how, in behavior therapy, we can assess the relative importance of these valued domains and harness them fully to our treatments. Our own work in this area is just beginning, but it provides an example of a possible direction.

Values Assessment: The Valued-Living Questionnaire

We have developed a short instrument called the Valued-Living Question-naire (VLQ; Wilson & Groom, 2002) that taps into 10 domains that are often identified as valued domains of living. Clients are asked to rate, on a scale of 1–10, the importance of the 10 domains, including (1) family (other than parenting and intimate relations), (2) marriage/couples/intimate relations, (3) parenting, (4) friendship, (5) work, (6) education, (7) recreation, (8) spirituality, (9) citizenship, and (10) physical self-care. We make considerable effort in the instructions to remove conventional constraints on answering, by emphasizing that not everyone values all of these domains, and that some areas may be more important, or important in different ways at different times in an individual's life. On the second page of the assessment, we ask clients to estimate, using the same 1–10 rating scale, how consistently they have lived in accord with those values over the past week. The instrument has shown good test–retest reliability (Groom & Wilson, 2003), and we are currently collecting validity data. Regardless of the merit of this instrument in terms of its psychometric properties, it provides a systematic means to approach values interventions, and so remains a sensible clinical tool.

Introducing the VLQ in Treatment

Because clients typically come to therapy with "a problem" such as depression or anxiety, they can sometimes be perplexed by our interest in the importance they place on these different valued domains. We explain to clients that the perspective we work from seeks to understand people's difficulties in the context of a whole 'life. Sometimes problems become so overwhelming that it is easy to lose contact with the "big picture." We do want to know how the client has struggled, but we seek an understanding of that struggle in the context of a whole person with hopes, desires, and aspirations. Our experience has been that clients find this aspect of treatment useful and important (Dahl, Wilson, & Nillson, in press; Greco, 2002; Heffner, Sperry, Eifert, & Detweiler, 2002; Orsillo, Roemer, Block, LeJeune, & Herbert, in press).

Examining VLQ Scores

We seek out domains of living in which the client feels a loss of freedom to act, and where that loss of freedom generates suffering. Our general strategy involves the two major components discussed in the previous section: behavioral activation and exposure (along with special cases of exposure, such as defusion and mindfulness). First, we look for valued activities in these domains for valued-events scheduling—values-directed behavioral activation. Second, we look for obstacles to increasing valued activity and target those with exposure and defusion strategies. Below are some profiles that we have observed clinically and that seem like fruitful ground for values discussions with our clients, as well as for theoretical analyses. The reader should keep in mind that these profiles may or may not underlie clinically relevant clusters. The therapist should assume a mindful posture with respect to interpreting profiles prior to interaction with the client.

Clinically and Theoretically Interesting Profiles

High Discrepancy between Rated Importance and Rated Consistency

Theoretically, this should be correlated with a lot of distress and what we think of as core pathological functioning from an ACT perspective. We view these discrepancies as an important source of distress that could be altered by increased engagement in discrepant domains. We have found clinically that clients experience these discrepancies as very disturbing. They tend to be associated with a great deal of negative self-evaluation, guilt, sadness, and anxiety. In the examination of these discrepant domains, it can be very difficult for our clients even to speak about them. If the client is sufficiently immobilized, even by the thought of activity in these discrepant domains, we have discovered a target for exposure and defusion exercises. We could move directly to advocating activity; but often exposure and defusion can generate more flexibility and a greater probability of successful engagement in the proposed activities.

Extreme High Total Importance and Consistency Scores

This appears to be pretty common, but bears examination. Such endorsement may be related to excessive concerns about social acceptance. If social acceptance is the central value directing a client's life, he or she will be likely to find it in conflict with other values. When we encounter extraordinary concerns about social acceptability, we may do exposure and defusion exercises around both instances in the client's history in which he or she experienced disapproval and also imagined future disapproval. We do so in order to help the client have a broader and more flexible repertoire with respect to thoughts about disapproval, as well as actual disapproval. We have also found clinically that these ratings change upon greater scrutiny. Sometimes clients answer these questions with little careful thought about the domain of interest. This does not necessarily involve deceit. The phenomenon appears to be more akin to an answer of "fine" when we ask people how they are doing. In the process of inquiring about the particular things valued within these domains, we have found that "fine" sometimes changes to something a bit less than fine. Problems can also be revealed by discussion of symptoms. When depressed clients talk about the costs of depression within their family, a high rating on consistency may drop.

Extreme Low Total Importance Score

We have seen this profile in a several client groups with whom we have worked. Among public health workers treated for chronic pain, we have found very low importance scores that upon examination reflected adaptation to the perceived impossibility of obtaining anything worthwhile within the domain (Dahl et al., in press). For example, in the area of education, when asked about low importance scores, some of the clients scoffed at being smart enough to pursue anything educational. Note that "not smart enough" is unrelated to how one experiences the importance of the domain. (Whether it is possible is a different question, and one that we will explore. Here, we are just looking for importance.) Some of these individuals valued this domain quite highly. "Not caring" was a way to distance themselves from disturbing thoughts about past and potential future disappointments. We have also seen this among some college and high school students at risk for academic failure (Ely & Wilson, 2003). Again, we assess for thoughts, memories, emotions, and other aspects of experience that the client experiences as barriers to moving forward in a given domain.

INTERVENING WITH MATERIAL FROM THE VALUES ASSESSMENT

Having collected the client's VLQ ratings, we examine them in detail. We want to understand the client's stake in the valued domain, whether across areas or in a single area. The intervention involves two key components. First, we want a deep sense of what it would mean to clients to make a difference in the selected domain. Second, we want clients to experience a personal commitment from the therapist to understand what they feel within that domain and to work with them to make a difference in that area of their life. The goal may not be completely achievable, but the aspiration should be made clear to the client.

What we are seeking is a client value that can inspire both the therapist and the client. Consider a case in which a woman presents for treatment for panic disorder with agoraphobia. Using the VLQ, we find a large discrepancy in rated importance and rated consistency in the domain of parenting. We find among the precipitants for treatment the fact that the woman's daughter will soon graduate from high school. Because the commencement is to be held in a large auditorium, the woman fears she will not be able to attend. We elicit from the woman other such events that she has missed in the past and that she fears missing in the future. We look for thoughts, memories, and emotions related to her role as a mother. If these topics are difficult, they become targets for exposure and defusion.

When flexibility increases, we press forward. When we are able to connect with the client around the central value, we repeat it to the client:

> "I can see how meaningful it would be to you to participate fully in your daughter's life. I can see how much it would mean to her and to you to really be there—not off in your head, checking your pulse, and monitoring the exit routes—but really *there*, with her at that moment she walks across the stage to get her diploma. What if our work here could be about making that possible?"

It may also be useful, in order to focus the treatment, to contrast this with a panic control agenda. To do so, we can ask the client to imagine that the therapist is able to offer two choices:

THERAPIST: I want to be sure that treatment connects to what you care about most. So, imagine I could offer you two choices. In this hand, I offer a guarantee of no panic attacks. And I mean none, never, ever. In order to get this, however, you have to give something up. You have to give up any meaningful relationship with your daughter. She graduates, moves away, and that is the end of it. You never really connect again. I am offering you another choice in this hand though. With this choice, you get to have an extraordinary, rich relationship with your daughter. You are there for this and many, many other important times: college, marriage, grandchildren—a lifetime of connection. But again, there is a cost: With this choice, you continue to have panic attacks but they do not stop you from doing any of the things you want to do. Which would you choose?

CLIENT: I don't like this. Can't I have both—I mean no panic and the relationship?

THERAPIST: Let me be clear. I am not saying that I can promise you either. I do not know the future. I am just asking you to *imagine* that I can absolutely guarantee either one or the other, but not both.

CLIENT: But I don't like it. I don't like the choice. I don't think I could do it.

THERAPIST: Yes, of course. I don't know anyone who has ever had a panic attack who likes them. There is not much there to be liked. And be clear that I am absolutely not asking whether you *can* do it. That is another issue, and we will cross that bridge when we come to it. I am only asking one thing: In a world where it was possible for you to make this choice and follow through, would you choose it?

CLIENT: OK. Well, I'd choose my daughter. But I *really* don't think I can do it.

THERAPIST: Yes, I get that you really think that, and it is absolutely OK to think that. In fact, I cannot imagine you would think anything else. There are a couple things that I can guarantee you. I guarantee that therapy will be difficult, but that we will not do anything difficult that does not connect directly to what you hold most dear in life. I hear how much your daughter means to you. To be willing to have panic in order to be there for your daughter inspires me. I want you to know that if you agree to this work, I will devote myself to working toward the realization of that value. So, if therapy could be about moving toward that relationship, would you be willing to have therapy be about that?

CLIENT: Yes, but I don't see how that can happen unless the panic attacks stop.

THERAPIST: Sure, and I am not asking you to take this on faith. Give me a period of time, and we will stop and evaluate how things are going. You will look at your own experience and tell me if it feels as though therapy is moving you in a direction that resonates with your deepest desires.

This intervention would be likely to occur within the first session or two. Although the interventions emerging from this session may focus on exposure, defusion, or behavioral activation, the seeds of the therapeutic contract have been planted in this short conversation.

Values and the Therapeutic Contract

ACT is a client-centered treatment in the sense that it is the client's values that direct the therapy. A solid therapeutic contract is consistent with such an approach. Clients should never feel that the treatment is being done to them. Equally, the therapist should never feel that he or she is doing something to the client. Exposure is often difficult for therapists, as well as clients. It is painful to see clients suffering while participating in work that the therapist asks them to do. Exposure in the context of values gives both the client and the therapist something meaningful to dignify the suffering that treatment produces.

Theoretically, it should make a difference that doing painful therapeutic work is explicitly chosen by the client. Data tell us that people prefer aversives that they control over aversives that they do not control (e.g., Zvolensky, Lejeuz, & Eifert, 1998). Animal studies have also demonstrated less activation of endogenous analgesia, less self-administered drug consumption, less fear, and less perseveration when painful events are controllable compared to when they are not controllable (Anisman, Hahn, Hoffman, & Zacharo, 1985; Anisman & Waller, 1974; Drugan, Ader, & Maier, 1985; Warren & Rosellini, 1988). Taken together, the basic behavioral science evidence suggests that we should make the client's choosing as salient as possible. In the therapeutic contract we are advocating here, the difficulty of treatment is made explicit. However, the adversity the therapist predicts is placed squarely in the context of what the client wants in life, and in so doing, there is a smaller chance that the client will feel victimized by the therapist when the treatment becomes painful. Nietzsche said that a person could stand almost any "how" if they have a "why." The why for the hard work that will follow is supplied by the client's own values and the control that derives from an uncoerced agreement to proceed.

Values, Motivation, and the Hard Work of Treatment

If you went to a dentist with a bad tooth, and the dentist looked around in your mouth, poked, prodded, and scraped, but only touched teeth that were healthy, the appointment would be painless but not particularly useful. Although the dentist may have kept you comfortable, if you paid the dentist for that appointment, your money was stolen, and you walk away with the same troublesome tooth. We use metaphors such as this to illustrate to clients the point that pain can be inherent in addressing problems. We do not undersell it. If it turns out to be less painful, no one will complain. But if it turns out to be very painful, which it may well be, clients should know at the outset. This should be part of the contract the client has made with the therapist. When the treatment gets painful we ask: "If this pain was between you and the life you want, would you be willing?"

Although there are phases of treatment in which the exploration of values is the focus of treatment, they ought to be touched upon in every session, even if only to remind the client of the valued domain being pursued. If the client's values are obscured by years of struggle with anxiety, depression, alcoholism, or the like, the therapist can still suggest that the therapy will be about revealing this obscured personal sense of life direction. Therapists should not allow clients to leave the session without it being entirely clear: The treatment is about them and a life they value.

Valued-Events Scheduling

In its simplest form, work with material generated by the VLQ might look like behavioral activation with deeply held personal values as the guiding force. Depending on the nature and intended duration of treatment, the scope of valued-events scheduling might be narrow or broad. In the domain of parenting, for example, as described with the agoraphobic case earlier, we might generate a list of activities that are consistent with the stated value. We might explore what depressed clients have been doing in their interactions with their children. Have they been withdrawn, disengaged, or unavailable? What have they not done that they would do, if only they were not anxious? How does it feel to be psychologically absent? What would it mean to the aforementioned client and to her daughter for her to be really present? As we examine these sorts of questions, we look for areas where clients' experiences are restricted—where they do not feel free to live their values fully. If obstacles emerge, such as "This is too painful" or "I just can't do it," we target those negative thoughts and emotions with acceptance, exposure, and defusion exercises. If clients cannot accept these thoughts *and* act effectively in their lives, initiating values-driven commitments will be impossible.

Values-Centered Exposure, Defusion, and Mindfulness

We have sometimes had difficulty getting clients fully engaged in the values work. In previous descriptions of this treatment (Hayes et al., 1999), we have given written assignments to clients, asking them to discuss their personal values. The problem we sometimes see with this approach is that when addressed directly, clients will produce a relatively lean, conventional endorsement of valued domains. In the area of parenting, for example, who does not want a rich relationship with their children? In order to help the client connect with these values in the context of avoided fearful thoughts and memories, we have devised some therapy sessions that incorporate experiential exercises and emotionally expressive writing as a bridge to discussion of valued ends that will ultimately direct the treatment. The sessions involve exposure, defusion, and mindfulness, all centered on creating more flexibility in a valued domain of living. Below is a session strategy constructed for use with the agoraphobic client described earlier, but it could be readily adapted to other client difficulties.

One of the obstacles expressed by this client upon initiation of the therapeutic contract was her certainty that she would not be willing to experience panic. The words "I can't do this!" occurred as a formidable psychological obstacle to making and keeping commitments to her daughter. In responding literally to the thought that she cannot tolerate panic, she must do what is necessary to avoid panic. To intervene, we chose an event from the client's history that was reminiscent of the upcoming graduation—a missed dance recital. We told the client that we were going to walk her through the missed recital in great detail. If the client balks at a similar exercise, we might ask, "If this exercise could make a difference for you and your daughter, could you be willing to do it? If this exercise could put you in that auditorium, completely present for that graduation, would you be willing?" Prior to the exercise, we gathered detailed information about the phenomenology of panic attacks for this woman—how they begin, thoughts that occur, and any other details that can enhance the exercise.

The form of this exercise is quite flexible. The function is to do exposure, acceptance, defusion, and mindfulness with respect to difficult and avoided psychological material, such as fears about the future and regrets about the past. Mindfulness and acceptance are used in the initial stages of the exercise in order to facilitate the exposure and defusion that occur later in the exercise. The purpose of this work is to generate sufficient flexibility to engage in more challenging *and* more personally meaningful activities. We begin the exercise by asking clients to sit upright, with their legs and arms uncrossed and their feet flat on the ground. This posture tends to remain reasonably comfortable and makes interference from the need to adjust positions less likely. The exercise is delivered in a slow, deliberate, and somewhat sedate tone of voice, with plenty of pauses. Eventually, the client is asked to imagine certain details of the experience. The following description offers a brief example:

> "I want you to notice the sound of my voice. I would like you to follow my instructions. If you find yourself drifting off, thinking of other things, or distracted in any other way, simply return to the sound of my voice. First, I want you to notice the different sounds you can hear around you. [Here, the therapist should pause and listen intently, then slowly catalogue the various sounds heard.] Perhaps you hear voices from other offices around us. Listen to the faint hum of the air-conditioning. As you draw your attention inward, see if you can picture the room around you. Try to picture where the chairs are, the carpet, the door. See what else you can notice as you imagine looking around the room. Drawing your attention further inward, notice the position of your body; notice the feel of your clothing, where it touches your skin. See if you can notice slight differences in the temperature of your skin in different places on your body. Notice your breathing. Notice the temperature of your breath. . . . Notice that it is warmer as you exhale and cooler as you inhale. Now take three very slow deep breaths and try to picture the path of the air as it enters and leaves your body. If you notice any tension anywhere in your body, imagine that each breath carries a bit of that tension away.
>
> "Now I want you to picture yourself on the night before your daughter's dance recital. You are in a room with your daughter. You are telling your daughter that you are very proud of her and that you will be there. I want you to picture her face as you say this. I want you to imagine allowing yourself to slip into the skin of the woman in this image—talking to her daughter. Notice the look on her face as you speak these words. 'I am proud and I will be there.' Notice things you feel, what you are thinking. Now I want you to imagine that you are at the dance studio on the night of the recital. Your daughter has already gone into the building. Look around and notice who else is there—other parents, dressed up, carrying cameras. As you move to-

ward the entrance, you notice your heart begin to beat more rapidly. It feels as though your temperature is beginning to rise. Notice the feeling of perspiration under your arms. You have a pretty good idea what is coming, but still . . . let yourself feel the weight of it. Imagine that you decide that you will not go in. Notice how sick you feel as you make that decision. Let yourself imagine your daughter's face as she scans the crowd looking for you. As you walk back to your car and sit down, let yourself notice how your body feels. Let yourself notice any emotions you are experiencing. Let yourself notice memories. Perhaps you remember other times that were like this. Let yourself notice any thoughts you are having.

"Now allow yourself to imagine that you are at home. Your daughter is there, and you tell her that you just couldn't stay. Picture the face of your daughter as you say this. Can you see the pain in her face? Notice how it feels as you see that. Notice the thoughts that you are having. Notice how your body feels. Let yourself picture your daughter. Let yourself notice the way her eyes fill with tears. Let yourself see her as she turns and walks away. Notice the thoughts that you are having. Notice how your body feels. Now stop and spend a moment; allow the thoughts, memories, emotions, and feelings in your body to be there. Just take a moment and allow yourself to feel them all."

After a few moments, ask the client to gently, slowly, open her eyes. Without further discussion, hand her the writing materials, ask her to begin writing, and leave the room. The therapist should say something like, "I would like for you to write for 15 minutes. Really let go—write your deepest thoughts and feelings. Also write about any memories, experiences, or worries that showed up during the exercise. Write in as much detail as you can. Allow yourself to really experience your thoughts and feelings. If you can't think of anything to write, just write the same thing over and over until something new shows up. Don't worry about what it looks like, or how things are spelled. If you wish, no one will read what you have written, although it might be helpful for us to talk about together." Without further discussion, hand the client some paper and a pen or pencil, and leave the room for 15 minutes. Ideally, the therapist could observe the client during the writing process. If an observation room is not available, however, the therapist should assess level of engagement during the debriefing process (writing process adapted with permission from J. Pennebaker, personal communication, 2001).

Debriefing the Exercise

After the writing period, the balance of the session is devoted to open, accepting, mindful exposure to whatever was generated in the exercise and writing. Themes that should be sought are clients' sense of what they hope for in the area of interest (parenting, in this instance). The questions eventually asked of the client include "What if it were necessary for you to be willing to feel this pain in order to succeed as a parent? Would it be worth it? Would you be willing?"

Success is not guaranteed. However, we can guarantee that pursuing parenting challenges will bring up thoughts of parenting failures, both recollected from the past and projected into the future. If one cannot accept thoughts, emotions, and memories related to failure, one must give up parenting challenges. If, by contrast, one can "make room" psychologically for feelings of failure, taking up challenges, and therefore success, becomes possible (not guaranteed, but possible).

Additional sessions of this exposure–values exercise involved the identical session structure. The only difference was that instead of focusing on memories of past failures, the additional sessions of this exposure–values exercise focused on thoughts of future failure. So, for example, a session involved an exercise where the identical thing happens on graduation night. It is important in doing this work, just as with any exposure work, that the duration of the session be dictated by the client's reaction to the material. Just as in an exposure session, we don't expose the client to the snake and then terminate the session at the point where he or she is most aroused and most wants to leave. Instead, we ride the wave of arousal and disposition to avoid the crest of the wave, and down the other side. Although these exercises are extraordinarily painful, the exposure they contain can generate the same flexibility we see when we do exposure to external phobic objects. Willingly remembering painful events in the service of a worthy cause fundamentally alters the client's relationship with those aversive events. This is suffering, but with a purpose. We have seen clients leave sessions such as these and spontaneously engage in activities that they have been avoiding for years. It is not so much the places and activities they fear, but their reactions to these places and activities. If we can use these technologies to build a broad and flexible repertoire with respect to clients' reactions, they become free to pursue the sort of activities we prescribe in the behavioral activation component of the treatment.

VALUES, CHOICE, AND FREEDOM

We conclude with a comment about the client who cannot decide what to do. At times, values seem to rage as if at war with one another. A recent case of this sort involved a woman trying to decide whether to stay in a 30-year marriage or to take her children and leave. Her question was "Should I or shouldn't I divorce?" The therapist's posture in session on this was "I believe that you could divorce with integrity, or divorce without integrity, or stay with integrity, or stay without integrity. My commitment is to coach you in doing whatever you do with integrity." Integrity, or the lack of it, is not to be found in the properties of the response. Instead, it lies in the functional relation between the response and deeply held values—or conversely, a functional relation to deeply held fears. We expect little benefit for someone who has lived without integrity in a marriage if he or she *leaves* the marriage blaming the partner for a screwed-up life. That will function in ways similar to *staying* and blaming the partner for a screwed up life (and will be equally nonvital).

Now, that said, there is suffering inherent in every choice, including the choice not to choose. We may cut off something of extraordinary value in a choice. We may feel that we are making a values-driven choice and find later that we were completely blind and acting in a self-righteous and mean-spirited way. (We sweat as we recollect such events in our own histories.) The possibility of one of these negative outcomes is psychologically inherent in the choice—it is why the choice is hard (and avoided). Now the issue of living with integrity falls back a step, and we need to examine the integrity of not choosing in the service of fear: Is that what we want our lives to stand for? We may need to do exposure and defusion in this frightening region, where delightful and tragic possibilities dance—that place on the brink of choice.

This is a hard place to stay. Two inclinations predominate. One is to back up from choosing and dwell in the land of should I–shouldn't I, making little lists in our head of the reasons we should and reasons we shouldn't in vain hope that the scales will finally tip decisively and tell us the truth about the choice we should make. A second option is to just choose—but in the service of ending the burden this frightening psychological space engenders. However, is that what we want our lives to stand for? We explore both of these options with clients. We first take imaginal trips in experiential exercises where we walk up to the edge of choice and experience the anxiety, the pressure; we then back up into rumination and worry and add up the pluses and minuses. We examine the vitality of that act. Then, again, we walk, in an experiential exercise, to the edge of choice. Again, feel the anxiety, notice the memories, how the body feels; this time, at the peak of anxiety, we choose a direction—explicitly in the service of ending the anxiety. And then, notice what happens. Relief, but also the thought, "What if I had chosen the other way?" In both of these scenarios, the choice occurs psychologically as a "must" and as a "must do correctly"—both psychological aspects of the choice that begs for defusion and exposure. They occur psychologically as a lack of freedom. There is a third path. Camus describes it best in "An Absurd Reasoning": "The real effort is to stay there, rather, in so far as that is possible, and to examine closely the odd vegetation of those distant regions. Tenacity and acumen are privileged spectators of this inhuman show in which absurdity, hope, and death carry on their dialogue" (1955, p. 8). What if we can, by defusion and exposure, create a psychological space where the client can stand rather than *have to* jump forward or backward? To us, that is the place from which choices with the most vitality emerge—that place where even *whether* to choose occurs psychologically as a choice.

THE ROLE OF VALUES IN ACCEPTANCE, MINDFULNESS, AND RELATIONSHIP

This chapter has focused on the potential relationship between values-oriented interventions and behavior therapy procedures. Throughout, we have attempted to make the connection between values and emerging issues in the behavior therapy movement. Values work has the potential to alter fundamentally our client's relationship with adversity. Answers to questions about acceptance are always context-dependent. When acceptance of adversity is placed in the context of making a difference in an important life domain, acceptance becomes more acceptable. Mindfulness can be practiced for its own sake, but we do therapy to make a difference in people's lives. Values work can provide targets for mindfulness when "mind fields" obstruct our clients' ability to move forward in their lives. Finally, in the domain of relationships, both the therapeutic relationship and other relationships in our clients' lives, focusing on values can make the hard work inherent in relationships possible.

If we are correct in our assessment of the need for such interventions, we are left with the task of producing a robust science of human purpose, meaning, and values. Such a science could potentially help us to open up our clients' lives. Individuals live in a psychological world. In that world, they "couldn't" have done anything except what they have been doing. When we teach mindfulness, or do exposure or defusion of other sorts, clients' psychological worlds expand. They come to inhabit a world with more flexibility and, therefore, more possibilities. It may seem odd to speak of liberation and behavior therapy in the same sentence. However, the client who has two options instead of one has been liberated in a very real sense. Such liberation is the aim of this work.

ACKNOWLEDGMENTS

Thanks to the Odd Edges Seminar members for a provocative and productive discussion of this work: Catherine Adams, Lisa Coyne, Tim Crawford, Chad Drake, Laura Ely, Hillary Hunt, Rhonda Merwin, Miguel Roberts, and Dianna Wilson. Special thanks also to Ragnaar Storaasli, JoAnne Dahl, Niklas Torneke, and Lisa Coyne for suggestions on earlier drafts of the manuscript.

REFERENCE

Anisman, H., Hahn, B., Hoffman, D., & Zacharo, R. M. (1985). Stressor invoked exacerbation of amphetamine-elicited perseveration. *Pharmacology, Biochemistry and Behavior, 23,* 173–183.

Anisman, H., & Waller, T. G. (1974). Effects of inescapable shock and shock-produced conflict on self selection of alcohol in rats. *Pharmacology, Biochemistry, and Behavior, 2,* 27–33.

Bach, P., & Hayes, S. C. (2002). The use of Acceptance and Commitment Therapy to prevent the rehospitalization of psychotic patients: A randomized controlled trial. *Journal of Consulting and Clinical Psychology, 70*(5), 1129–1139.

Barlow, D. H. (2002). *Anxiety and its disorders: The nature and treatment of anxiety and panic* (2nd ed.). New York: Guilford Press.

Barlow, D., Craske, M., Cerny, J., & Klosko, J. (1989). Behavioral treatment of panic disorder. *Behavior Therapy, 20,* 261–282.

Beck, A. T., Rush, A. J., Shaw, B. F., & Emery, G. (1979). *Cognitive therapy of depression.* New York: Guilford Press.

Borkovec, T., Mathews, A., Chambers, A., Ebrahimi, S., Lytle, R., & Nelson, R. (1987). The effects of relaxation training with cognitive or nondirective therapy and the role of relaxation-induced anxiety in the treatment of generalized anxiety. *Journal of Consulting and Clinical Psychology, 55,* 611–619.

Bouton, M. E., Mineka, S., & Barlow, D. H. (2001). A modern learning theory perspective on the etiology of panic disorder. *Psychological Review, 108,* 4–32.

Bruder-Mattson, S. F., & Hovanitz, C. A. (1990). Coping and attributional styles as predictors of depression. *Journal of Clinical Psychology, 46,* 557–565.

Camus, A. (1955). *The myth of Sisyphus and other essays.* New York: Vintage.

Christensen, A., Jacobson, N. S., & Babcock, J. C. (1995). Integrative behavioral couple therapy. In N. S. Jacobson & A. S. Gurman (Eds.), *Clinical handbook of couple therapy* (pp. 31–64). New York: Guilford Press.

Cooper, M. L., Russell, M., Skinner, J. B., Frone, M. R., & Mudar, P. (1992). Stress and alcohol use: Moderating effects of gender, coping, and alcohol expectancies. *Journal of Abnormal Psychology, 101,* 139–152.

Dahl, J., Wilson, K. G., & Nillson, A. (in press). Acceptance and commitment therapy and the treatment of persons at risk for long-term disability resulting from stress and pain symptoms. *Behavior Therapy.*

DeGenova, M. K., Patton, D. M., Jurich, J. A., & MacDermid, S. M. (1994). Ways of coping among HIV-infected individuals. *Journal of Social Psychology, 134,* 655–663.

Drugan, R. C., Ader, D. N., & Maier, S. F. (1985). Shock controllability and the nature of stress-induced analgesia. *Behavioral Neuroscience, 99,*791–801.

Ellis, A. (1962). *Reason and emotion in psychotherapy.* New York: Stewart.

Ely, L. J., & Wilson, K. G. (2003, August). *ACT for academic success.* Paper presented at the World Conference on ACT, RFT, and the New Behavioral Psychology, Linköping, Sweden.

Ferster, C. B. (1973). A functional analysis of depression. *American Psychologist, 28,* 857–870.

Foa, E. B., & Riggs, D. S. (1995). Post-traumatic stress disorder following assault: Theoretical considerations and empirical findings. *Current Directions in Psychological Science, 4,* 61–65.

Forsyth, J. P., & Eifert, G. H. (1998). Phobic anxiety and panic: An integrative behavioral account of their origin and treatment. In Joseph J. Plaud & G. H. Eifert (Eds.), *From behavior theory to behavior therapy* (pp. 38–67). Boston: Allyn & Bacon.

Fox, R., Rotatori, A. F., Macklin, F., & Green, H. (1983). Assessing reinforcer preference in severe behaviorally disordered children. *Early Child Development and Care, 11,* 113–121.

Geller, I. (1960). The acquisition and extinction of conditioned suppression as a function of the base-line reinforcer. *Journal of the Experimental Analysis of Behavior, 3,* 235–240.

Greco, L. A. (2002, November). Creating a context of acceptance in child clinical and pediatric settings. In G. H. Eifert (Chair), *Balancing acceptance and change in the treatment of anxiety disorders.* Symposium presented at the annual meeting of the Association for the Advancement of Behavior Therapy, Reno, NV.

Groom, J. M., & Wilson, K. G. (2003, May). *Examination of the psychometric properties of the Valued Living Questionnaire (VLQ): A Tool Acceptance and Commitment Therapy (ACT).* Paper presented at the annual meeting of Association for Behavior Analysis, San Francisco.

Hayes, S. C., Barnes-Holmes, D., & Roche, B. (Eds.). (2001). *Relational frame theory: A post-Skinnerian account of human language and cognition.* New York: Plenum Press.

Hayes, S. C., Strosahl, K. D., & Wilson, K. G. (1999). *Acceptance and commitment therapy: A experiential approach to behavior change.* New York: Guilford Press.

Hayes, S. C., Wilson, K. G., Gifford, E. V., Follette, V. M., & Strosahl, K. (1996). Experiential avoidance and behavioral disorders: A functional dimensional approach to diagnosis and treatment. *Journal of Consulting and Clinical Psychology, 64,* 1152–1168.

Heffner, M., Sperry, J., Eifert, G. H., & Detweiler, M. (2002). Acceptance and commitment therapy in the treatment of an adolescent female with anorexia nervosa: A case example. *Cognitive and Behavioral Practice, 9,* 232–236.

Higgins, S. T., Wong, C. J., & Badger, G. J. (2000). Contingent reinforcement increases cocaine abstinence during outpatient treatment and 1 year of follow-up. *Journal of Consulting and Clinical Psychology, 68,* 64–72.

Houlihan, D., Rodriguez, R., & Levine, H. D. (1990). Validation of a reinforcer survey for use with geriatric patients. *Behavioral Residential Treatment, 5,* 129–136.

Jacobson, N. S., Dobson, K. S., Truax, P. A., Addis, M. E., Koerner, K., Gollan, J. K., et al. (2000). A component analysis of cognitive-behavioral treatment for depression. *Prevention and Treatment, 3,* 295–304.

Kabat-Zinn, J. (1995). *Whereever you go, there you are: Mindfulness meditation in everyday life.* New York: Hyperion.

Kanfer, F. H., & Phillips, J. S. (1970). *Learning foundations of behavior therapy.* Oxford: Wiley.

Kessler, R. C., McGonagle, K. A., Zhao, S., Nelson, C. B., Hughes, M., Eshleman, S., et al. (1994). Lifetime and 12-month prevalence of DSM-III-R psychiatric disorders in the United States: Results from the National Comorbidity Study. *Archives of General Psychiatry, 51,* 8–19.

Kessler, R. C., McGonagle, K. A., Zhao, S., Nelson, C. B., Hughes, M., & Eshleman, S. (1994). Lifetime and 12-month prevalence of DSM-III-R psychiatric disorders in the United States: Results from the National Comorbidity Study. *Archives of General Psychiatry, 51,* 8–19.

Leitenberg, H., Greenwald, E., & Cado, S. (1992). A retrospective study of long term methods of coping with having been sexually abused during childhood. *Child Abuse and Neglect, 16,* 399–407.

Lewinsohn, P. M., Sullivan, J. M., & Grosscup, S. J. (1980). Changing reinforcing events: An approach to the treatment of depression. *Psychotherapy: Theory, Research and Practice, 17,* 322–334.

Linehan, M. M. (1987). Dialectical behavior therapy for borderline personality disorder: Theory and method. *Bulletin of the Menninger Clinic, 51,* 261–276.

Marlatt, G. A. (2002). Buddhist philosophy and the treatment of addictive behavior. *Cognitive and Behavioral Practice, 9*, 44–49.

Martell, C. R., Addis, M. E., & Jacobson, N. S. (2001). *Depression in context: Strategies for guided action.* New York: Norton.

Miller, I. W., & Norman, W. H. (1979). Learned helplessness in humans: A review and attribution-theory model. *Psychological Bulletin, 86*, 93–118.

Monti, P. M., Kadden, R. M., Rohsenow, D. J., & Cooney, N. (2002). *Treating alcohol dependence* (2nd ed.). New York: Guilford Press.

Moser, A. E., & Annis, H. M. (1996). The role of coping in relapse crisis outcome: A prospective study of treated alcoholics. *Addiction, 91*, 1101–1114.

Northup, J. (20000. Further evaluation of the accuracy of reinforcer surveys: A systematic replication. *Journal of Applied Behavior Analysis, 33*, 335–338.

Öst, L. (2001). Single-session exposure treatment of injection phobia: A case study with continuous heart rate measurement. *Scandinavian Journal of Behaviour Therapy, 14*, 125–131.

Orsillo, S. M., Roemer, L., Block, J., LeJeune, C., & Herbert, J. D. (in press). ACT with anxiety disorders. In S. C. Hayes & K. Strosahl (Eds.) *Acceptance and commitment therapy: A clinician's guide.* New York: Guilford Press.

Polusny, M., & Follette, V. M. (1995). Long-term correlates of child sexual abuse: Theory and review of the empirical literature. *Applied and Preventive Psychology, 4*, 143–166.

Purdon, C. (1999). Thought suppression and psychopathology. *Behaviour Research and Therapy, 37*, 1029–1054.

Roemer, L., & Orsillo, S. M. (2002). Expanding our conceptualization of and treatment for generalized anxiety disorder: Integrating mindfulness/acceptance-based approaches with existing cognitive-behavioral models. *Clinical Psychology: Science and Practice, 9*, 54–68.

Segal, Z. V., Williams, J. M. G., & Teasdale, J. D. (2001). *Mindfulness-based cognitive therapy for depression: A new approach to preventing relapse.* New York: Guilford Press.

Seligman, M. E., & Beagley, G. (1975). Learned helplessness in the rat. *Journal of Comparative and Physiological Psychology, 88*, 534–541.

Seligman, M. E., & Maier, S. F. (1967). Failure to escape traumatic shock. *Journal of Experimental Psychology, 74*, 1–9.

Seligman, M. E., Maier, S. F., & Geer, J. H. (1968). Alleviation of learned helplessness in the dog. *Journal of Abnormal Psychology, 73*, 256–262.

Tighe, T. J., & Tighe, L. S. (1969). Some observations of reinforcer preference in children. *Psychonomic Science, 14*, 171–172.

Warren, D. A., & Rosellini, R. A. (1988). Effects of Librium and shock controllability upon nocioception and contextual fear. *Pharmacology, Biochemistry and Behavior, 30*, 209–214.

Wilson, G. T. (1996). Acceptance and change in the treatment of eating disorders and obesity. *Behavior Therapy, 27*, 417–439.

Wilson, K. G. (1997). The revolution to come. *Behavior Therapy, 28*, 597–600.

Wilson, K. G., & Blackledge, J. T. (1998, May). *Implications of relational frame theory for psychopathology and psychotherapy.* Paper presented at the annual meeting of the Association for Behavior Analysis, Orlando, FL.

Wilson, K. G., Hayes, S. C., Gregg, J., & Zettle, R. D. (2001). Psychopathology and Psychotherapy. In S. C. Hayes, D. Barnes, & Roche, B. (Eds.), *Relational frame theory: A post Skinnerian account of human language and cognition* (pp. 211–237). New York: Plenum Press.

Wilson, K. G., & Groom, J. (2002). *The Valued Living Questionnaire.* Available from the first author at Department of Psychology, University of Mississippi, University.

Wilson, K. G., & Luciano, C. (2002). *Terapia de Aceptión y Compromiso: Un Tratamiento Conductual Orientado a los Valores [Acceptance and commitment therapy: A values-oriented behavioral treatment].* Madrid: Editorial Psychología Pirámide.

Zvolensky, M. J., Lejuez, C. W., & Eifert, G. H. (1998). The role of offset control in anxious responding: An experimental test using repeated administrations of 20% carbon dioxide-enriched air. *Behavior Therapy, 29,* 193–209.

7

Finding the Action
in Behavioral Activation

*The Search for Empirically Supported
Interventions and Mechanisms of Change*

Christopher Martell, Michael Addis, *and* Sona Dimidjian

Behavioral activation (BA) was originally proposed as a behavioral treatment for major depressive disorder in the early 1970s by the work of Peter Lewinsohn (1975) and colleagues. The approach lost momentum in the 1980s but emerged again in the late 1990s, with the work of Jacobson and colleagues (Jacobson, Martell, & Dimidjian, 2001; Jacobson et al., 1996; Martell, Addis, & Jacobson, 2001). In this chapter, we address the history and current investigations of BA. We provide an overview of the treatment rationale and theory, and briefly present selected interventions used in the treatment. We discuss preliminary, speculative hypotheses about possible mechanisms of change and active ingredients in BA, and the relationship of these to the new behavior therapies in particular.

BEHAVIORAL ACTIVATION AND
BEHAVIORAL AND COGNITIVE THERAPY
Origins within Behavior Therapy

Lewinsohn (1975) and colleagues postulated that a decrease in pleasant events or an increase in aversive events is a mechanism that leads to depression. The treatment developed, therefore, included teaching clients to monitor the number of pleasant events in which they engaged, and to use activity scheduling to increase pleasant events. Ferster also conceptualized depression from a behavioral perspective. Ferster's (1973) radical behavioral theory emphasized the importance of a functional analysis of behavior. Depressive behaviors conceptualized as avoidance behaviors were an essential feature of his model.

Lewinsohn's (1975) work differed slightly from behavioral activation as conceptualized by Jacobson and colleagues (Jacobson et al., 2001; Martell et al., 2001). Lewinsohn and colleagues prescribed broad classes of pleasant events based on the particular absence of pleasant events for individual clients. The current approach to BA emphasizes a functional analysis of contingencies of reinforcement operating for a particular individual, without assuming that engaging in activities that are formally pleasant will function as reinforcing for the person. The subtle distinction between the form of a behavior and the function of the behavior places the current application of BA into the behavior analytic tradition more than the behavior therapy tradition. Whether this distinction between the Jacobson and colleagues version of BA and the Lewinsohn version is significant in practice has yet to be demonstrated.

Assimilation into Cognitive Therapy

While a minority of researchers and clinicians continued to apply the activation strategies proposed by Lewinsohn in a purely behavioral context, most incorporated behavioral strategies into a broader cognitive-behavioral context. Behavior change was conceptualized as a means for producing cognitive change rather than as an important mechanism in its own right. For example, Beck's cognitive therapy approach includes activation early in treatment, but the work is seen as a means of testing dysfunctional cognitions (e.g., scheduling and structuring activities combats the automatic thought, "I'm lazy and unproductive") (Beck, Rush, Shaw, & Emery, 1979).

Other cognitive therapists have suggested that the greater the intensity of depression, the more a therapist would use behavioral rather than cognitive interventions (Freeman, 1990). Although Beck and colleagues (1979) originally spoke of the behavioral aspects as auxiliary, more recently, DeRubeis, Tang, and Beck (2001) have stated that the impact of the behavioral components of cognitive therapy "should not be underestimated" (p. 355).

ARE COGNITIVE INTERVENTIONS NECESSARY?

The recent reemphasis on BA within the cognitive therapy tradition (e.g., DeRubeis et al., 2001) follows the findings of the Jacobson and colleagues

(1996) component analysis of cognitive therapy for depression. In this study, 150 participants who met the diagnosis of major depressive disorder (MDD) were randomly assigned to one of three treatment conditions: standard cognitive therapy, behavioral activation with modification of automatic thoughts, and behavioral activation alone. This study found no differences in acute treatment outcome between behavioral activation alone in the treatment of MDD and a full cognitive therapy protocol including schema work. In this study, behavioral activation consisted of therapeutic techniques from the Beck and colleagues (1979) manual, with strict proscriptions against doing cognitive therapy. Importantly, no differences were also found in relapse rates among the three treatments over a 2-year follow-up (Gortner, Gollan, Dobson, & Jacobson, 1998).

The Jacobson et al. (1996) component analysis study demonstrated the robust nature of the behavioral elements of cognitive therapy for depression. It is interesting to note that several of the therapists involved in that study originally considered doing behavioral activation alone as withholding treatment, and questioned the ethics of doing so. The results of the study, however, demonstrated that behavioral activation could be a sufficient treatment for MDD. The study demonstrated that BA was no less effective than cognitive therapy in the treatment of depression, a finding consistent with other research in the area of depression (e.g., Emmelkamp, 1994). The component analysis study suggests that cognitive interventions may not be necessary for all depressed clients, and calls into question the need for cognitive restructuring. It also served to increase attention to the role of behavioral activation in cognitive therapy.

What the Component Analysis Study Did Not Do

The Jacobson and colleagues (1996) study failed to find significant differences among treatments, but due to the lack of a control group, results could not demonstrate than any of the therapies were better than no treatment at all. A component analysis that tests broad classes of interventions, such as behavioral activation and other behavioral techniques, automatic thoughts, and core belief work, can only begin to answer questions about the active ingredients of a therapy package. Such a study raises many questions.

The component analysis study was able to demonstrate that a protocol that consisted of "not doing cognitive interventions" was no less effective than including the cognitive interventions. Logically, this does not necessarily mean that activation is the key ingredient in the cognitive therapy treatment. It did not prove or disprove either a behavioral or cognitive *model* of depression. Nor did it definitively answer questions regarding the active ingredients of cognitive therapy or mechanisms of change.

It seems unlikely that general or arbitrary increases in activity per se would be sufficient to alleviate the symptoms of MDD. Some clients present with histories of being very busy, yet still very depressed. It also seems unlikely that simple and arbitrary behavioral prescriptions (e.g., instructing clients to buy a stationary bicycle and ride for a specified amount of time) would work for a majority of clients. In BA, increases of activity are based on a functional analysis in the context of a larger treatment structure and are, therefore, not applied arbitrarily.

The University of Washington Treatment for Depression Study

Jacobson and colleagues set out to answer a number of questions raised by the component analysis study with a larger treatment study comparing cognitive therapy (Beck et al., 1979), BA (Martell et al., 2001), fluoxetine (Paxil) with clinical management (Fawcett, Epstein, Fiester, Elkin, & Autry, 1987), and pill placebo. Details of the development of this study have been published elsewhere (Dimidjian & Hollon, 2000; Jacobson & Gortner, 2000). The current clinical trial has been under way since 1997.

The treatment for depression study is both a replication and extension of the component analysis study. Several additions to the study make it a needed extension of the earlier component analysis study. First, pharmacological treatments (antidepressant medication, or ADM) were included to replicate the methodology used in the Treatment of Depression Collaborative Research Program (TDCRP; Elkin et al., 1989). Second, the study included a placebo control group. Third, all of the cognitive therapists participating in the study were considered experts. Finally, behavioral activation was approached differently in the recent study than in the component analysis study. The new study updated BA as a solo treatment based squarely in the theory of behavior analysis and contextualism. The theoretical underpinnings of BA were more carefully articulated in this study, emphasizing a behavior analytic framework. These changes in particular align BA with some of the new behavior therapies considered in this volume. Results of the recently completed trial indicated that BA was comparable in outcome to ADM; in addition, BA demonstrated significantly better retention and brought a significantly greater percentage of patients to full remission as compared to ADM. Both BA and ADM significantly outperformed cognitive therapy, which was not significantly different than pill-placebo (Dimidjian et al., 2003).

THEORETICAL UNDERPINNINGS OF BEHAVIORAL ACTIVATION

In the current investigation, the BA is based on Ferster's (1973) theory of depressive behaviors as responses to avoidance contingencies. The target in BA became avoidance behaviors, particularly inactivity and ruminating. According to Ferster, depression can develop under contingencies that require a high number of responses prior to reinforcement. Under these conditions, individuals respond primarily to deprivation rather than develop a behavioral repertoire that provides access to positive reinforcers in the natural environment. Therefore, behaviors that relieve deprivation are increased because they are negatively reinforced. For example, an individual feeling a need for social interaction may respond to the need (deprivation) by calling a friend and complaining about feeling lonely. This interaction may alleviate the social deprivation, therefore reinforcing the complaining behavior. However, the individual has not actively engaged his or her environment to provide positive reinforcement through an interpersonal exchange. The friend may over time be less likely to initiate contact with someone who telephones primarily when he or she is feeling lonely. The rejection by the friend may then continue the pattern of feeling lonely, responding to that need, and calling someone to complain, and so on. In addition, behaviors that were reinforced in one context may be overgeneralized to inappropriate contexts. For example, if the other person showing empathy has reinforced telling someone how bad one feels, an individual may engage in the behavior of talking (or thinking) about how badly one feels even in the absence of reinforcement. The talking (or thinking) may continue and be intermittently reinforced. In other words, the negative thinking, or complaining, of a depressed individual may be similar to a pigeon pecking circles that are reddish in color after training to terminate shock by pecking a red circle.

Jacobson and colleagues (2001) proposed that activation is effective, because it increases opportunities for clients to engage in behaviors that will be positively reinforced in their natural environment. It is necessary, therefore, for the BA therapist to focus on behavior that is meaningful for a particular client. Meaningful activity increases, because it is positively reinforced and allows a person to attain goals. Many activities are reinforced because they alleviate distress, or allow a client to escape or avoid aversive feelings. While aversive life circumstances may well be avoided, bad feelings are a part of life and may serve an instructive function for many individuals. Avoidance of negative feelings can lead to behaviors that may exacerbate rather than alleviate symptoms of depression, whereas working toward the attainment of goals or engaging in a proactive manner may relieve symptoms (negative reinforcement) but also increase the proactive behavioral repertoire via positive reinforcement. Undermining avoidance and focusing instead on the attainment of goals overlaps with other of the new behavior therapies covered in this volume.

The current model also focused on routine regulation, which has been associated with mood. Depressive or manic episodes are often triggered by dysregulation in routine for people with bipolar disorder (Ehlers, Frank, & Kupfer, 1988). Such routine disruptions may also be indicated in unipolar depression. BA focuses on helping clients to establish and maintain a regular routine in order to address this problem. Major life events often cause disruptions in routine; for instance, job loss is a classic example, when an individual has had structure determined by employment and suddenly is at a loss as to managing time. Thus, the activation approach serves to help clients to adhere to a plan and to a routine.

BA therapy, therefore, looks at events taking place and client responses to those events. The therapist will specifically look for escape or avoidance behaviors that may become secondary problems to depressive symptoms and exacerbate such symptoms for the client. The treatment encourages clients to work from the "outside-in" and to commit to changing behavior regardless of private (internal) states, such as feeling depressed or lethargic. When clients complain that they lack motivation, the BA therapist agrees, stating that being poorly motivated fits with being depressed. Therefore, clients are asked to commit to action without feeling motivated, in order to see whether the motivation follows, and if it does not, to examine what other positive outcomes of action may have occurred.

SPECIFIC ELEMENTS OF BEHAVIORAL ACTIVATION

BA is designed to be an idiographic therapy. However, the therapist would not act willy-nilly in order to meet the needs of a particular client. A protocol was developed for treatment and has recently been published (Martell et al., 2001). The principal elements of the treatment are described below.

Treatment Targets

The primary targets in BA consist of four main problems (1) inertia, which is often characteristic of depression; (2) avoidance behaviors; (3) routine disruption; and (4) passive ruminative thinking.

Course of Treatment

Therapy progresses through a logical course of treatment. Initially, the therapist focuses on establishing rapport and presenting the BA model to the client. The bulk of treatment consists of monitoring the relationship between activity and mood through functional analysis. In some cases, the client will be helped to apply new coping strategies to the major life issues he or she is facing. The final sessions are focused on preparing for termination and relapse prevention.

Intervention Strategies

There are five primary strategies on which the BA therapist relies. The first is the standard set by Lewinsohn so many years ago. This part of the treatment involves the use of activity logs to assess client activity and to schedule guided activities that may increase a client's pleasure or mastery of certain situations. The assumption is that activity leads to activity, whereas inactivity and lethargy will also be self-perpetuating. Activity logs can be used for several purposes. Martell and colleagues (2001) identified seven uses, but these are certainly not exhaustive. Creativity on the part of the BA therapist is always encouraged, provided that such creative use of the techniques does not conflict with the overall behavioral theory of the treatment. The seven uses identified in Martell and colleagues include (1) gathering a baseline of activity, (2) understanding the range of the client's feelings, (3) complete mastery and pleasure ratings, (4) observing the breadth or restriction of activity, (5) guiding activity, (6) monitoring avoidance behaviors, and (7) evaluating progress toward life goals.

Three strategies are used to combat client avoidance behaviors. The first two are simple acronyms used to help clients monitor their reaction to life events and experiment with alternatives to avoidance. Clients are instructed to notice when an event is a trigger for negative feelings and leads to avoidance by remembering the word TRAP (signifying trigger, response, and avoidance pattern). When they recognize the avoidance pattern they are instructed to get out of the TRAP and get back on TRAC(k) by using "alternative coping" (AC) instead of the avoidance pattern. A third acronym, ACTION is used to suggest to clients that they can (A) assess the function of their behavior, (C) choose either to continue in avoidance behaviors or change their behavior, (T) try the behavior chosen, (I) integrate any new behaviors into a routine prior to determining the outcome, (O) observe the results of their chosen behavior, and (N) never give up, but continue to take such a trial-and-error approach to their circumstance.

The treatment protocol developed by Jacobson and colleagues (2001) tries to account for clients' negative, ruminative thinking using functional analysis rather than resorting to cognitive interventions. BA therapists primarily ask clients to examine what behaviors they may be avoiding by engaging in such ruminative thinking. Thus, clients are encouraged to attend to the function, not the content of ruminative behavior. Clients are also shown that by focusing on their negative thinking, they are often not fully engaging in situations at hand. An example is a young man who wanted to spend more time with his family. On a holiday weekend, he arranged to have his father and sisters join him for dinner at a restaurant. He reported that he did not enjoy the interaction. When the therapist examined what had actually happened, it was clear that the man had been in mere physical proximity to his family. Yet, he was busy ruminating about how bad it was that he did not have a good relationship with his two sisters, and that he was a bad sibling. Instead of questioning these beliefs, which would be a valid and important cognitive-behavioral therapy intervention, the therapist asked him what color clothing people were wearing. He did not know. The therapist also asked what various people ordered for dinner. Again, the man did not know. As questions about the details of the family's behavior were asked and the young man was unable to answer, the therapist pointed out how much interaction with the family the man had missed while ruminating about how little he got to see them. Although this man thought that he was engaging in multiple behaviors at once (i.e., conversing, spending time with his family, eating dinner, and being immersed in thought), it was clear that ruminating behavior trumped the other behavior. Without attempting to find a behavioral alternative to treating such ruminations, therapists would be quick to question the client's beliefs about his role in his family.

Clients are also taught to set goals and to carry out behaviors that will bring them closer to their goal. Goals may be immediate, such as consistently getting up when the alarm rings and making coffee, or longer term, such as finding a better job. In each case, the client discusses the necessary steps to achieving the goal with the therapist, then carries out the steps between sessions. In the following session, the client reports on the success of his or her attempts, and the assignment is modified to overcome any difficulties that the client experienced when following the steps. Clients are instructed to act toward their goals, and not according to a mood. They may even act in ways that are inconsistent with their mood. For example, a client with a goal of awaking with the alarm and making coffee may feel like staying in bed, but may get out of bed and turn on the coffee maker instead, since it is acting toward the goal. This is akin to opposite action in dialectical behavior therapy (DBT; Linehan, 1993) or to the idea of "Fake it until you make it" in Alcoholics Anonymous.

UNANSWERED QUESTIONS

As the efficacy of BA continues to be demonstrated in clinical trials, it will likely continue to remain in the forefront of treatments for depression. Demonstrating that the treatment works, however, is a good beginning. There continue to be questions that the treatment outcome studies have not yet answered. First, the success of BA does not sufficiently confirm the behavioral theory of depression. Second, the idea that BA should be a practical and easily learned and disseminated treatment has yet to be confirmed. Third, we do not as yet understand the mechanisms of change in BA. Finally, although the treatment has been stripped down to a handful of techniques, BA may be further dismantled to understand both practical and theoretical implications.

There are different assumptions made in BA and cognitive therapy about the processes that underlie therapeutic change. In BA, it is assumed that an increase in positive reinforcement produces change. Cognitive therapy assumes that there are cognitive mechanisms associated with change. In cognitive therapy, behavior change is seen primarily as a means to change a belief. BA focuses on changing behavior and talks about change from the "outside-in," whereas cognitive therapy considers attitude change as a necessary component for lasting emotional or behavioral change. The motto used with BA clients is "Activity breeds activity."

Despite these different assumptions, BA shares processes with cognitive therapy that may contribute to success of treatment. The collaborative therapeutic relationship is an important aspect of BA and cognitive therapy. In BA, clients are asked to work with the therapist as if he or she were a coach. The therapist and client work as a team to develop strategies that the client can try, and both observe and discuss the results of the client's attempts.

Addis and Carpenter (2000) suggest that clients' "buying into" the treatment rationale is critical, regardless of the therapeutic techniques used. There is a strong emphasis in both BA and cognitive therapy on presenting the therapy rationale to clients. For example, both provide reading material on the therapeutic rationale to clients in the first session.

BA maintains the general session structure that is required of cognitive therapy. Therapist and client collaborate on an agenda each session, and clients are asked to prioritize items. Therapists also check on the client's mood. Therapists do not make frequent summaries, as cognitive therapists do, because to do so is thought to be irrelevant to the therapeutic task. No attempts are made to provide insight or new beliefs, so there is little to summarize, with the exception of a brief overview of topics that have been discussed during the session. The goal of BA is to get the client active outside of the therapy session, ultimately. This is accomplished through between-session assignments or homework, another factor common to the two treatments. Finally, in BA, clients are asked to complete the Beck Depression Inventory (BDI; Beck, Ward, Mendelson, Mock, & Erbaugh, 1961) prior to each session, as is commonly done in cognitive therapy.

Despite these commonalities, most of the possible BA component processes seem specific to BA or are shared with some of the newer behavior therapies covered in this volume.

Possible Active Ingredients Unique to BA

Several of the following components seem relatively unique to BA.

Activity Rule

One thing is consistently pointed out to clients in BA: Activity breeds activity, and inactivity breeds inactivity. Clients are taught this idea and coached to test this out. Behavior that fits with this rule is reinforced by their therapists and, in many cases, reinforced in their natural environment. The possibility exists, then, that BA succeeded at teaching depressed clients to follow a new rule or algorithm. Whereas clients had been following the rule that could basically be stated as "When feeling blue, shut down," they were taught to take a different approach that could be stated as "When feeling blue, get active." This possibility may explain what keeps clients working through the process in BA.

Functional Analysis

Clients in BA are trained to conduct a functional analysis of their behavior, looking closely at antecedents and consequences of their behavior. They are taught to "view their lives as a rich tapestry" and to try to understand the detail. Conducting such analyses and making changes to reach desired outcomes would be consistent with the theory behind BA. As Hollon (2001) suggests, BA may provide concrete, simple treatment algorithms that focus on behavior change that can be effective in reducing affective distress.

Scheduling Activities

This technique is standard in BA and has been since the beginning of this approach by Lewinsohn. Lejuez, Hopko, LePage, Hopko, and McNeil (2001) completed a study of a short-term BA treatment that consisted solely of having clients set activity targets for the week and monitor success as achieving the activity goals in an activity log. Using an $N = 1$ design, they demonstrated that the treatment was efficacious in the amelioration of depressive symptoms. This provides initial evidence of the power of simple activation.

Graduated Activities

BA relies heavily on breaking tasks into their component parts, so that clients can achieve success in a graduated fashion. Ferster (1973) stated that the "most general way of increasing the perceptual repertoire is to begin with simple activities whose reinforcement is reliable but not so invariant that there are not some circumstances where the performance is appropriate and others where it is not" (p. 863). By "perceptual repertoire," Ferster was referring to discrimination between occasions when behavior will likely be reinforced and when it will not. Ferster hypothesized that for depressed persons, there were disruptions in the perceptual repertoire. Furthermore, Ferster (1981) suggested that "a schedule of reinforcement in which a relatively fixed and large amount of activity is required for reinforcement may be a cause of depression" (p. 183). It makes sense, therefore, to break tasks down, so that clients may obtain immediate reinforcement of discrete actions and observe the connection between their activity and the reinforcing consequences.

Possible Active Ingredients Common to Other Behavior Therapies

Behavioral activation is a change-oriented therapy. Observing the techniques used in the treatment, however, reveals similarities to newer behavior therapies, particularly those that are more contextualistic. It is possible that BA shares common elements with these therapies, although it was not specifically designed to do so. Four of these ingredients are described here.

Explicit Targeting of Avoidance

This aspect of the current conceptualization of BA is not completely unique in treatment for depression, though it is consistent with other contextual approaches (e.g., Ferster, 1973; Hayes, Strosahl, & Wilson, 1999; Zettle & Hayes, 1987). As treatment was being conducted in the study, it was noted that much of the client behavior observed appeared to function as avoidance behavior. This was consistent with Ferster's understanding of the function of many depressed behaviors. No other treatment of depression has specifically targeted avoidance. Encouraging approach behaviors rather than avoidance is similar to behavioral treatments for anxiety.

By specifically targeting avoidance behavior, BA is similar to other techniques that block experiential avoidance. It may be more accurate, however, to say that BA targets escape and avoidance behaviors. Both escape and avoidance are negatively reinforced, and avoidance can be thought of as escaping a situation related to a higher probability of aversive events. Behaviors such as rolling over and staying in bed an extra hour or two when one is depressed may function as a means of escaping aversive feelings. They may also function as avoidance of targets that induce aversive feelings, such as a demanding boss or the absence of a lover or partner in one's home.

Opposite Action

The principle use of opposite action (Linehan, 1993) is teaching clients to block avoidance with increased activity. When clients complain of feeling fatigued, for example, they are asked whether sleeping makes them feel more refreshed or more lethargic. If they say that they feel refreshed when they awaken, the therapist will say that may indicate that they were truly in need of sleep. However, if they feel more fatigued, then the need for sleep may be avoidance behavior. The client would then be encouraged to refrain from sleeping or retiring to the sofa, and to get engaged in an activity despite the feeling of fatigue. Again, this may either relieve the feelings of fatigue or simply get certain tasks accomplished in the midst of negative feelings. Clients are taught to conduct a functional analysis of sleep behavior and to engage in activities that help them accomplish a goal, regardless of whether they feel like acting in this way.

Acceptance

In BA, clients are told that the treatment is generally geared to make them feel better. However, the treatment also takes into account the fact that a variety of feelings, negative and positive, are part of life. Clients are taught to interrupt the cycle of avoidance that keeps them depressed. By acting from the "outside-in" rather than trying to feel a certain way prior to acting, clients learn to accept their feelings and move forward in life in spite of them. Both client and therapist take an empirical approach to activity. After conducting a functional analysis, the client engages in behaviors that may lead to improved mood. However, the behaviors may have no effect on mood at all but still be useful, because life situations may be improved. For example, one client complained of feeling particularly depressed and blue in her damp, messy, dark house. One activity that she had been avoiding was cleaning her house, so that she could feel better in her environment. She began cleaning her office and took a number of boxes off windowsills. She then noticed that her windowsills were dirty with old paint and grime. She removed the paint and dirt and was amazed at the amount of light that came flooding into her office. In this case, the dual effect of the cleaner room and increased light did improve this client's mood somewhat. The point was, however, that she could still have felt depressed, but it would be better to be depressed in a pleasant environment than in an environment that led to discomfort. She had been waiting to feel motivated prior to cleaning her office. In BA, she learned to change her behavior without needing to change her mood. The combination of acceptance elements in the change process is similar to some of the new behavior therapies (Hayes et al., 1999; Jacobson & Christensen, 1996; Linehan, 1993).

Like other acceptance procedures, BA teaches clients that they can feel their feelings, even the aversive feelings, and take constructive action nevertheless. Although we suggest that, over time, acting in this manner may break the depressive cycle and improve mood, we also stress that feelings are just feelings, and that life can be lived fully even in the presence of negative feelings.

Mindfulness

Because depressed clients often spend a great amount of time ruminating about their problems, and because such ruminating can lead to deeper depression or longer episodes (Nolen-Hoeksema, Morrow, & Fredrickson, 1993), this behavior needed to be addressed in BA. Dealing with the content of ruminations would have been a cognitive intervention and was therefore not used in BA clinical trials. Instead, therapists treated the process of rumination and worked with clients to identify and target the function of rumination as opposed to the content. Therapists also taught clients to block rumination by attending to their experience rather than to ruminate. In attention to experience, clients are asked what activities they avoid by ruminating and are then asked to engage in those activities. When clients complain that they cannot keep on track with the activity because they are preoccupied with their ruminations, they are asked to attend to their experience. Therapists ask clients to pay attention to the sights, smells, tastes, and tactile sensations that make up the experience.

For example, the client who complained that having dinner with his family did not make him happy, as he planned, admitted that he had actually been busily ruminating about his depression while his family enjoyed dinner conversation. Then, on another visit, he tried to pay attention to the sound of their voices, to be able to notice which one talked the loudest, the colors in their clothes, changes in facial expressions as they talked and so on. He returned having really engaged in the experience and stated that he had felt more connected with his family. The BA therapist's many detailed questions necessitated that the client pay attention to his experiences so that he could describe them in therapy. In these ways, BA may parallel components of the more explicit training in mindfulness and attention to the moment that is present, as in some of the other new behavioral and cognitive therapies in this volume, such as DBT, acceptance and commitment therapy (ACT), or mindfulness-based cognitive therapy (MBCT).

Depathologizing Client Thinking or Behaving

As a contextual treatment, BA is a therapeutic attempt to see the client as a whole and to address problems broadly, without pathologizing client thinking or behaving. The "symptoms" of depression experienced by the client are considered reactions to the contextual shifts in the client's life that signal that something has gone awry. The problem with depression, from a BA perspective, is not the "blues" or the negative affect that is often experienced. Rather, it is the downward spiral in behavior toward less productive activity in both thinking and acting. Clients are encouraged to engage in productive behaviors despite their mood, disengaging them from mood dependence. Thus, while BA is in many ways a return to some of the earlier behavior approaches, it does so with a broader contextualistic quality that shares features with other approaches discussed in this volume.

IS BEHAVIORAL ACTIVATION EASILY LEARNED?

Researchers often find it difficult to train therapists to adhere to treatment protocols, and the amount of supervision usually offered to ensure therapeutic competence and adherence may hinder the exportability of treatment to the general clinical community (Hollon, 1999). If BA proves to be as effective as the entire cognitive therapy package, then a treatment that may be much easier to learn could be used in the treatment of MDD. Despite the relative simplicity of the model, it may be some time before this question is adequately addressed, since the research demands of the current randomized controlled trials lead to substantial care in the supervision of BA therapists. BA therapists in the clinical outcome study were provided with ongoing case consultation on a weekly basis, both individually and in a group format. This level of supervision and consultation is not realistic in the clinical community at large, where busy schedules may limit consultation to a small group of practitioners who generally share theoretical orientations but are not necessarily experts in a particular protocol.

SUMMARY

Although BA has resurfaced in the literature as a stand-alone treatment for depression, the mechanisms by which it is effective are as yet unknown. Initially seen as a component of cognitive therapy, the component analysis study (Jacobson et al., 1996) introduced the exciting and provocative finding of no difference between BA and cognitive therapy in the treatment of depression. This discovery lent additional support to years of data showing that behavioral and cognitive interventions are at least equally efficacious, and that the addition of cognitive components to behavior therapy does not necessarily add to the treatment (e.g., Beidel & Turner, 1986; Latimer & Sweet, 1984; Zettle & Hayes, 1987). BA may be easier to learn, especially for those with elementary behavioral training, but this is yet to be demonstrated conclusively.

Clearly, there is room for further analysis of the mechanisms of change in BA. This component of cognitive-behavioral therapy can be broken down into its various components and reviewed for further understanding of the process. This chapter has highlighted a number of exciting and important avenues for future investigation.

REFERENCES

Addis, M. E., & Carpenter, K. M. (2000). The treatment rationale in cognitive behavioral therapy: Psychological mechanisms and clinical guidelines. *Cognitive and Behavioral Practice, 7*(2), 147–155.

Beck, A. T., Rush, A. J., Shaw, B. F., & Emery, G. (1979). *Cognitive therapy of depression.* New York: Guilford Press.

Beck, A. T., Ward, C. H., Mendelson, M., Mock, J. E., & Erbaugh, J. K. (1961). An inventory for measuring depression. *Archives of General Psychiatry, 4*, 561–571.

Beidel, D. C., & Turner, S. M. (1986). A critique of the theoretical bases of cognitive-behavioral theories and therapy. *Clinical Psychology Review, 6,* 177–197.

DeRubeis, R. J., Tang, T. Z., & Beck, A. T. (2001). Cognitive therapy. In K. S. Dobson (Ed.), *Handbook of cognitive-behavioral therapies* (2nd ed., pp. 349–392). New York: Guilford Press.

Dimidjian, S., & Hollon, S. (2000, November). *Designing and implementing controlled, clinical trials on the treatment of depression: Lessons from the University of Washington Treatment for Depression Study.* Paper presented at the meeting of the Association for Advancement of Behavior Therapy, New Orleans, LA.

Dimidjian, S., Hollon, S., Dobson, K., Schmaling, K., Kohlenberg, R., McGlinchey, J., Markley, D., Atkins, D., Addis, M., & Dunner, D. (2003, November). *Behavioral activation, cognitive therapy, and antidepressant medication in the treatment of major depression: Design and acute phase outcomes.* Presented at the 37th annual convention of the Association for Advancement of Behavior Therapy, Boston.

Ehlers, C. L., Frank, E., & Kupfer, D. J. (1988). Social zeitgebers and biological rhythms: A unified approach to understanding the etiology of depression. *Archives of General Psychiatry, 45,* 948–952.

Elkin, I., Shea, M. T., Watkins, J. T., Imber, S. D., Sotsky, S. M., Collins, J. F., et al. (1989). National Institute of Mental health Treatment of Depression Collaborative Research Program: General effectiveness of treatments. *Archives of General Psychiatry, 46,* 971–982.

Emmelkamp, P. M. G. (1994). Behavior therapy with adults. In. A. E. Bergin & S. L. Garfield (Eds.), *Handbook of psychotherapy and behavior change* (4th ed., pp. 379–427). New York: Wiley.

Fawcett, J., Epstein, P., Fiester, S. J., Elkin, I., & Autry, J. A. (1987). Clinical management—imipramine/placebo administration manual. *Psychopharmacological Bulletin, 23,* 309–324.

Ferster, C. B. (1973). A functional analysis of depression. *American Psychologist, 28,* 857–870.

Ferster, C. B. (1981). A functional analysis of behavior therapy. In L. P. Rehm (Ed.), *Behavior therapy for depression: Present status and future directions* (pp. 181–196). New York: Academic Press.

Freeman, A. (1990). Cognitive therapy. In A. S. Bellack & M. Hersen (Eds.), *Handbook of comparative treatments for adult disorders* (pp. 64–87). New York: Wiley.

Gortner, E. T., Gollan, J. K., Dobson, K. S, & Jacobson, N. S. (1998). Cognitive-behavioral treatment for depression: Relapse prevention. *Journal of Consulting and Clinical Psychology, 66*(2), 377–384.

Hayes, S. C., Strosahl, K. D., & Wilson, K. G. (1999). *Acceptance and commitment therapy: An experiential approach to behavior change.* New York: Guilford Press.

Hollon, S. D. (2001). Behavioral activation treatment for depression: A commentary. *Clinical Psychology: Science and Practice, 8*(3), 271–274.

Jacobson, N. S., & Christensen, A. (1996). *Integrative couple therapy: Promoting acceptance and change.* New York: Norton.

Jacobson, N. S., Dobson, K., Truax, P. A., Addis, M. E., Koerner, K., Gollan, J. K., et al. (1996). A component analysis of cognitive-behavioral treatment for depression. *Journal of Consulting and Clinical Psychology, 64*(2), 295–304.

Jacobson, N. S., & Gortner, E. (2000). Can depression be de-medicalized in the 21st century: Scientific revolutions, counter-revolutions and the magnetic field of normal science. *Behaviour Research and Therapy, 38,* 103–117.

Jacobson, N. S., Martell, C. R., & Dimidjian, S. (2001). Behavioral activation for depression: Returning to contextual roots. *Clinical Psychology: Science and Practice, 8*(3), 255–270.

Latimer, P. R., & Sweet, A. A. (1984). Cognitive versus behavioral procedures in cognitive behavior therapy: A critical review of the evidence. *Journal of Behavior Therapy and Experimental Psychiatry, 15*, 9–22.

Lejuez, C. W., Hopko, D. R., LePage, J. P., Hopko, S. D., & McNeil, D. W. (2001). A brief behavioral activation treatment for depression. *Cognitive and Behavioral Practice, 8*(2), 164–175.

Lewinsohn, P. M. (1975). The behavioral study and treatment of depression. In M. Hersen, R. M. Eisler, & P. M. Miler (Eds.), *Progress in behavior modification* (Vol. 1, pp. 19–65). New York: Academic Press.

Linehan, M. M. (1993). *Cognitive-behavioral treatment of borderline personality disorder.* New York: Guilford Press.

Martell, C. R., Addis, M. E., & Jacobson, N. S. (2001). *Depression in context: Strategies for guided action.* New York: Norton.

Nolen-Hoeksema, S., Morrow, J., & Fredrickson, B. L. (1993). Response styles and the duration of episodes of depressed mood. *Journal of Abnormal Psychology, 102*(1), 20–28.

Zettle, R. D., & Hayes, S. C. (1987). A component and process analysis of cognitive therapy. *Psychological Reports, 61*, 939–953.

8

Mindfulness, Acceptance, Validation, and "Individual" Psychopathology in Couples

Alan E. Fruzzetti *and* Kate M. Iverson

Predominant models of psychopathology typically view the word *individual* as redundant when placed next to *psychopathology*. In most models, psychopathology resides inside the skin of the individual. These models may be linear in nature (e.g., broken brains, broken receptor cells, broken cognitions, broken personalities, broken defenses), or they may be interactional, describing interactions between the person and his or her environment (e.g., diathesis–stress or other models in which *levels* of individual and environmental factors interact, leading to disorder in the individual). However, psychopathology in both the behavioral and family systems traditions has long been understood simply as problematic individual behaviors (including thoughts, feelings, wants, sensations, and overt actions) that occur in, and are in ongoing transaction with, the person's social and family environment. In other words, the individual acts on his or her world, and the world acts on the individual, each influencing the other.

In a linear or interactional model, we typically think of individual psychopathology as the set of problematic emotional, cognitive, sensory, motivational, and overt responses of the individual to life situations. But it is also possible to see the context of these problematic behaviors as part of the "disorder" as well, or to see the entire transaction as the "problem."

Thus, alternative models do exist in which the individual's problematic responses are not artificially disaggregated from the interpersonal or family context in which they develop and function currently. For example, if a person is sad, we may define the "problem" as *inside* the person (e.g., she "is not producing enough serotonin" or has "maladaptive cognitions" or is not "active enough") or *outside* the person (e.g., "the environment is very punishing" or "she was abused" or "her partner is consistently critical of her"). However, to achieve a more comprehensive conceptualization, we may describe the situation, problem, or transaction to include *both* parts (e.g., "in situation x [which focuses on the present, especially on interpersonal contingencies such as how a spouse or partner or parent responds to her disclosure of emotion, wants, thoughts], she has these particular thoughts, desires, urges, engages in these particular behaviors, and feels sad"). For both theoretical and empirical reasons, we think there is a lot of utility in trying to understand many problems of individual psychopathology as transactional (cf. Fruzzetti, 1996).

The purposes of this chapter are (1) to explicate a specific, transactional model of many forms of psychopathology, one that includes both the role of specific individual behaviors (e.g., self-disclosure, emotion regulation and self-management) and the role of specific spouse/partner or family member behaviors (e.g., mindfulness, acceptance, and validation); and (2) to describe intervention strategies that are implied by this model to treat both the individual's problem behaviors (psychopathology) and the problematic partner responses (unmindful/reactive/nonaccepting/nonvalidating behaviors) that engender and/or maintain "distressed" partner behavior. Together, these may provide a more comprehensive model of the "problem" and provide a framework with more clinical utility for intervention. Although this model may be applicable to many types of relationships (e.g., parents and children, couples, friendships), we focus mostly on married or cohabiting partners or couples, largely because more research has been focused on these particular relationships.

THE ROLE OF COUPLE AND FAMILY INTERACTIONS IN INDIVIDUAL PSYCHOPATHOLOGY

The idea that behavior (broadly defined to include not only overt actions but also emotions, cognitions, sensations, wants, etc.) occurs in a context that is meaningful is not new, of course. Binswanger's (1956) existential notions of the person-in-the-world (*umwelt, mitwelt,* and *eigenwelt*), Skinner's behavioral model of humans operating on the world (1953), and many family systems models of psychopathology (e.g., Guttman, 1986) all suggest a central role for partners, parents, and other significant persons as contexts for all individual behaviors, including problematic ones. Although it has long been known that distressed individual behavior, such as depression, tends to be associated with relationship problems (e.g., Fruzzetti, 1996; Weissman & Paykel, 1974), the nature of this association is varied and complex.

Summary of the Evidence

Couple and family factors have been demonstrated to be very relevant to individual psychopathology for a variety of disorders, including depression, anxiety disorders, substance abuse, schizophrenia, borderline personality disorder, and many other disorders. For example, after controlling for quality of relationships with other family members and friends, Whisman, Sheldon, and Goering (2000) found that marital/partner satisfaction was associated with nearly 70% of the disorders assessed by the Ontario Health Survey Mental Health Supplement (including high rates of association with anxiety disorders and depression, in particular).

A comprehensive review of the dozens of studies demonstrating linkages between couple and family functioning and psychopathology is beyond the scope of this chapter. It is important to note, however, that couple factors have been shown to be relevant to individual psychopathology, and vice versa, in a number of different ways: (1) development of psychopathology (e.g., Addis & Jacobson, 1996; Cascardi, O'Leary, Lawrence, & Schlee, 1995; O'Leary, Christian & Mendell, 1994; Whisman & Bruce, 1999); (2) maintenance of distress and disorder (e.g., Biglan et al., 1985; Hooley & Hoffman, 1999; Hooley, Orley, & Teasdale, 1986); (3) demonstration of the efficacy of couple treatment for psychopathology (e.g., depression; Beach & O'Leary, 1992; Jacobson, Dobson, Fruzzetti, Schmaling, & Salusky, 1991); (4) relapse versus maintained recovery after treatment (e.g., Jacobson, Fruzzetti, Dobson, Whisman, & Hops, 1993); and (5) demonstration of the utility of couple interventions to augment individual treatment (e.g., Campbell, 2003). Clear relationships between couple interactions or couple and family functioning and individual psychopathology have been shown for suicidal behaviors, depression, anxiety disorders, substance abuse, sexual dysfunction, borderline personality disorder, and a variety of other clinical and subclinical problems.

Conflict in Couple Interactions and Individual Distress

Conflict has been the focal point for the preponderance of couple research, which typically has demonstrated that certain types of conflict (e.g., violence and aggression, high criticality and negativity) are associated with increased depression, higher rates of suicidality, poorer course of disorder or rate of recovery, higher relapse rates, and so on (e.g., Fincham & Beach, 1999). Most often, conflict has been considered problematic both to relationships and to the well-being of the individuals in them. Consequently, solving problems and resolving conflict have been central goals of many treatment programs (e.g., Jacobson & Margolin, 1979), and the absence of conflict has been implicitly adopted as a marker for a good relationship. The absence of conflict in and of itself may not adequately describe a good relationship: Those relationships in which partners do not argue, but also do not disclose to one another or are punished for doing so, would not be healthy. Clearly, both conflict and intimacy behaviors are relevant. For example, Arkowitz-Westen and Fruzzetti (2004) found that even after covarying out conflict and invalidating behaviors, validating behaviors still predicted higher relationship satisfaction in a cross section of clinic and community couples.

It may be more useful to consider conflict a set of behaviors that includes constructive disagreement and negotiation at one end of the spectrum, and destructive and aggressive interactions, and ignoring or avoidance behaviors at the other end, rather than as a linear dimension ranging from high/problematic to low/healthy (e.g., Fruzzetti, 1996; Markman, 1991). Moreover, when viewed this way, the more destructive types of conflict (e.g., hostile, avoidant) seem to be the ones largely associated with individual psychopathology, while constructive conflict, albeit rarely examined, would be presumed to be associated with partner well-being, or with improvements in functioning.

Intimacy in Couple Interactions

There is increasing evidence that a good, healthy relationship is not simply the absence of conflict (e.g., Campbell & Fruzzetti, 2004). Rather, a healthy relationship for both partners includes constructive conflict and high levels of intimacy (e.g., Fruzzetti, 1996). Clearly, the "benefits" or "goodies" (reinforcers) in relationships are intimacy and closeness. We define "intimacy" as a pattern of interacting in which one person is able to disclose accurately her or his thoughts, emotions, wants, and so on, and in response to those disclosures, the other person expresses acceptance and understanding through validation, which in turn leads to the experience of closeness and of being understood and/or supported (see also Fruzzetti & Jacobson, 1990). Of course, these behaviors are mutual and reciprocal. Thus, intimacy behaviors include accurate self-disclosures plus those responses that demonstrate awareness of the partner, understanding of the partner, and support of the partner. We call responses that communicate acceptance and understanding *validating* (discussed further below). Thus, the self-disclosure/validating response cycle describes the core of intimate interactions.

There is increasing research support for the importance of intimacy in partner (individual) well-being. For example, lack of intimacy may be associated with depression (Waring & Patton, 1984) and is associated with problematic parenting practices, which are in turn associated with individual distress (Sayrs & Fruzzetti, 2004). Similarly, in a study of 30 chronically distressed inpatients and outpatients (diagnosed with depression, substance abuse, personality disorders, etc.), only partner validation predicted improvements longitudinally (Thorp & Fruzzetti, 2004).

It is this process of partner acceptance and validation on which we focus our attention. Specifically, we must consider how acceptance and validation, versus nonacceptance and invalidation, might be integrally related to individual dysfunctional behavior and psychopathology.

Self-Disclosure, Emotion Regulation, and Validation

The role of emotion and problems in emotion regulation are increasingly understood to be a core part of psychopathology developmentally (e.g., Southam-Gerow & Kendall, 2002), and of adult psychopathology (e.g., Fruzzetti & Fruzzetti, 2003; Keltner & Kring, 1998; Linehan, 1993). Although sometimes emphasized in different ways, interpersonal responses (e.g., a lack of validating responses, or the presence of invalidating responses) are key factors in the development, maintenance, treatment, and relapse of psychopathology. This is largely because regulating emotion in turn regulates the individual's cognitive, physiological, and overt behavioral repertoires (Fruzzetti, Lowry, Mosco, & Shenk, 2003; Southam-Gerow & Kendall, 2002).

Emotion Regulation and Dysregulation

Emotion regulation includes a variety of specific behaviors and "processes by which individuals influence which emotions they have, when they have them, and how they experience and express these emotions" (Gross, 1998, p. 275). Emotion regulation processes necessarily are in the service of the individual's larger, long-term goals (Thompson, 1994), rather than only in the service of immediate "escape-oriented" or short-term goals (although short- and long-term goals are sometimes consonant). Conversely, emotion dysregulation occurs when the individual is not able to accept (notice or bring into awareness, discriminate, tolerate at least long enough to change it effectively, experience, label accurately, express accurately) the relevant emotional experience. Instead, the individual engages in some form of escape behavior (emotionally, cognitively, physiologically, or overtly) that is typically problematic in some way. Therefore, emotion dysregulation is quite different from simply being upset or having a lot of emotional intensity or arousal, which can be managed in a very healthy way without problematic escape responses. Thus, emotion dysregulation occurs when the intensity or arousal of the person is functionally related to escape-oriented consequences (Fruzzetti et al., 2003).

Paradoxically, then, emotion regulation includes both acceptance and change strategies (Fruzzetti et al., 2003; Linehan, 1993a). Specifically, emotion regulation behaviors include (1) behaviors employed to help an individual *accept* his or her emotion (notice, understand, discriminate, label accurately, experience safely, express, and connect cognitively to antecedent stimuli), and (2) behaviors that help a person *change* his or her emotion (change the particular type of emotion experienced, or alter the intensity or duration of the emotion, often by modulating attention or by titrating actual contact with the relevant emotional stimuli).

Self-Disclosure Followed by Validation

Almost all of the behaviors relevant to regulating emotions occur in a social context (with interpersonal behaviors most often being the antecedent stimuli for high emotional arousal), are learned in a social context, and may therefore be inhibited or interrupted (or engendered or reinforced) by social processes. For example, children learn to label their emotions according to social conventions when attentive, empathic caregivers notice the emotionally relevant antecedent, connect it to children's expression of arousal, and validate their experiences, while providing an accurate label to those private experiences. Children and adults further develop acute emotion discrimination by discussing situations and subsequent sensory experiences, other emotional responses, thoughts, motivational tendencies, and so on, again with significant others validating their experiences and shaping their response repertoire. In addition, self-regulation skills such as modulating attention, titrating exposure to arousing stimuli, and so on, are mostly taught by others via modeling or direct instruction, which, again, is experienced as validating (cf. Linehan, 1993a; Southham-Gerow & Kendall, 2002).

This process in which some private behavior (sensation, want, emotion, thought, urge, etc.) is expressed, verbally or nonverbally, and is at least in part validated, is essential to healthy development and healthy psychological processing. We call the identification, expression, and management of private experiences simply "accurate self-expression," which is promoted by validating responses. Not only does understanding and validation promote healthy relationship functioning but it also facilitates arousal reduction and effective psychological processing of the various responses people have to situations or stimuli in the world (cf. Swann, 1997). The alternative, problematic process occurs when these valid experiences are expressed but the other person responds critically, rejecting the validity or legitimacy of the person's experience or the legitimacy of his or her subsequent actions. This inhibits future expression and adds further emotional arousal to the mix (Fruzzetti et al., 2003), both central processes in the development or maintenance of psychopathology.

Of course, this is not really a new perspective. For example, Thich

Nhat Hanh notes that in the ancient Buddhist writings of the *Lotus Sutra*, "compassionate listening brings about healing" (1998, p. 79). Modern researchers have demonstrated explicitly the benefits of validating responses and the problematic consequences of invalidating responses. For a more complete description of the processes through which invalidating responses (and a lack of validating ones) lead to the development and maintenance of psychopathology, see Linehan (1993a), Southam-Gerow and Kendall (2002), or Fruzzetti and Boulanger (2004).

Thus, although validation has been used to label a variety of inter- and intrapersonal processes, for our purposes, validation is the expression of understanding (and implicitly or explicitly acknowledging the legitimacy) of a target experience or behavior (emotion, want, thought, sensation, action, etc.) of another person. However, acceptance of our *own* private responses or reactions to the other person's expression (our own emotions, desires, attributions, and other reactions to the person's disclosure) is required in order to move our attention to the other person and to understand his or her experience. In turn, of course, acceptance requires mindful engagement to keep attention focused, prevent judgments (or to let them go quickly), and thus keep arousal in check. Otherwise, our own reactions can interfere and we may get "stuck" on our own experience (e.g., having judgments, increased emotional reactivity). Thus, our own lack of mindfulness permits nonacceptance, which leads to nonunderstanding of the other and increases the likelihood of invalidation, or at least a lack of validating responses. Conversely, mindfulness promotes acceptance, which allows understanding, facilitates validation, reduces arousal in the other person, and may facilitate in turn his or her own affect and self-regulation.

Now we must consider the varying ways of conceptualizing acceptance in more detail, and how it relates both to the person engaging in the accepting and validating behaviors, and to the partner whose behaviors (feelings, wants, requests, thoughts, etc.) are being accepted and validated.

ACCEPTANCE

The term "acceptance" has been employed to describe a variety of different psychological processes and interactional behaviors, many of them represented in this volume. Acceptance in couples is complicated because it requires us not only to understand acceptance as a psychological phenomenon within a person, but also to understand something about the transactional process, or interpersonal context, of that individual acceptance. Let us begin with a description of the individual behaviors that are integral to the phenomenon of acceptance in general before turning to acceptance of partner behaviors.

Definitions

First, acceptance is something a person does (or does not do) in response to his or her own *private* experience; that is, we accept (or do not) a thought, sensation, emotion, experience of arousal, desire or want, or other stimulus inside our skin. This private experience, of course, is only the proximal stimulus to accepting or nonaccepting responses. The experience is itself connected to an antecedent stimulus or multiple antecedent stimuli, which may be private (inside the person) or public (something happening outside the person).

In common language, it is often the case that we are not very precise in describing what it is that we are "accepting." For example, a person might feel very hot while standing in line in the sun, waiting to buy a ticket to a positively anticipated event. She might have the thought, "I'm so hot, and I'm really uncomfortable." She might have an immediate urge to seek shade, go home, or otherwise escape her discomfort, which would, of course, preclude her getting the tickets at this time. For our purposes, as long as she stays in line and is uncomfortable, she is willing to tolerate her distress in the service of her goal (anticipated event) and thus is accepting her discomfort. Thus, behavioral tolerance (not actively working on change) is one form of acceptance. Similarly, she could stay in line and simultaneously marshal resources to change or minimize that discomfort (e.g., by fanning herself or asking a friend in line with her to get her a cold drink). Because she is still acting in a way that is consistent with her overarching (genuine) wants and goals, she is still accepting her discomfort. Thus, in this view, acceptance does not preclude also putting energy into change, although that energy must not preclude or significantly diminish continuing to work effectively toward genuinely held goals. Once the uncomfortable/ unwanted experience changes to something more comfortable or wanted, of course, the person is no longer demonstrating active accepting behavior (e.g., if the woman in line cools off by fanning herself while still in line). By integrating or synthesizing change strategies (minimizing discomfort) with acceptance strategies (distress tolerance), the woman may effectively be able to attain her goals, with or without discomfort. These are examples of acceptance in a synthesis with change, which is assumed to be effective or healthy in intimate relationships as well.

Of course, tolerating distress is not the only way to be accepting (although tolerance is required, by definition, as long as the experience is distressing or uncomfortable); that is, a person may notice different aspects of the situation, or the relationship between the situation and the discomfort, and create a new stimulus that is less distressing (or not distressing at all). This kind of acceptance involves transforming the initial stimulus for distress into a different stimulus, with different responses. For example, a person may be very distressed that the candy machine has taken his or her money without delivering any candy. After several attempts to shake the machine (nonacceptance), the person may realize that candy is not a very healthy lunch and see the broken candy machine as an opportunity to eat lunch in a more healthy way. Thus, the person may transform the stimulus from one of discomfort ("damn machine took my money") to one of contentment ("Brand X has no protein, vitamins, etc., anyway, so it really isn't a good lunch for me; I'll see if my friend is free, and we'll go get a quick, healthier lunch that's much more satisfying"). The person may still think it is not fair that the machine took the money, but this is no longer a focal point for his or her energy and attention. This is an example of pure acceptance: The change in discomfort is never the goal per se; rather, living in a way that is more consistent with one's values or more likely to achieve one's goals is the target. Moving one's attention toward these goals may (or may not) alter the experience of discomfort or displeasure, but the person will be, overall, more content.

Acceptance in synthesis with change is a different way of considering acceptance. In this view, at least some acceptance is necessary for effective change to occur; that is, the person must be able to recognize the experience of discomfort or displeasure, connect it to some aspect of the situation, and act effectively while still experiencing discomfort. Although change may be the primary motivation, at least minimal acceptance (awareness that the "problem" exists and how it is relevant, and sufficiently low arousal to allow self-control over subsequent actions) is required to change it effectively. Alternatively, if the person does not "accept" the experience or situation in any way and purely acts to escape or change it, there is an increased likelihood that the change-oriented behaviors will be problematic. For example, if one partner is very angry that the other is coming home late and is not in any way accepting, he or she may become extremely aversive very quickly in order to change the situation. Although that may get the other partner to come home (or to stay out longer), the chances of them having a nice evening together are minimized in the process. Alternatively, accepting that the other partner intends to come home late may lead either to pure acceptance (taking advantage of the evening alone to go out with a friend, appreciating the partner's extra efforts at work, etc.) or to acceptance/change (describing how much the working partner would be missed, how disappointed one is, and so forth, which might lead the partner to bring work home and at least join the other for dinner).

Thus, for our purposes, acceptance has several components or defining features: (1) The phenomenon in question is within the person's awareness; (2) the person, regardless of the valence of the experience (pleasant or unpleasant, initially desired or not), is not *presently* focused exclusively on organizing his or her resources to change the experience or the stimulus (or stimuli) that elicited the experience; and (3) the person has an understanding (regardless of its accuracy or veracity) of the relationship between the present private experience and some stimulus, or stimuli, that preceded it. Thus, there are two levels of acceptance: (1) acceptance in balance with change, and (2) pure acceptance. In addition, pure acceptance ranges from simple tolerance to genuine or radical acceptance, in which the experience is transformed from one that is negative to one that is neutral or even positive.

Individual Mindfulness as a Means to Acceptance

Mindfulness as a means to, or form of, acceptance is an ancient concept. For example, mindfulness practice is "at the heart of the Buddha's teachings" (Nhat Hanh, 1998, p. 59), and mindfulness itself has been considered a kind of miracle due to its ability to transform experiences and actions (Nhat Hanh, 1975, 1998). In fact, there are seven "miracles of mindfulness" that all involve attention, understanding, and transaction or transformation (Nhat Hanh, 1998): (1) mindfulness as a means of experiencing (full awareness, contacting) whatever and whomever is in our presence; (2) mindfulness as a means of facilitating others' presence (awareness); (3) mindfulness as means of nourishing or supporting whatever or whomever is the object of your attention; (4) mindfulness of another as a means of ameliorating his or her suffering; (5) mindfulness as a means of "looking deeply," or observing the relationships and interdependence among us; (6) mindfulness as a means of understanding, or becoming aware of connections between individuals and their histories, environments, and us; and (7) mindfulness as a means of transformation of suffering into being, into effective action, into acceptance, into freedom, and/or into peace and joy.

Marsha Linehan (1993a, 1993b) successfully translated these principles of mindfulness into nonspiritually based individual psychological skills, with significant treatment effects across dozens of studies. Although she was among the first behavior therapists to do so, other researchers and treatment developers also have adapted these principles effectively (e.g., many of the authors in this volume). Definitions or descriptions of mindfulness generally include awareness and attention, present-focus, sensitivity to a subset of available stimuli, awareness of connections between self and the external world, and a lack of escape urges from present-experience "mindless" compulsivity (cf. Brown & Ryan, 2003).

Linehan's mindfulness skills (1993b) include two separate, albeit connected, subsets: the "what" skills (what to do to be mindful) and the "how" skills (how to engage in these behaviors). Specifically, the "what" skills include (1) observing or just noticing, or becoming aware of what is present (inside the person or outside); (2) describing what has just been observed, with care to the use of language that is truly descriptive; and (3) participating fully in the behavior (feeling, thinking sensing, acting), without a lot of self-conscious mental activity; letting go of extraneous verbalizations (e.g., descriptions, evaluations, judgments). The idea is that a person can be doing only one of these activities at one time (observing *or* describing *or* participating).

The "how" skills, according to Linehan (1993b) include (1) being nonjudgmental, or forgoing right–wrong, should–shouldn't, and good–bad evaluations; (2) focusing attention in the present on one thing at a time; and (3) putting energy only into actions or activities that are consistent with one's values and life goals (e.g., "describing" a fire burning out of control would not be mindful, whereas getting to safety, helping to warn others, or attempting to extinguish it safely would be mindful). We now explicate an application of mindfulness principles and skills to individual behavior in couple and family interactions.

Individual Mindfulness in Interpersonal Situations

Mindfulness of another person requires the integration of mindfulness of one's own experience with being mindful of another person. In ordinary pleasant or neutral (nonreactive) situations, of course, this is somewhat easier to do. For example, consider that partner A and partner B are happy with each other presently: If during dinner partner A says, "I noticed that the new restaurant that we have been looking forward to trying has finally opened. Maybe we can go there some time this week or next," partner B likely can readily discern that the new restaurant is open and that partner A is interested in trying it out soon. Partner A likely would simply respond with some acknowledgment (validation of partner B's desire/request) and maybe (depending on other factors) agree to go to the restaurant. However, if partner B regularly blames partner A for the couple's financial difficulties and often thinks that partner A is not careful enough with money, is not appreciative enough of how much overtime partner A works to try to keep things stable financially, and that partner A is not committed to paying off their debt, the interaction could unfold quite differently. For example, partner B might start to be judgmental of partner A, which likely leads to anger that partner A made this request, which in turn might lead partner B to criticize partner A (e.g., "I can't believe you are asking me to go to that new, expensive restaurant given the terrible financial situation we're in. You're so selfish, never thinking about how hard I have to work to keep us afloat"). Partner B is not being mindful and is, of course, invalidating partner A in number of ways (e.g., invalidating the legitimacy of partner A wanting to go out to dinner; invalidating partner A globally by making a judgmental accusation such as "selfish," etc.). Being able to respond effectively in these kinds of situations requires a number of acceptance and mindfulness skills. First, the ability to accept our own experiences is required before we can understand and "accept" another person, or another person's behaviors. Accepting our own experiences typically includes a number of separate skills that we discuss next: awareness of one's own emotional reactivity, accurate identification of emotions, and self-validation.

Awareness of Rising Reactivity

The first skill involves an awareness of the fact that one's own emotional arousal is rising, and an ability to connect this rising reactivity to its proximal stimulus (whatever the other person just expressed or described) in a *nonjudgmental* (e.g., descriptive) way. For example, partner B may have noticed increased feelings of anxiety related to finances when partner A brought up a potentially expensive activity. Although this process seems straightforward, it is often very difficult for some people to associate increased reactivity with its proximal stimulus, because primary and secondary emotions may not be accurately identified; that is, they may quickly blame the other person, escalate emotionally, begin to remember past problems, and see the other person's motivation, personality, or judgment of the situation as the stimulus.

Accurate Identification of the Primary Emotion

The ability to label accurately the emotion associated with rising arousal is essential to effective responding. If the emotion is labeled inaccurately, not only will the individual mislead him- or herself into pursuing an ineffective path (responding to the "wrong" emotion) but also the partner will similarly be misled and likely be ineffective in his or her response (either defensive/reactive or inadvertently invalidating). The accurate, normative, authentic, and effective emotional response may be considered the person's *primary* emotion, whereas reactions (learned, often escape-oriented) to the primary emotion may be considered secondary emotions (Greenberg & Safran, 1987; 1989). Secondary emotional responses may be quite rapid and may overwhelm primary emotions, especially if the couple has a history of fighting about the current topic (Fruzzetti & Jacobson, 1990). Mindfulness requires attentional focus on the primary emotion, ignoring any secondary emotional responses or noticing and letting them go by returning attention to the primary emotion. In this example, anxiety, fear, or worry were partner A's primary emotions, whereas anger likely was a secondary emotional response.

Secondary emotional reactions may be learned and become rather automatic (e.g., Greenberg & Safran, 1987) or may be mediated by judgments. Judgments, in turn, lead to rising arousal. The mindful practice of letting go of judgments is very useful in facilitating noticing, discriminating, and labeling primary emotions. In high-conflict situations, anger is a likely secondary emotion (Fruzzetti & Fruzzetti, 2003; Fruzzetti & Levensky, 2000): Judgments about the other person may exacerbate this anger focus, and rising anger often promotes more negative judgments. This process is often incendiary for the partner as well (being judged, being the target of anger), resulting in the well-known process in the couples' literature of negative escalation (e.g., Weiss & Heyman, 1990), which is associated with negative outcomes for relationships and the individuals in them.

Self-Validation

Accurate labeling of emotion is self-validating in and of itself. In addition, understanding the chain and noticing (and describing) the relationship between the antecedent stimulus and the subsequent emotion is also self-validating. In this process, one implicitly says, "It makes sense that I feel this way," without blaming or judging the other person (stimulus).

For individuals who have a lot of judgments and/or rapidly rising reactivity, mindfully describing the situation (stimuli) and their sensations, thoughts, wants, and emotions in temporal order can be helpful. In this way, mindful description may truncate judgments, facilitate self-acceptance and self-validation, and subsequently make listening to and understanding the other person possible.

It is important to point out that being mindful does not require consistent agreement with the other person, not does it mean the mindful person cannot have very strong feelings. For example, partner B might feel very anxious and be very committed to *not* spending money on the restaurant. However, partner B could communicate this descriptively, without judgment, and without invalidating partner A's desires (e.g., "I am so worried about our finances! I know you'd like to try the restaurant—that makes sense, it looks like a nice place—but I would much rather wait until we're out of debt").

Relational Mindfulness as a Means to Acceptance

Remember Context and Long-Term Goals and Values

Making judgments contributes to high emotional arousal, and high arousal interferes with memory and effective problem solving. Therefore, it may be very useful for partners to practice reminding themselves that "this is my partner, my love" or "I love this person, this person loves me, and we both want to work this out together" as a means of interfering with escalating negative reactions. Practicing this kind of self-talk until it is automatic can be very helpful. Similarly, purposefully selecting locations (favorite sofa) or objects (wedding rings, scrapbooks) to become associated with closeness and successful conflict resolution (utilizing associational learning or classical conditioning strategies) can make it easier to reduce reactivity, stay nonjudgmental, and participate effectively in the current task. These activities promote acceptance of one's own experiences and goals, as well as the ability to manage oneself effectively in the service of those goals.

Practicing and Enjoying Being Together

Another application of mindfulness in relationships involves partners staying present and enjoying being together in everyday situations and activities. It is often the case in distressed relationships, or with distressed individuals, that there is so much pain or unpleasantness that a veneer of tension or fear can permeate many situations or interactions, even potentially pleasing ones. It is common for partners then to semiwithdraw, paying attention only to their own experience or individual activity, or to focus on just "getting through" whatever it is they are doing (a kind of noncontact with the world, or anhedonia). Mindfulness is an antidote to this dilemma. Relationally, we call being in this noninteractive, nonmindful state being "passively together," in which awareness of the other person is very limited. Two people might both be watching the same film or television show, sitting at the same dinner table, going to sleep in the same bed, and so forth, but each may be entirely focused on what he or she is doing, with barely any attention on the other person or on being together. Conversely, being "actively together" means that the person deliberately focuses a subset of attention or awareness on the other, utilizing relational mindfulness strategies and skills. Thus, watching a film together might include (1) an awareness that "we are both here, together, watching this movie," and (2) awareness of the other person's reactions to the film. Similar awareness of going to sleep in the same bed, taking a walk together, and so forth, can transform the experience from one that is solitary and tense to one that is more relaxed and connected. Moreover, being actively together does not require a lot of verbal communication, nor does it require mutuality in that moment (i.e., one person can be mindful of the other even if the other is not noticing or doing the same). Finally, it is also possible to be "interactively together," which requires that each partner's attention and awareness essentially be focused on the other and the transaction. This may be verbal or nonverbal and requires mutual participation and full engagement in the moment rather than simply engaging in something that involves the other partner. This can be done in conversation, sitting together on the sofa, during breakfast, on the telephone, during sexual activity, or in virtually any situation that does not require a lot of attention to the noninterpersonal aspects of the task itself (e.g., driving, cooking, and watching a film require attention to those activities, whereas dinner table conversation allows exclusive focus on each other and on the interaction). Practicing being actively or interactively together may be useful not only for relationship enhancement in general by promoting intimacy but it also may facilitate the ability to be mindful when the situation is tense or difficult, which can in turn promote understanding and validation, minimizing emotional distance and emotion dysregulation.

Awareness/Mindfulness of Partner

Once a person can manage his or her own reactivity in a conflict situation, it is possible to observe and to listen mindfully. Relationship mindfulness employs the same skills as individual mindfulness (e.g., Linehan, 1993b), but the object of mindful attention is the other person, in order to facilitate understanding and subsequent validation. Thus, this involves (1) observing or noticing the other's facial expression, suffering or joy, emotion, wants, opinions, reactivity, and so on; (2) describing these behaviors and how they are connected (descriptively, not interpretively) to one's own behaviors and the situation; describing the relations between the other person's feelings, wants, and so on, and one's own behavior or the situation; describing one's own responses as one listens mindfully (e.g., "It makes sense that you'd feel *x* when I said *y*"); and (3) participating in the transaction (noticing the relationship between what one partner experiences or expresses and the other's responses). Again, similar to individual mindfulness, this includes staying nonjudgmental, staying present in the conversation (not thinking about or bringing up things from past arguments), and staying effective (e.g., remembering that the other person is someone one loves, considering changing something in response to the other's needs or requests).

The ability to listen mindfully (not mitigated by one's own reactivity or judgments) and understand the partner's experiences and expressions makes it possible to communicate that understanding and alleviate suffering in the partner. Of course, there are many different levels of legitimacy and understanding, and many different ways to validate that legitimacy and communicate understanding. We now turn our attention to the different ways to validate.

VALIDATING AND INVALIDATING BEHAVIORS

Evidence from both self-report and observational studies indicates that couples' emotional communication has an enormous impact on relationship quality. Validation is at the core of couples' communication, because it communicates acceptance and understanding, and results in lowered arousal and vulnerability; conversely, invalidating behaviors communicate criticism, contempt, dismissiveness, illegitimacy, and disregard, and result in increased arousal and vulnerability (Fruzzetti & Fruzzetti, 2003; Swann, 1997). Relationships are complex, particularly when one or both partners are experiencing both individual and relationship distress. Thus, a successful intimate relationship meets and balances both partners' needs at a personal and relational level, and is rich in both disclosure and validating responses. Validation communicates understanding and acceptance, and consequently builds trust and intimacy. After regulating one's own emotion, listening mindfully to the other until nonjudgmental understanding is reached, acceptance can be communicated via validation. At its most basic level, validation is anything that communicates acceptance and understanding of the other person's thoughts, wants, emotions, actions, goals, or other behaviors in a clear and nonjudgmental manner. Because we typically define ourselves according to our thoughts, emotions, wants, and other behaviors, validation communicates acceptance of the person as a valued human being. Validating is saying, "I respect and accept who you are as an individual today and how you have become the person you are today."

Of course, as with individual acceptance, there are two levels of acceptance of another person: (1) acceptance in balance with change; and (2) pure acceptance. Thus, acceptance is possible both when change is not a desired outcome at all, and when change remains a desired goal. This is an essential point, because acceptance is defined frequently as the opposite of change. Here, acceptance can be an effective, integral part of change, or it may stand alone (signifying no change goals whatsoever).

Targets of Validation

Any behavior of the other person can be validated (legitimized, understood, acknowledged). We can validate our partner's emotions, what we actually see or hear, or what we imagine our partner may be feeling after listening mindfully to the situation or stimuli. We can also validate wants and desires or goals, as well as thoughts, beliefs, and opinions. It is important to be mindful that we do not have to have the same wants, sensations, emotions, or other experiences as others to validate them: The fact that they want what they want, feel what they feel, think what they think, and are doing what they are doing means that the behavior is valid in some way. However, the way that we validate communicates the ways that things are (and are not) valid or legitimate, or specific ways that the other person's behavior makes sense. Thus, we must consider these different ways of communicating understanding and note how important it is to match the validating response to the ways in which the other's behavior is actually valid.

Types of Validation

The following section describes different types of validating responses, and is an integration of research on couple behaviors (e.g., Fruzzetti, 1995, 2001) and an explication of validation in psychotherapy (Linehan, 1997).

Mindful Listening

What we earlier described as relationship or partner mindfulness is actually a basic, and essential, component of validating the other. This includes empathic attention that may be nonverbal or minimally verbal. Mindful listening means *really* paying attention, not distracted by one's own reactivity, and involves communicating that attention to the other person. Behavioral indicators of mindful listening include eye contact or gaze, head nodding, not engaging in other activities, and facial expressions that express interest. It is not enough to listen: It is also essential to communicate that attention. For couples, this often includes turning the television off, putting the newspaper down, or going to a quiet place where self-expression or self-disclosure and mindful listening are easier.

Reflecting and Acknowledging

This includes empathically reflective comments, especially of the other person's expressions of private experiences, such as emotions, wants, and thoughts, as well as just acknowledging "what is" actually present. The person communicates understanding by saying/reflecting back or otherwise acknowledging what he or she hears the other saying. Individuals do not have to repeat their partner's statements back word for word (and probably should not, because it sounds rote and disingenious), but instead should convey the essence of their partner's expression. Behavioral indicators of this include verbalizing what is observed, such as saying, "I can see you are upset," "You look tired," or "Sounds like you are feeling sad."

There are no interpretations in this type of validating response, and one can validate in this way even when disagreeing with the content. For example, partner A might say, "You're late again. You obviously don't listen to me and don't care about what I want." Even if partner B thinks he does listen and does care about partner A, he can still validate some important things here: "You're right, I'm late. And I can see you're really upset with me." This validating response may well begin to help abate partner A's high negative arousal, and might therefore make further effective communication possible, which may lead to enhanced closeness and individual well-being (rather than distance, isolation, negative mood, and distress).

Paradoxically, effective validating responses can facilitate effective *invalidating* responses. For example, after validating partner A's feelings, partner B may be able to invalidate some of partner A's thoughts (assuming they are not accurate descriptions of partner B): "It makes sense that you're upset with me for being late: I didn't call, and wasn't very sensitive to what you wanted to do. But I do care about what you want, and I'm committed to communicating better with you about our plans. Here's what I'll try to do from now on . . . " Thus, it is important to note that this kind of validation does not have to include complete agreement with the partner; rather, is an expression of accurate understanding of his or her perspective or experience, reflecting or acknowledging the other's feelings descriptively and nonjudgmentally.

Clarifying and Summarizing

This involves gentle, empathic attempts to understand what the partner is feeling privately, even though not yet clarified by the partner him- or herself. This can involve summarizing the partner's perspective or even asking questions of clarification. Behavioral indices of clarifying and summarizing include offering ideas about what the partner is thinking, feeling, or wanting based on the situation, knowledge about his or her prior responses to these kinds of situations, or an understanding of common responses to these kinds of situations. Asking questions about what the other might be thinking, wanting, or feeling, or questions about the situation, may also be validating.

Putting Problem Behavior in a Larger Context

This type of validating response is appropriate when a person has done something problematic and is at risk for high negative arousal, negative self- (or other-) judgments, and is therefore at risk for further problem behavior. It involves recontextualizing the problem behavior to include a broader array of "context," including past events or behaviors that were less problematic, or acknowledging the person's limited repertoire (e.g., due to learning history, biological limitations), but without blaming him or her and still acknowledging one's own role (when relevant). Putting problem behavior into a larger context does not mean ignoring or minimizing the problem; rather, it involves balancing the problem behavior by also noticing legitimate other factors or behaviors. For example, if a person said some very nasty things last night, a validating response might be, "Yes, what you said was very hurtful. But I was no saint in this discussion either. And rather than just leaving the house like you used to do, you stuck around, calmed yourself down, and you're willing to work on some repairs."

Normalizing

This type of validating response involves finding the "of course" in a given situation. In other words, it normalizes the partner's behavior. This communicates to the partner that his or her behavior (action, emotion, want, etc.) is understandable and normative. Behavioral indicators of normalizing behaviors include statements such as "I would feel that way too" or "Of course, you responded that way; that makes perfect sense," or "It makes complete sense that you would feel that way; anybody would." This requires finding the clearly normative or "legitimate" parts of a partner's disclosures and letting him or her know you or anyone would feel that way given the situation. For example, if one partner comes home late and is exhausted because traffic was slow due to a snowstorm, the other could say, "It is so exhausting when the snow is blowing and visibility is low, and you have to crawl along. Anybody would be tired after an hour of that."

Expressing Equality and Respect

This is characterized by practicing willingness, empathic or radical genuineness (e.g., Linehan, 1997), and involves acceptance of the partner as a person of worth and equal value. This also involves not treating the person as fragile (not "walking on eggshells") and a willingness to allow ordinary suffering (knowing that the person will be OK). Thus, validation at this level includes a willingness to stay with or even enhance the strength of the person's "negative" emotion, treating the other as an equal and competent person. For example, if one's partner is sad because a close friend has died, one can be sad with the partner rather than trying to cheer him or her up. Similarly, if one partner has done something problematic, the other would neither avoid acknowledging the problem, nor minimize it.

Reciprocating (Matching) Vulnerability

This involves allowing oneself to be vulnerable when the other is vulnerable. The person is willing to match the other person's level of vulnerability through his or her own vulnerable self-disclosures. For example, if one partner says, "I am sad because we have been fighting a lot lately and I do not feel as close to you," a validating statement would be, "I've been feeling sad, too, that we have not been close." This type of validating response typically has the form of self-disclosure, but its function is to reassure, or validate, the safety in the other's vulnerability and the mutual importance of the relationship. Even though the validating person is also disclosing, the focus of this part of the interaction stays on the first partner.

Responding with Action

Sometimes a validating response involves action rather than words. For example, if one partner says she's hungry, the other can make her breakfast. If one person discloses that he's sad, the other can sit close or give him a hug. Validating with action demonstrates a clear understanding of what has been expressed.

TRUE (RADICAL) ACCEPTANCE
AND CLOSENESS IN RELATIONSHIPS

Conflict sometimes leads to successful problem solving, and desired changes in one or both persons' behavior can be implemented. This can be quite useful. However, some "problems" cannot be solved easily, and ongoing attempts to change the other person, and frustration about the lack of change, can be very corrosive to the relationship and to the individuals involved. For example, it is common for couples to struggle chronically over how much closeness to have; ironically, this conflict significantly erodes closeness and intimacy. Similarly, chronic displeasure over nonchange (e.g., "He still leaves dirty clothes on the floor [or other undesirable behavior] after all these requests to pick them up") can be corrosive. Interestingly, the lack of acceptance on the part of one partner may be at least as corrosive as the lack of change in the other; this polarization is itself a part of the problem. The question is, what does one do after exhaustive efforts have been made to facilitate change (or even to demand it), and change still has not occurred? True or radical acceptance may provide one answer. Individual and relational mindfulness can be employed to resolve these kinds of difficulties, to facilitate true acceptance, and sometimes even to transform conflict into closeness and ameliorate the suffering of individual partners.

Step 1: Individual Mindfulness

In this step, the person has to become aware that his or her attempts to solve the problem (e.g., requesting, demanding, nagging the other to change) have become problems themselves. The "solution" is the "the problem," and the person no longer wants to live this way, expending a lot of energy trying to change something that, realistically, is not going to change at all, or at least not this way. This also involves the acknowledgment that giving up the struggle for change likely means that the person will not get something desired, and must therefore balance short- and long-term ("big picture") desires.

If the conclusion to this mindful exploration includes statements such as (1) "I don't like the consequences for me, my partner, and/or my relationship of my efforts to get him or her to change," and (2) "Maybe I can tolerate his or her not changing," then the person may be willing to stop engaging in the previous (failed) attempts at change.

Step Two: Behavioral Tolerance

In this step, the person decides to cease and desist previous change-oriented behaviors that were the stimulus for negative escalation, and tolerate the behavior in question. The partner stops targeting partner change, stops putting energy into changing the other. This requires changing one's own overt behaviors, and no longer asking, demanding, nagging, or otherwise attempting to get the other person to change. It also requires tolerating one's own disappointment (acknowledging that one is forgoing a desired outcome, and even grieving that loss) and possibly letting go of anger and judgments about the partner (or oneself). This step alone may have a salutary effect on the partner and, in turn, on the couple's interactions (perhaps reducing conflict and offering more opportunities for closeness).

Step 3: Pattern Awareness

Even after one partner stops the corrosive and ineffective attempts to get the other to change, thoughts about the change goals might still be present, as well as judgments and negative emotion about the status quo (lack of desired change). Becoming aware of the pattern includes noticing the costs to oneself, the partner, and the relationship of "hanging on" to desires for change and judgments about the partner resulting from a lack of change. In this intermediate step, the focus turns from tolerating disappointment or anger to ceasing to complain (or other change-focused activity), to noticing the full range of toxicity that has resulted from an "extreme" focus on changing the partner's behavior. Noticing the consequences of ongoing disappointment and anger, such as increased vulnerability for more conflict due to higher arousal states (e.g., not asking for change overtly, but thinking about it, being frustrated by the lack of it), consequent emotional distance, and so forth, is part of the task in this step. It also includes the realization that this focus on change interferes with mindful participation in the relationship, leading to distance and unhappiness for both partners. These observations may lead to increased motivation for true or more radical acceptance.

It may be possible for partners to engage in conversations about their patterns, and these conversations may provide opportunities for a lot of increased understanding. When both partners are discussing each other's behaviors descriptively, seeing things not as one person's faults but as a transaction, as a dance that includes both partners, defensiveness may abate and heightened empathy and understanding (with concomitant validation) may follow.

Step 4: True or Radical Acceptance and Synthesis of Conflict into Closeness

In this step, the person may realize that the behavior of the partner that he or she formerly defined as a "problem" actually has other "meanings"; that is, by looking more deeply and mindfully (cf. Nhat Hanh, 1998) it is possible to see the behavior descriptively in its historical context (e.g., how the person reasonably came to do these things, including one's own role in the development of the behavior), and descriptively in its present, larger context (e.g., the partner is often late in part because he or she works hard, not just because he or she is insensitive to requests to come home earlier). Remembering the larger goals (i.e., "This is my partner, my life") can facilitate willingness to engage in this kind of interaction. Similarly, employing the other strategies of mindfulness and relationship mindfulness described earlier can prevent rapidly rising reactivity that otherwise could lead to further conflict in the old, repetitious, corrosive style. Alternatively, providing descriptions (or accurate self-disclosures) helps the formerly "offending" party to validate, providing healing (and reinforcing a more three-dimensional, non-problem-focused view of the behavior in its context). The goal is to describe more fully, less judgmentally; to understand the origins of the target behavior descriptively; to pay attention to what is, rather than what is not; to listen mindfully to the partner and respond with respect, compassion, and acceptance of his or her experience (validate); to let go of focus on difference; to participate together in the relationship without the "gaps" in closeness that result from nonacceptance; to transcend the "I" and achieve a "we" via participation, willingness, and reciprocity.

With repeated experience describing rather than judging, disclosing rather than demanding, and listening, participating, and validating rather than avoiding or attacking, the former conflict can be transformed into genuine understanding and closeness.

CONCLUSIONS

Problematic relationship patterns have long been associated with not only relationship dissatisfaction and dissolution but also individual distress and psychopathology. Employing a transactional model of relationships that includes both conflict and closeness may have salutary effects on relationships and on the well-being of individuals in those relationships. Moreover, validating partner experiences of wanting, feeling, and so on may play a central role in how those private experiences are processed, and may therefore play an integral part in the alleviation of psychopathology in couples. This transaction between accurate self-description or self-disclosure and partner validation needs further study. The steps suggested provide alternatives to chronic conflict, distance, and distress, utilizing both pure acceptance and a synthesis of acceptance and change strategies.

REFERENCES

Addis, M. E., & Jacobson, N. S. (1996). Reasons for depression and the process and outcome of cognitive-behavioral psychotherapies. *Journal of Consulting and Clinical Psychology, 64*, 1417–1424.

Arkowitz-Weston, L., & Fruzzetti, A. E. (2004). *Beyond negativity: The role of acceptance and validation in predicting couple relationship quality.* Unpublished manuscript, University of Nevada, Reno.

Beach, S. R. H., & O'Leary, K. D. (1992). Treating depression in the context of marital discord: Outcome and predictors of response of marital therapy versus cognitive therapy. *Behavior Therapy, 23*, 507–528.

Biglan, A., Hops, H., Sherman, L., Freidman, L. S., Arthur, J., & Osteen, V. (1985). Problem-solving interaction of depressed women and their husbands. *Behavior Therapy*, *16*, 431–451.

Binswanger, L. (1956). Existential analysis and psychotherapy. In E. Fromm-Reichmann & J. L. Moreno (Eds.), *Progress in psychotherapy* (pp. 144–168). New York: Grune & Stratton.

Brown, K. W., & Ryan, R. M. (2003). The benefits of being present: Mindfulness and its role in psychological well-being. *Psychological Science*, *14*, 822–848.

Campbell, L., & Fruzzetti, A. E. (2004). *Cohesion as ersatz intimacy: Its role in individual and couple well being*. Unpublished manuscript, University of Nevada, Reno.

Campbell, T. L. (2003). The effectiveness of family intervention for physical disorders. *Journal of Marital and Family Therapy*, *29*, 263–281.

Cascardi, M., O'Leary, K. D., Lawrence, E. E., & Schlee, K. A. (1995). Characteristics of women physically abused by their spouses and who seek treatment regarding marital conflict. *Journal of Consulting and Clinical Psychology*, *63*, 616–623.

Fincham, F. D., & Beach, S. R. H. (1999). Conflict in marriage: Implications for working with couples. *Annual Review of Psychology*, *50*, 47–77.

Fruzzetti, A. E. (1995). *The closeness–distance family interaction coding system: A functional approach to coding couple interactions*. Coding manual, University of Nevada, Reno.

Fruzzetti, A. E. (1996). Causes and consequences: Individual distress in the context of couples interactions. *Journal of Consulting and Clinical Psychology*, *64*, 1192–1201.

Fruzzetti, A. E. (2001). *Validating and Invalidating Behavior Coding Scale manual (Version 3.1)*. Reno: University of Nevada.

Fruzzetti, A. E., & Fruzzetti, A. R. (2003). Borderline personality disorder. In D. K Snyder & M. A. Whisman (Eds.), *Treating difficult couples: Helping clients with coexisting mental and relationship disorders* (pp. 235–260). New York: Guilford Press.

Fruzzetti, A. E., & Jacobson, N. S. (1990). Toward a behavioral conceptualization of adult intimacy: Implications for marital therapy. In E. A. Blechman (Ed.), *Emotions and the family: For better or for worse* (pp. 117–135). Hillsdale, NJ: Erlbaum.

Fruzzetti, A. E., & Levensky, E. R. (2000). Dialectical behavior therapy for domestic violence: Rationale and procedures. *Cognitive and Behavioral Practice*, *7*, 435–447.

Fruzzetti, A. E., & Boulanger, J. (2004). *A behavioral approach to understanding borderline personality and related disorders*. Unpublished manuscript, University of Nevada, Reno.

Fruzzetti, A. E., Lowry, K. Mosco, E., & Shenk, C. (2003). Emotion regulation: Rationale and strategies. In W. T. O' Donohue, J. E. Fisher & S. C. Hayes (Eds.), *Empirically supported techniques of cognitive behavior therapy: A step-by-step guide for clinicians* (pp. 152–159). New York: Wiley.

Greenberg, L. S., & Safran, J. D. (1987). *Emotion in psychotherapy*. New York: Guilford Press.

Greenberg, L. S., & Safran, J. D. (1989). Emotion in psychotherapy. *American Psychologist*, *44*, 19–29.

Gross, J. J. (1998). The emerging field of emotion regulation: An integrative review. *Review of General Psychology*, *2*, 271–299.

Guttman, H. A. (1986). Epistemology, systems theories and the theory of family therapy. *American Journal of Family Therapy*, *14*, 13–22.

Hooley, J. M., & Hoffman, P. D. (1999). Expressed emotion and clinical outcome in borderline personality disorder. *American Journal of Psychiatry*, *156*, 1557–1562.

Hooley, J. M., Orley, J., & Teasdale, J. D. (1986). Levels of expressed emotion and relapse in depressed patients. *British Journal of Psychiatry*, *148*, 642–647.

Jacobson, N. S., Dobson, K., Fruzzetti, A. E., Schmaling, K. B., & Salusky, S. (1991). Marital therapy as a treatment for depression. *Journal of Consulting and Clinical Psychology*, *59*, 547–557.

Jacobson, N. S., Fruzzetti, A. E., Dobson, K., Whisman, M., & Hops, H. (1993). Couple therapy as a treatment for depression: II. The effects of relationship quality and therapy on depressive relapse. *Journal of Consulting and Clinical Psychology, 6,* 516–519.

Jacobson, N. S., & Margolin, G. (1979). *Marital therapy: Strategies based on social learning and behavior exchange principles.* New York: Brunner/Mazel.

Keltner, D., & Kring, A. M. (1998). Emotion, social function, and psychopathology. *Review of General Psychology, 2,* 320–342.

Linehan, M. M. (1993a). *Cognitive-behavioral treatment of borderline personality disorder.* New York: Guilford Press.

Linehan, M. M. (1993b). *Skills training manual for treating borderline personality disorder.* New York: Guilford Press.

Linehan, M. M. (1997). Validation and psychotherapy. In A. Bohart & L. S. Greenberg (Eds.), *Empathy and psychotherapy: New directions to theory, research, and practice* (pp. 343–392). Washington, DC: American Psychological Association.

Markman, H. J. (1991). Constructive marital conflict is NOT an oxymoron. *Journal of Family Psychology, 4,* 416–425.

O'Leary, K. D., Christian, J. L., & Mendell, N. R. (1994). A closer look at the link between marital discord and depressive symptomatology. *Journal of Social and Clinical Psychology, 14,* 1–9.

Skinner, B. F. (1953). *Science and human behavior.* New York: Free Press.

Southham-Gerow, M. A., & Kendall, P. C. (2002). Emotion regulation and understanding: Implications for child psychopathology and therapy. *Clinical Psychology Review, 22,* 189–222.

Swann, W. B. (1997). The trouble with change: Self-verification and allegiance to the self. *Psychological Science, 8*(3), 177–180.

Nhat Hanh, T. (1975). *The miracle of mindfulness: A manual on meditation.* Boston: Beacon Press.

Nhat Hanh, T. (1998). *The heart of the Buddha's teaching: Transforming suffering into peace, joy, and liberation.* Berkeley, CA: Parallax Press.

Thompson, R. A. (1994). Emotion regulation: A theme in search of definition. *Monographs of the Society for Research in Child Development, 59,* 24–52.

Thorp, S. R., & Fruzzetti, A. E. (2004). *Predicting course of disorder in psychiatric outpatients: The impact of validation and invalidation by cohabiting partners.* Unpublished manuscript, University of Nevada, Reno.

Waring, E. M., & Patton, D. (1984). Marital intimacy and depression. *British Journal of Psychiatry, 145,* 641–644.

Weiss, R. L., & Heyman, R. E. (1990). Observation of marital interaction. In F. D. Fincham & T. N. Bradbury (Eds.), *The psychology of marriage: Basic issues and applications* (pp. 87–117). New York: Guilford Press.

Weissman, M. M., & Paykel, E. S. (1974). *The depressed woman: A study of social relationships.* Chicago: University of Chicago Press.

Whisman, M. A., & Bruce, M. L. (1999). Marital dissatisfaction and incidence of major depressive episode in a community sample. *Journal of Abnormal Psychology, 108,* 674–678.

Whisman, M. A., Sheldon, C. T., & Goering, P. (2000). Psychiatric disorders and dissatisfaction with social relationships: Does type matter? *Journal of Abnormal Psychology, 109,* 803–808.

9

Acceptance, Mindfulness, and Trauma

Victoria M. Follette, Kathleen M. Palm,
and Mandra L. Rasmussen Hall

Understanding the long-term effects of trauma continues to be a complex and controversial topic. Recent literature has debated not only the prevalence rates of abuse experiences but also whether the impact of such experiences are indeed "traumatic." While these debates are important and have led to a higher standard of research in the field of traumatic stress, it remains clear that, in the normal course of life experiences, one will face a number of life stressors that have an important influence on psychological well-being. The range of events that have been labeled traumatic runs the gamut from combat experiences, rape, and child physical and sexual abuse to natural disasters and motor vehicle accidents, to name just a few examples. Similarly, the outcomes associated with these experiences have spanned a range of intra- and interpersonal problems. Posttraumatic stress disorder (PTSD), depression, anxiety, substance abuse, relationship difficulties, and suicide are among the psychological sequelae that have been associated with trauma (Polusny & Follette, 1995). In our work, we have avoided a syndromal approach to the problems associated with trauma and have focused on a more behavior analytic approach to understanding trauma symptoms (Follette, 1994; Pistorello & Follette, 2000). In particular, our work has at its core an emphasis on mindfulness, acceptance, and relationship. In this chapter, we present an integrative behavioral approach for survivors of trauma.

Our treatment of trauma survivors is guided by a fundamental principle of a contextual behavioral approach: Behavior is best understood in terms of its function rather than its form. For example, if a trauma survivor reported self-mutilation, instead of solely attending to the behavior or a particular diagnosis, we would focus on the how that behavior functions in the person's environment. Given the variety of clinical presentations observed in trauma survivors, understanding the behaviors in context provides the most useful opportunity for case conceptualization. We take a pragmatic approach to treatment planning that is based on an analysis of the client's strengths and vulnerabilities. As is true with all the new behavior therapies described in this text, we focus on both observable and nonobservable behavior in assessing the client's concerns. While this might be seen as stating the obvious, in many professional and public realms, the misconception remains that behaviorists are not concerned with thoughts and feelings.

We believe that a functional analysis of client problems is essential in planning treatment for trauma survivors. As explicated in Naugle and Follette (1998), not doing so puts the client and therapist at risk of focusing on the trauma as the cause of all the client's complaints, when other factors may also be relevant. Conversely, we believe that it is equally true that ignoring a client's history, including a history of trauma, is not only potentially invalidating but also inadequate, in that important etiological variables may be overlooked. We examine both distal and proximal variables in the case conceptualization process. For example, in the case of a history of child sexual abuse, the therapist would consider the environment in the family of origin, including any sources of positive emotional support in addition to the abuse. It is also important to take into account current stressors such as couple issues or work–school stress that might be significant in understanding the client's issues (Follette, Ruzek, & Abueg, 1998). This is one of the primary dialectics that underlie our treatment approach. Specifically, we balance both the trauma history and current stressors in forming a contextual conceptualization of the case. Additionally, we attend to issues involving the therapeutic relationship, including validation, at all stages of the treatment process. The central importance of these concerns, not simply as an adjunct to therapy, but as an ongoing treatment concern, is discussed in more detail later in this chapter.

AN INTEGRATIVE BEHAVIORAL APPROACH

In our work with trauma survivors, primarily women with a history of interpersonal victimization, we have found it useful to integrate several therapies with differing emphases depending on the individual client's needs. In order to avoid theoretical eclecticism in the integration of these treatments, it is important to understand how these concepts fit within a clinical conceptualization and theoretical framework that guide treatment. The use of a combination of dialectical behavior therapy (DBT; Linehan, 1993), acceptance and commitment therapy (ACT; Hayes, Strosahl, & Wilson, 1999), and functional analytic psychotherapy (FAP; Kohlenberg & Tsai, 1991) has provided us the maximum flexibility in tailoring treatment to clients' needs, without sacrificing an overarching philosophical approach to therapy (Palm & Follette, 2000). These therapies are principle-driven and theoretically consistent, with explicated mechanisms of change. We also use a somewhat modified version of exposure therapy (Foa & Rothbaumm, 1998) to address specifically some aspects of posttraumatic symptomology, such as intrusions and flashbacks. In the early phases of treatment, our primary agenda is to assist the client in developing the requisite skills for actively engaging the treatment, which will focus on the problems associated with emotional avoidance. Attention to the therapeutic relationship is essential in providing a foundation for the very difficult work that we ask of the client (Hembree & Foa, 2003).

This chapter presents a general overview of our therapy approach, with an explanation of how these concepts relate to the behavioral treatment of trauma symptomology. Specifically, this chapter (1) presents experiential avoidance as one theoretical conceptualization of a variety of clinical problems that may also explain the long-term correlates of trauma; (2) describes the concepts of acceptance and mindfulness, including a brief discussion of three contemporary behavioral treatments that incorporate these practices in therapy; and (3) discusses a modified treatment approach for trauma survivors that incorporates mindfulness and acceptance practices into traditional exposure treatment.

EXPERIENTIAL AVOIDANCE

Researchers have suggested that functional classification of psychopathology, compared to a more traditional syndromal approach, increases identification of underlying change processes and strengthens treatment utility (Hayes, Wilson, Gifford, Follette, & Strosahl, 1996). Understanding that topographically different behaviors have functional similarity yields powerful implications for treatment. This approach allows for the treatment of functionally relevant specified behaviors (e.g., hypervigilance; attempts to avoid specific thoughts, feelings, or activities; detachment from others) rather than the amelioration of collections of symptoms (e.g., PTSD).

Experiential avoidance is conceptualized as a functional diagnostic dimension that may organize the topographies of several different forms of psychopathology, including substance abuse, anxiety disorders, obsessive–compulsive disorder, and PTSD. Specifically, experiential avoidance is "the phenomenon that occurs when a person is unwilling to remain in contact with particular private experiences (e.g., bodily sensations, emotions, thoughts, memories, behavioral predispositions) and takes steps to alter the form or frequency of these events and the contexts that occasion them" (Hayes et al., 1996, p. 1154). While some forms of avoidance may sometimes serve a useful function, for example, not thinking about an argument with one's partner while conducting a therapy session, we are interested in efforts to escape, avoid, or control thoughts, emotions, memories, and other private experiences that interfere with living a valued life. For example, a person with agoraphobia may engage in a number of overt efforts to avoid symptoms of panic; however, in doing so, she is not able to be involved in important functions she values, such as attending her children's school activities or pursuing work opportunities.

Similarly, experiential avoidance may provide a useful way of understanding the long-term correlates associated with a history of trauma. While trauma survivors' emotional responses, thoughts, and memories are themselves not pathological, attempts to avoid or eliminate those experiences may become so (Follette, 1994; Hayes, 1994). Empirical support for this idea can be seen in the suppression literature. Studies demonstrate that efforts to control one's mood and thoughts may paradoxically cause those experiences to continue (Salkovskis & Campbell, 1994; Wegner, Erber, & Zanakos, 1993), and may also lead to engaging in maladaptive behaviors. Polusny and Follette (1995) suggest that individuals with a history of trauma may seek to avoid or escape negative private events, such as distressing thoughts and feelings about their trauma histories, by engaging in behaviors such as dissociation, substance abuse, and self-injury. While these behaviors may provide survivors of trauma with short-term relief from negative internal events, clearly, they can be associated with other difficulties. For example, substance abuse may be highly reinforced by the temporary reduction of aversive private experiences, including memories of the trauma, painful emotions, sexual dysfunction, and thoughts such as "I'm worthless" or "I can't handle feeling like this." However, substance abuse can contribute to further problems, such as interpersonal difficulties, withdrawal symptoms, depression, revictimization, and risk of exposure to human immunodeficiency virus (HIV). These problems often create more aversive thoughts and feelings from which to escape, either through continued drug use or more lethal means (e.g., suicide, parasuicide; see Polusny & Follette, 1995, for a more detailed discussion). Moreover, a number of other problems such as depression, anxiety, and relationship distress may also be mediated by avoidance (Hayes et al., 1996).

ACCEPTANCE AND MINDFULNESS
IN THE TREATMENT OF TRAUMA

Psychotherapy Outcome Research

While broad-based outcome research related to the treatment of trauma is still in a relatively early phase of development (e.g., compared to depression), there is a growing literature on acknowledged therapies for the treatment of trauma. Most of these approaches focus on decreasing distress related to reminders of the traumatic event and minimizing behavioral inhibition. The treatment outcome literature for trauma has been primarily in the areas of cognitive-behavioral therapy (CBT), eye movement desensitization reprocessing (EMDR), and psychotropic medications (Foa, Keane, & Friedman, 2000). While these treatment approaches have shown promising results and seem to be generally equivalent (Hembree & Foa, 1993), there remain a number of areas for treatment enhancement for trauma survivors. For example, issues related to comorbidity, mechanisms of change, and differential response patterns are not fully understood.

McFarlane and Yehuda (2000) note that upon close examination of treatment outcome data, therapy gains do not seem to be dependent on confrontation of the feared event. For example, stress inoculation therapy (SIT), which focuses on current stressors, is more efficacious at posttreatment than exposure (Foa et al., 1999). Furthermore, Foa and colleagues (1999) did not find significant differences between CBT, SIT, or supportive counseling at follow-up. Other researchers and clinicians have found that exposure to the feared event alone is not effective for some people (Becker & Zayfert, 2001; Cloitre, Koenen, Cohen, & Han, 2002). However, Foa's exposure-based CBT, which is based on emotional processing theory, has considerable empirical support and continues to set a standard in the field (Jaycox, Zoellner, & Foa, 2002).

Roth, Newman, Pelcovitz, van der Kolk, and Mandel (1997) reported that, in addition to reports of PTSD symptoms, emotion regulation problems and interpersonal difficulties were reported with equal, if not greater, frequencies among patients with PTSD. An inability to regulate emotional responses and difficulties in interpersonal relationships may be part of the pre- and posttraumatic factors that maintain poor functioning among individuals with PTSD. Furthermore, Cloitre and colleagues (2002) argue that these factors may lead to complications in using exposure-based treatments, especially for child abuse survivors. Not addressing impairments in emotion regulation and interpersonal difficulties early in treatment may lead to symptom exacerbation, high dropout rates, and compliance problems (Pitman et al., 1991; Scott & Stradling, 1997; Tarrier et al., 1999; as cited in Cloitre et al., 2002).

Researchers have identified some differential characteristics between treatment responders and nonresponders to exposure-based treatment.

Skills deficits in distress tolerance and emotion regulation, vulnerability to dissociation under stress, and inability to maintain a good working relationship with a therapist are all factors associated with nonresponse to treatment (Chemtob, Novaco, Hamada, Gross, & Smith, 1997; Cloitre & Koenen, 2001; Jaycox & Foa, 1996). Cloitre and colleagues (2002) found that skills training in affective and interpersonal regulation before conducting exposure resulted in significant improvements in functioning. In particular, they found that improvements in emotion regulation and positive therapeutic alliance during skills training were significant predictors of PTSD symptomatology reduction during exposure. Significant changes in affect regulation and anger expression occurred only during the skills training phase of the study, whereas PTSD symptoms decreased only during exposure. These findings suggest that including skills training in emotion regulation and interpersonal effectiveness before conducting exposure may lead to better outcomes than doing exposure alone.

Becker and Zayfert (2001) have described a treatment approach for PTSD that integrates the theory and techniques of DBT (Linehan, 1993) with manualized exposure-based CBT for PTSD. They base their treatment model on the observation that a large number of individuals with PTSD exhibit a wide range of problems similar to those experienced by individuals with borderline personality disorder (BPD), including intense negative emotion, rapid cycling of negative emotion, and chaotic life situations. They suggest that DBT increases therapist confidence in delivering exposure treatment in the face of complex clinical presentations by (1) providing a set of skills to individuals who may traditionally become overwhelmed by exposure, and (2) offering a nonpejorative stance from which the therapist can maintain effective delivery of treatment. This is hypothesized to allow the therapist to "make sense of avoidance behaviors without becoming frustrated; conceptualize seemingly manipulative behaviors as unskilled attempts to get valid needs met; and maintain a positive orientation toward patients even when they behave in ways that would elicit negative emotional reactions" (Becker & Zayfert, 2001, p. 110). They assert that integrating DBT with exposure treatment may allow "exposure intolerant" individuals with PTSD to deal with a wide range of difficulties that interfere with exposure, including intense negative emotion, suicidal ideation, and dissociation, before proceeding with exposure treatment. They suggest that this approach facilitates successful completion of exposure treatment in a population of individuals with PTSD who would otherwise drop out of treatment.

Becker and Zayfert's (2001) utilization of DBT theory and techniques in treating a challenging subpopulation of individuals with PTSD is well explicated and is an exciting development in the exposure treatment literature. These researchers emphasize that manualized CBT for PTSD is the core treatment of their model, whereas DBT is added as a supplement to

enhance the core treatment. However, in our view, there is some philosophical tension that occurs in the combination of these two treatments. These
researchers emphasize the importance of DBT's dialectical balance of acceptance and change in understanding and treating the complex presentation of PTSD. They also recognize the potentially invalidating nature of
CBT techniques, particularly cognitive restructuring. However, in response,
they incorporate validation as a strategy for reducing any invalidation experienced by the client, *while* continuing to implement cognitive restructuring as a key component in the treatment. Furthermore, manualized exposure treatment for PTSD is based on the core principle that exposure to a
feared stimulus leads to eventual habituation to that stimulus (see Foa &
Rothbaum, 1998). In other words, the goal of exposure is to reduce the frequency and/or intensity of the client's emotional response to the trauma,
subsequently reducing PTSD symptomatology. While this may be helpful,
implementing strategies to change or control private experience at all may
be problematic in the treatment of avoidance in individuals with posttraumatic symptomology. Thus, there exists a fundamental tension between the
blending of cognitive change strategies and acceptance in Becker and
Zayfert's model.

Conceptual Issues in Acceptance and Mindfulness

Hayes (1994) defines acceptance as "making contact with the automatic or
direct stimulus functions of events, without acting to reduce or manipulate
those functions, and without acting on the basis solely of their derived or
verbal functions" (pp. 30–31). In other words, acceptance involves three
processes: noticing private events that are experienced, letting go of efforts
to avoid or change those private events, and responding to actual events
that have occurred rather than to the private experiences elicited by those
events. Therefore, acceptance involves the conscious abandonment of behaviors that function as experiential avoidance, and the willingness to experience one's own emotions and thoughts as they occur.

Individuals who have enduring patterns of avoidance behavior will
likely have difficulty abandoning those behaviors for a number of reasons.
The coping patterns are frequently overlearned behaviors that have provided some relief from very painful stimuli. Additionally, the majority of
the clients we treat have large lacunae in their coping repertoires that include deficits in emotion regulation skills that interfere with adopting new,
more effective behaviors. An important aspect of emotion regulation that
may impact the course of psychological health is the ability to flexibly adjust emotion regulation strategies to the specific context (Gross & Munoz,
1995; Southam-Gerow & Kendall, 2002). Many people with trauma histories struggle with this flexibility of responding across contexts. For example, women who were sexually abused as children may have learned to dis-

sociate during the abuse. While dissociation may have been a useful survival technique at the time of the abuse, its long-term use can lead to greater psychological distress, problems in intimate relationships, parasuicidal behavior, and increased risk for revictimization (Wagner & Linehan, 1998).

Mindfulness is an important tool in developing emotion regulation skills (Linehan, 1993). As treatment progresses, mindfulness continues to be essential in helping the client engage in the acceptance work. In other words, individuals can use mindfulness strategies to increase awareness and flexibility of responding to emotional experiences, as well as to practice experiencing thoughts and feelings they typically avoid. Mindfulness exercises provide instructions on how to attend to and identify thoughts, feelings, and memories, without acting to alter those private experiences. They also teach increased awareness of emotional responses and the effectiveness of those responses in the current context. With acceptance as a primary goal, we use DBT, ACT, and FAP in our work with trauma survivors. While these therapies are more thoroughly explicated in other chapters in this text, we provide a brief overview of these treatments as they relate to our work.

DBT

DBT is an influential and innovative treatment that was developed to treat suicidal and parasuicidal behavior in individuals diagnosed with BPD (Linehan, 1993). This therapy uses techniques that emphasize experience of (rather than escape from) difficult emotion, along with effective action toward a life worth living. While borrowing some concepts from various principles associated with Eastern religions, this treatment is primarily informed by a biosocial theory of personality functioning. It describes how ineffective emotion regulation systems develop through "biological irregularities combined with certain dysfunctional environments, as well as their interaction and transaction over time" (Linehan, 1993, p. 42). Therefore, human beings may have a biological vulnerability to emotion dysregulation and in certain contexts, for example, invalidating environments, have inadequate learning opportunities that support the acquisition of regulation skills that are effective in contexts outside of the dysfunctional environment. For example, Wagner and Linehan (1998) discuss child sexual abuse in and of itself as an extreme example of invalidation; additionally, the circumstances surrounding the abuse are often prototypical examples of an invalidating family environment.

The dialectical philosophical position of DBT reflects the overall approach of acceptance and change. Linehan quotes Levins and Lewontin (1985; as cited in Linehan, 1993), who state: "Parts and wholes evolve in consequence of their relationship, and the relationship itself evolves. These are the properties of things that we call dialectical: that one thing cannot exist without the other, that one acquires its properties from its relation to the other, that the properties of both evolve as a consequence of their interpretation" (p. 3). Thus, emphases on acceptance and validation in DBT counterbalance the focus on change (Robins, 2002). Linehan introduced mindfulness practice partly as a vehicle to promote greater self-acceptance. Since clients, especially those with a trauma history, often have difficulty with self-acceptance and validation, mindfulness training has become an essential component of our approach.

Linehan describes mindfulness practice as an "instance of exposure to naturally arising thoughts, feelings, and sensations" (1993, p. 354). Mindfulness skills are taught as the "core" skills of DBT, and emphasize focused attention and awareness through observing, describing, and participating fully in both public and private experience (Linehan, 1993). Other behaviors that are taught in DBT skills training include emotion regulation, distress tolerance, and interpersonal effectiveness. Given the variety of problems frequently observed in clients with a trauma history (Polusny & Follette, 1995), the utility of incorporating these strategies into our treatment approach seems quite apparent. However, we want to reiterate that there may be many factors that lead to the development and maintenance of the difficulties observed in clients with a trauma history, not the least of which are factors associated with the family environment.

ACT

ACT (Hayes et al., 1999) is based on a theory of psychopathology, which posits that some types of psychopathology are forms of ineffective self-regulatory coping strategies, often involving experiential avoidance. This understanding of psychopathology is based on relational frame theory (RFT; Hayes, Barnes-Holmes, & Roche, 2001), which describes how language produces a unique situation in which direct experience is fused with cognition. In such instances, human beings respond to the literal content of thoughts as "truth" rather than responding to the thought as an experience. For example, thoughts such as "I can't do this" or "This will never get better" are responded to as reality. This "cognitive fusion" can then lead to efforts to avoid situations or emotions that give rise to these thoughts, or to escape such thoughts at the time they occur. While some avoidance of private experience may be necessary for healthy functioning and may in fact serve as effective coping (e.g., taking a walk to distract from work-related stress), routine avoidance of unpleasant private experiences may result in increased psychological distress when the avoidance interferes with effective living (Hayes et al., 1996).

From an ACT perspective, the fusion between self and language processes creates suffering. Acceptance is fostered through defusing language (Hayes et al., 1999). Mindfulness meditation, metaphors, and other experiential exercises undermine this fusion and rigid adherence to rules, while teaching healthy distancing and nonjudgmental awareness. Addressing these processes in therapy helps clients behave in ways consistent with their values and goals.

FAP

The therapeutic relationship described in FAP in and of itself can be used as a tool to facilitate change (Kohlenberg & Tsai, 1991) and FAP can be used as an enhancement to other treatment modalities (Kohlenberg, Kanter, Bolling, Parker, & Tsai, 2002). The primary focus of FAP is on clinically relevant behaviors (CRBs) that occur in the therapy session. A detailed analysis of the importance of attending not only to client problems that occur in session but also to client improvements and interpretations of behavior is provided in Kohlenberg and Tsai (1991). As these authors note, therapy provides multiple opportunities for the therapist to model behavior and respond contingently to different client behaviors. The therapist can relay to the client his or her reactions to the client's reports of past and current difficulties. For example, the therapist can respond to a client's report of her trauma history by modeling the identification and labeling of his or her own emotions. These types of interventions can serve many functions, including building the therapeutic relationship, providing a validating response to the client's report of a traumatic event, and beginning basic skills building with the client.

Acceptance and Skills Enhancement

Our treatment approach integrates elements of ACT, DBT skills training, FAP, and modified exposure therapy in the treatment of emotion skills deficits and experiential avoidance in individuals with histories of trauma who present with complex sets of problems. Treatment components include a functional behavioral assessment of symptomatology. If this assessment reveals a circumscribed set of symptoms that would be most appropriately addressed by a standard, empirically supported treatment, we take that treatment approach first. Our therapy is more suited for individuals who have a more complex set of problems, and includes skills training, acceptance-based therapy, and exposure, when indicated. The practices of acceptance and mindfulness are emphasized throughout treatment. Additionally, the therapeutic relationship is itself used as an agent of change using the principles of FAP. This approach offers a coherent theoretical framework from which to deliver treatment, as well as a treatment alternative to the change or control of private experience. Although the phenomena of emotion regulation and acceptance appear to contradict each other topographically, both concepts coexist in a dialectical framework. In other words, neither emotion regulation nor acceptance alone is a sufficient place from which to engage the world. Emotion regulation skills are necessary for individuals to modulate the frequency and intensity of their emotions in order to safely and fully experience the wide range of trauma-related thoughts, feelings, and memories they have been working so diligently to avoid. The remainder of this chapter provides an overview of our treatment model.

Contextual Behavioral Assessment

A contextual behavioral approach is a useful way to understand posttraumatic symptomology. The value of this perspective is that it fosters the examination of individuals in the context of both historical and environmental factors in order to understand how clinically relevant behaviors develop, function, and are then maintained. This is particularly important in the case of trauma, in that the clinician is vulnerable to overattributing the importance of a trauma history in either the development or maintenance of the presenting complaints. This approach does not invalidate the importance of the client's trauma history; rather, it provides a richer analysis of the problems and allows for a more idiographic approach to treatment planning. As described earlier, researchers have suggested that functional classification of psychopathology, compared to a more traditional syndromal approach, increases identification of underlying change processes in mental health problems and strengthens treatment utility (Hayes et al., 1996). Consequently, this approach allows for the treatment of specified behaviors (e.g., hypervigilance; attempts to avoid specific thoughts, feelings, or activities; detachment from others) rather than the amelioration of collections of symptoms (e.g., PTSD). Naugle and Follette (1998) provide a detailed explanation of this type of analysis.

Skills Training

As previously described, many survivors of trauma do not have the requisite skills to emotionally engage the process of therapy, including exposure. There may be such a rich reinforcement history of avoidance and escape that the task of emotional experiencing, particularly around trauma cues, may be nearly impossible without some strengthening of the client's basic coping resources. The task of reducing emotional dysregulation in some trauma survivors requires simultaneously increasing client capabilities around emotion. Although we believe that eliminating ineffective avoidance behaviors without also helping the client develop a repertoire of more effective behavioral responses to intense emotion is not a sufficient treatment solution, there is some controversy about this issue, and data are needed to verify this point. In order to achieve an effective balance, it is useful for individuals to learn to (1) observe, describe, and fully participate nonjudgmentally in their private and public experience (mindfulness skills); (2) tolerate and accept distressing private events as they are in the moment, without engaging in behavior to make the situation worse (distress tolerance skills); (3) identify and label emotions, understand how emotions function, reduce vulnerability to negative emotion, increase experience of positive emotion, and behave opposite to urges associated with a given emotion (emotion regulation skills); and (4) engage others effectively when making requests or saying "no" in the face of difficult private experience (interpersonal effectiveness skills). Mindfulness skills are the core skills that foster the acquisition of all the other skills (Linehan, 1993). Developing capabilities in these domains allows clients to engage in experiential acceptance of private events, without attempting to avoid or escape those events.

Acceptance-Based Exposure

Acceptance-based exposure is aimed at expanding the standard exposure treatments developed by Foa and Rothbaum (1998) and Resick and Schnicke (1993) to include a broader and more functional conceptualization of avoidance and the treatment of trauma-related phenomena. Standard exposure treatment has been empirically supported for the treatment of PTSD, specifically targeting a reduction in symptomatology and emotional responding related to memories of a circumscribed traumatic event. However, standard exposure appears most successful among individuals with one or two isolated traumatic experiences, who meet full criteria for PTSD. The population of individuals with a mixed-symptom presentation will benefit from a modified approach.

Acceptance-based exposure emphasizes (1) assessing the function of both private and public behavior, looking for behaviors that function as avoidance of private experience; (2) identifying classes of private experience most routinely avoided, including thoughts, feelings, physical sensations, memories, and so on; (3) assessing whether the effort to change or control aversive private experience is a workable solution; (4) exposing clients to specified classes of aversive private experience, while coaching them on accepting the experience as it is in the moment rather than avoiding the experience; (5) emphasizing the importance of living in accordance with identified life values rather than making choices in life based on the content of aversive private events; and (6) helping clients to clarify their own set of life values and make behavioral commitments toward those values.

Approaching exposure from an acceptance-based perspective targets a broader range of avoidance behavior and a larger set of aversive stimuli, allowing for greater generalization of exposure effects. Acceptance-based exposure offers a comprehensive treatment approach that addresses the myriad stimuli avoided by individuals with histories of multiple traumatic events, including understanding current avoidance strategies in the context of historical environments that may have shaped experiential avoidance.

Specific Therapeutic Techniques and Exercises

Mindfulness exercises are particularly useful in treatment sessions to facilitate focused attention for both the client and therapist, as well as provide opportunities to practice acceptance in the moment. Clients often arrive at sessions distracted by daily life events, and they may have difficulty being psychologically present. Mindfulness exercises can be used at the beginning of session as a way to help the client focus on present experience and prepare for the work ahead, at various times throughout the session as a way to facilitate acceptance of thoughts, feelings, and memories, and as part of regular homework assignments to foster generalization of acceptance and skills acquisition.

Mindfulness exercises may involve having the client get comfortable in her chair, close her eyes (however, a number of trauma survivors are uncomfortable with this, and the exercises may be done with the eyes open), and then notice various sensations; for example, her breathing, her legs pressing against the chair, or tension in her body. The therapist typically continues the exercises by having the client notice thoughts, memories, or emotions she is experiencing. She is instructed to experience exactly what is happening in the moment, without avoiding or clinging to any of it (Linehan, 1993). The rationale is that, with enough practice, the client will be able to have different thoughts, feelings, and memories throughout the day, without focusing on any one experience and becoming distressed. Instead of talking "about" mindfulness, the goal is to help the client to observe her private experiences in session, experiencing them as they come and go in the moment.

Additionally, the client may be engaging in behaviors that preclude her receiving adequate social support. If the therapist notices such behaviors during session, he or she can identify those behaviors and discuss with the client how the behaviors affect the therapist in session. As elaborated in Chapter 5 on FAP, the therapist and client can then explore how the interaction is similar to, or different from, others in her life, and identify alternative behaviors that may be more effective in developing valued relationships. In the process of discussing these interactions, the client is encouraged to practice mindfulness of her thoughts and feelings as they occur.

Therapist Training and Supervision

While supervision and clinical training have been discussed frequently in the psychotherapy literature, there is much less information on these topics in the behavior therapies, particularly as they relate to acceptance and mindfulness practices. Our clinical research team strongly adheres to a point of view that our conceptualization of therapy is not simply a treatment approach but is rather a general life philosophy. In our supervision meetings, we regularly address the roles of emotion and mindfulness, both didactically and experientially (Follette & Batten, 2000). Thus, we believe that it is essential that the therapist have a repertoire that includes the ability to label, express, and elicit emotion, as well as practice mindfulness skills. In regard to mindfulness, some researchers emphasize that the best way to learn mindfulness is through direct practice (Segal, Williams, & Teasdale, 2002). Given that research has shown that experiential learning is more effective than instruction (Bennett-Levy et al., 2001), it seems probable that therapists who practice mindfulness regularly may more thoroughly understand the barriers and benefits of mindfulness for their clients, and may thus be more effective teachers. Nevertheless, there is little empirical research documenting any of these hypotheses, and future outcome research should also address these supervision–therapist variables.

FUTURE DIRECTIONS AND CONCLUSION

The theory of experiential avoidance is a useful way to explain the variety of behavior problems that have been associated with a trauma history. Expanding on an acceptance-based treatment approach, using theoretically consistent behavioral treatments, provides an opportunity to respond to a wide range of behaviors that are functionally related but may be topographically divergent. Our treatment model focuses on the acquisition of skills related to emotional functioning, exposure to a number of private experiences that have been avoided, and the identification of goals associated with living a valued life. An important theme woven throughout the therapy is the practice of mindfulness. While psychotherapy outcome literature illustrating the incremental effectiveness of mindfulness appears promising, further empirical examination of this practice is needed. First, few researchers have adequately operationally defined mindfulness. A greater understanding of the specific behaviors included in the construct of mindfulness and how those behaviors function to promote acceptance and psychological health is essential. Second, once mindfulness has been better defined, researchers must develop measurement strategies to assess the occurrence of mindful behaviors, as well as changes in mindfulness during treatment. Third, a clearer understanding and more thorough assessment of mindfulness will allow researchers to examine how (or whether) changes in these behaviors are associated with decreases in psychopathology.

The inclusion of the concept of acceptance has radically changed Western cognitive-behavioral therapy. Practitioners and clients seem to be benefiting from the enthusiastic espousal of mindfulness and acceptance approaches (see Segal et al., 2002). However, while Eastern philosophy encourages experiential examination of the effectiveness of these practices, hypothesis-testing remains a valued and useful practice in Western culture. Therefore, it is necessary for researchers in the newer behavior therapies to operationally define and empirically examine core constructs such as acceptance and mindfulness as mechanisms of change in evaluating psychotherapy outcomes.

Creative and flexible responding of treatment developers in the treatment of trauma is essential in moving our interventions to the next level of effectiveness. Certainly, significant advances have been made in trauma therapy, particularly among behavior therapists. However, a number of our clients either do not respond to treatment or have additional problems that are not addressed by current protocols. Instead of limiting our repertoire in responding to difficult client problems by repeatedly intervening in the same way, psychologists are accepting the current limitations of psychotherapy and investigating alternative ways to respond. We expect no less of ourselves than we do of our clients. As scientists–practitioners, our lives stand for moving the field forward in ways that make a difference in the world.

REFERENCES

Becker, C. B., & Zayfert, C. (2001). Integrating DBT-based techniques and concepts to facilitate exposure treatment for PTSD. *Cognitive and Behavioral Practice, 8,* 107–122.

Bennett-Levy, J., Turne, F., Beaty, T., Smith, M., Paterson, B., & Farmer, S. (2001). The value of self-practice of cognitive therapy techniques and self-reflection in the training of cognitive therapists. *Behavioural and Cognitive Psychotherapy, 29*(2), 203–220.

Chemtob, C. M., Novaco, R. W., Hamada, R. S., Gross, D. M., & Smith, G. (1997). Anger regulation deficits in combat-related posttraumatic stress disorder. *Journal of Traumatic Stress, 10,* 17–35.

Cicchette, D., Ackerman, B. P., & Izard, C. E. (1995). Emotions and emotion regulation in developmental psychopathology. *Development and Psychopathology* [Special issue]: *Emotions in developmental psychopathology, 7*(1), 1–10.

Cloitre, M., & Koenen, K. (2001). Interpersonal group process treatment for CSA-related PTSD: A comparison study of the impact of borderline personality disorder on outcome. *International Journal of Group Psychotherapy, 51,* 379–398.

Cloitre, M., Koenen, K. C., Cohen, L. R., & Han, H. (2002). Skills training in affective and interpersonal regulation followed by exposure: A phase-based treatment for PTSD related to childhood abuse. *Journal of Consulting and Clinical Psychology, 70*(5), 1067–1074.

Foa, E. B., Dancu, C. V., Hembree, E. A., Jaycox, L. H., Meadows, E. A., & Street, G. P. (1999). A comparison of exposure therapy, stress inoculation training, and their combination for reducing posttraumatic stress disorder in female assault victims. *Journal of Consulting and Clinical Psychology, 67*(2), 194–200.

Foa, E. B., Keane, T. M., & Friedman, M. J. (Eds.). (2000). *Effective treatments for PTSD: Practice guidelines from the International Society for Traumatic Stress Studies*. New York: Guilford Press.

Foa, E. B., & Rothbaum, B. O. (1998). *Treating the trauma of rape*. New York: Guilford Press.

Follette, V. M. (1994) Survivors of child sexual abuse: Treatment using a contextual analysis. In S. C. Hayes, N. S. Jacobson, V. M. Follette, & M. J. Dougher (Eds.), *Acceptance and change: Content and context in psychotherapy* (pp. 255–268). Reno, NV: Context Press.

Follette, V. M., & Batten, S. V. (2000). The role of emotion in psychotherapy supervision: A contextual behavioral analysis. *Cognitive and Behavioral Practice, 7*, 306–312.

Follette, V. M., Ruzek, J. I., & Abueg, F. R. (Eds.). (1988). *Cognitive-behavioral therapies for trauma*. New York: Guilford Press.

Gross, J. J., & Munoz, R. F. (1995). Emotion regulation and mental health. *Clinical Psychology: Science and Practice, 2*(2), 151–164.

Hayes, S. C. (1994). Content, context, and types of psychological acceptance. In S. C. Hayes, N. S. Jacobson, V. M. Follette, & M. J. Dougher (Eds.), *Acceptance and change: Content and context in psychotherapy* (pp. 13–32). Reno, NV: Context Press.

Hayes, S. C., Barnes-Holmes, D., & Roche, B. (2001). *Relational frame theory: A post-Skinnerian account of human language and cognition*. New York: Plenum Press.

Hayes, S. C., Strosahl, K., & Wilson, K. G. (1999). *Acceptance and commitment therapy: An experiential approach to behavior change*. New York: Guilford Press.

Hayes, S. C., Wilson, K. G., Gifford, E. V., Follette, V. M., & Strosahl, K. (1996). Experiential avoidance and behavioral disorders: A functional dimensional approach to diagnosis and treatment. *Journal of Consulting and Clinical Psychology, 64*, 1152–1168.

Hembree, E. A., & Foa, E. R. (2003). Interventions for trauma-related emotional disturbances in adult victims of crime. *Journal of Traumatic Stress, 16*(2), 187–199.

Jaycox, L. H., & Foa, E. R. (1996). Obstacles in implementing exposure therapy for PTSD: Case discussions and practical solutions. *Clinical Psychology and Psychotherapy, 3*, 176–184.

Jaycox, L. H., Zoellner, L., & Foa, E. B. (2002). Cognitive-behavioral therapy for PTSD in rape survivors. *Journal of Clinical Psychology, 58*, 891–906.

Kohlenberg, R., Kanter, J. W., Bolling, M. Y., Parker, C., & Tsai, M. (2002). Enhancing cognitive therapy for depression with functional analytic psychotherapy: Treatment guidelines and empirical findings. *Cognitive and Behavioral Practice, 9*, 213–229.

Kohlenberg, R. J., & Tsai, M. (1991). *Functional analytic psychotherapy*. New York: Plenum Press.

Levins, R., & Lewontin, R. (1985). *The dialectical biologist*. Cambridge, MA: Harvard University Press.

Linehan, M. M. (1993). *Cognitive-behavioral treatment of borderline personality disorder*. New York: Guilford Press.

McFarlane, A. C., & Yehuda, R. (2000). Clinical treatment of posttraumatic stress disorder: Conceptual challenges raised by recent research. *Australian and New Zealand Journal of Psychiatry, 34*(6), 940–953.

Naugle, A. E., & Follette, W. C. (1998). A functional analysis of trauma symptoms. In V. M. Follette, J. I. Ruzek, & F. R. Abueg (Eds.), *Cognitive-behavioral therapies for trauma* (pp. 48–73). New York: Guilford Press.

Palm, K. M., & Follette, V. M. (2000). Counseling strategies with adult survivors of sexual abuse as children. *Directions in Clinical and Counseling Psychology, 11*, 49–60

Pistorello, J., & Follette, V. M. (2000). A behavior analytic conceptualization of the long-term correlates of child sexual abuse. In M. Dougher (Ed.), *Behavior analytic approaches to clinical psychology*. Reno, NV: Context Press.

Pitman, R., Altman, B., Greenwald, E., Longre, R. E., Macklin, M. L., Poire, R. E., et al. (1991). Psychiatric complications during flooding therapy for posttraumatic stress disorder. *Journal of Clinical Psychiatry, 52*, 17–20.

Polusny, M. A., & Follette, V. M. (1995). Long-term correlates of child sexual abuse: Theory and review of the empirical literature. *Applied and Preventive Psychology, 4*, 143–166

Resick, P. A., & Schnicke, M. K. (1993). *Cognitive processing therapy for rape victims: A treatment manual*. Thousand Oaks, CA: Sage.

Robins, C. J. (2002). Zen principles and mindfulness practice in dialectical behavior therapy. *Clinical Psychology: Science and Practice, 9*(1), 50–57.

Roth, S., Newman, E., Pelcovitz, D., van der Kolk, B., & Mandel, F.S. (1997). Complex PTSD in victims exposed to sexual and physical abuse: Results from the DSM-IV field trial for posttraumatic stress disorder. *Journal of Traumatic Stress, 10*(4), 539–555.

Salkovskis, P. M., & Campbell, P. (1994). Thought suppression induces intrusion in naturally occurring negative intrusive thoughts. *Behaviour Research and Therapy, 32*, 1–8.

Scott, M. J., & Stradling, S. G. (1997). Client compliance with exposure treatments for posttraumatic stress disorder. *Journal of Traumatic Stress, 10*, 523–526.

Segal, Z. V., Williams, J. M. G., & Teasdale, J. D. (2002). *Mindfulness-based cognitive therapy for depression: A new approach to preventing relapse*. New York: Guilford Press.

Southam-Gerow, M. A., & Kendall, P. C. (2002). Emotion regulation and understanding: Implications for child psychopathology and therapy. *Clinical Psychology Review, 22*(2), 189–222.

Tarrier, N., Pilgrim, H., Sommerfield, C., Faragher, B., Reynolds, M., Graham, E., et al. (1999). A randomized trial of cognitive therapy and imaginal exposure in the treatment of chronic posttraumatic stress disorder. *Journal of Consulting and Clinical Psychology, 67*, 13–18.

Wagner, A. W., & Linehan, M. M. (1998). Dissociative behavior. In V. M. Follette, J. I. Ruzek, & F. R. Abueg (Eds.), *Cognitive-behavioral therapies for trauma* (pp. 191–225). New York: Guilford Press.

Wegner, D. M., Erber, R., & Zanakos, S. (1993). Ironic processes in the mental control of mood and mood-related thought. *Journal of Personality and Social Psychology, 65*, 1093–1104.

10

Generalized Anxiety Disorder

*Bringing Cognitive-Behavioral Therapy
into the Valued Present*

T. D. Borkovec *and* Brian Sharpless

Understanding generalized anxiety disorder (GAD) and developing interventions for its amelioration could contribute significantly to the understanding and treatment of all adult emotional disorders. GAD has a fairly high prevalence rate, is often associated with multiple additional Axis I diagnoses, and is a frequent comorbid condition for other anxiety and mood disorders. Moreover, worry is pervasive across all anxiety and depression problems. Most importantly, GAD is arguably a "basic" anxiety disorder (Brown, Barlow, & Liebowitz, 1994), out of which often emerge other anxiety and mood disorders. Compatible with such a view, psychological treatment of GAD results in dramatic declines in comorbid Axis I conditions (Borkovec, Abel, & Newman, 1995). Learning about the nature, functions, and origins of this disorder and its cardinal feature of worry could increase our understanding of human psychopathology and of human beings in general.

Worry primarily involves thinking or talking to oneself (Borkovec & Inz, 1990). Such abstract, internal, verbal behavior represents one of the most evolved systems characterizing human beings, allowing us to experiment with ideas, consider alternative choices, and evaluate the motives and consequences of each choice before implementing one of them, and without fearing that the environment will punish us for considering them. Thought is also perhaps the most important psychological experience that composes both our moment-to-moment sense of self and our sense of being voluntary creatures. Thus, learning about worry could teach us a considerable amount about human ways of being.

We have been attempting to acquire basic knowledge about GAD and worry, and to develop effective forms of psychological intervention for over two decades. Our directions are grounded in basic empirical knowledge from our own work and that of other psychological investigators, and from logical deductions drawn from prior research and theory within both the anxiety area and the broader psychological literature. In doing so, we are fulfilling our responsibility as behavior therapists to the commitment made by the field at its organized dawning in the 1960s to develop new therapies through the application of empirical knowledge and known principles of behavior. Where relevant, we also gain concurrent validity for this work by citing parallels within the Western philosophical tradition at large. Our work is relevant to the topic of this book, because we have added several key components to traditional cognitive-behavioral therapy (CBT) approaches over the years, including teaching clients to focus on the present moment, to value tasks based on their intrinsic value rather than solely their eventual outcomes, and to deepen interpersonal and emotional contact with events. Before describing some of our specific interventions, we begin with general comments about the nature of human anxiety, which provide a context relevant to our development of GAD interventions.

THE NATURE OF HUMAN ANXIETY

Anxious Sequences

Linear views of anxiety involve the specification of two sequential events. An immediate evaluative response occurs upon detection of internal or external stimuli that have threatening meaning. Strategic control of this response is not possible; its occurrence is based on past associative learning (e.g., classical aversive conditioning) and is automatic. In response to this response, the individual engages in a sequence of secondary defensive responses whose goal is to eliminate the threat and whose occurrences maintain anxious meanings. The defensive responses (e.g., avoidance) are initially strategic but become increasingly habitual over repeated experiences and preclude functional exposure to the feared stimulus. This way of viewing anxiety and subsequent coping was originally explicated by Mowrer's (1947) two-stage theory of fear, an empirically based theoretical account of the neurotic paradox based on animal conditioning research. From such a view emerged the varieties of exposure therapies that exist today. Its implication is that reduction in anxious meanings (the immediate evaluative response) would best come about by repeated exposures to feared stimuli while defensive responses (negatively reinforced by the removal of aversive stimuli) are prevented. At a more general level, its implication is that meaning is action: What a stimulus means partly depends on how we have behaved toward it previously; James–Lange theory is alive and well (Fehr & Stern, 1970). While our automatic reactions may be problematic, the problem and its solution really reside in our reactions to our reactions. The latter thus serve as the best focus for interventions. Worry is an example of a defensive secondary reaction, a negatively reinforced cognitive avoidance response (Borkovec, Alcaine, & Behar, 2004). The treatment implication is that change in anxious meanings will best occur if we strategically change our habitual secondary reactions, including worry, to our immediate evaluative reactions.

Anxiety Is Anticipatory

Anxiety is always anticipatory; it has to do with the possibility of future bad things happening. The verbal content of worry especially refers to threatening futures that are quite often very distant in time (Borkovec, Robinson, Pruzinsky, & DePree, 1983). An important implication is that clients with GAD (or other people, when they are worrying) are phenomenologically spending their time in an illusory world of future-oriented thoughts that contain negative emotional material. They are living many lives, with their bodies and minds reacting to mentally constructed realities as if those realities were actually happening. The consequence is a life of nearly constant anxiety, little joy, and little contact with present-moment information. So interventions would usefully aim at increasing the person's contact with present reality and the accurate processing of adaptive information that present reality contains. Present-moment experiencing, ability to shut off thought, and the generation of positive affect would be specific goals of such interventions.

Reality, Unreality, and the Primary Motivational Goal of GAD

Given current thinking in epistemology and the philosophy of science, it would be difficult to posit the existence of neutral facts or an absolutely true and accessible reality independent of conceptual frameworks. Perception of the world is largely an act of creation that brings order and meaning to the "blooming buzzing confusion" of sensory data. While this view is foundational in cognitive therapy (CT; Clark & Steer, 1996), this claim goes back at least to Kant (1781/1996). We do not ever receive the world as it is "in itself" (Kant's noumenal realm); all is filtered through our "hardwired" perceptual capacities. Taking this further, Kierkegaard (1843/1990) prefigured perceptual psychologists such as Helmholtz and Irvin Rock, writing that "all observation is not just a receiving, a discovering, but also a

bringing forth, and insofar as it is that, how the observer himself is consti-
tuted is indeed decisive" (p. 59). As applied to modern Western science,
Kuhn's (1962/1996) conception of a paradigm indicates that what we believe in our theories affects both what we are able to perceive and how we
process information. These preconceptions can blind us to new information
when they become fixed, stuck, or outside of awareness (Bernstein, 1983;
Gadamer, 1960/1975). GAD clients are in a similar situation to that of a
paradigmatic scientist in their dominant and rigid perspective on life (i.e.,
"The world is a potentially dangerous place; I might not be able to cope
with whatever comes down the road; therefore, I need to anticipate all possible dangers in order to avoid catastrophes").

Basic research demonstrates the power of preconceptions, even at
basic perceptual and attentional levels (e.g., Bruner & Postman, 1949;
Mikulas, 2002; Palmer, 1999). Such interpretive elements are essential but
can be nonadaptive if their content lacks congruence with what is going on
in the present-moment environment (Bargh & Chartrand, 1999). Importantly, such interpretations are heavily influenced by how they relate to
current goals (Bargh & Chartrand, 1999) that may be activated by the environment without awareness as much as 95% of the time (Baumeister,
Bratlavsky, Muraven, & Tice, 1998; Baumeister & Sommer, 1997). Analo-
gously, social psychological research documents the importance of self-
fulfilling prophecies, wherein individuals remember and interpret information in other people's personal histories in ways that support the individual's
current beliefs and assumptions (Snyder, 1984). In a self-maintaining process, people often overestimate the amount of feedback that confirms their
self-conceptions, attend to and remember social feedback that is confirmatory more than disconfirmatory and, when receiving feedback that discon-
firms their self-conceptions, interpret this information to minimize the
impact of disconfirming evidence (Swann & Read, 1981).

This does not necessarily entail a strict relativism in which no criteria
exist with which to evaluate different ways of living. Perspectives vary
along a dimension of appropriateness and adaptiveness, and clients with
GAD have been shown to have particularly inaccurate views that cause
them considerable misery. So increasing their awareness of, and flexibility
in observing, the present moment and providing more adaptive perspectives
(especially those that encourage approach to life rather than avoidance) are
central goals of our therapy.

Interacting Response Systems and Stuck Habits

The idea that humans are interacting systems is not new and can be found
in Hippocrates' theory of temperaments/humors, Plato's *Republic*, and
Stoic thought. In our theory and therapy, it has been useful to conceptualize
human beings as having evolved several layers of processing systems that

constantly interact moment to moment as they are recruited together in a nonlinear dynamical process in response to a constantly changing environment. Humans do not ordinarily go immediately from one state to another (e.g., from tranquility to panic); rather, the systems interact upon detection of significant stimuli in a spiraling process designed to accomplish the prime directive for living organisms to approach what is good for them and avoid what is bad. Thus, when we speak of maintaining secondary reactions (reactions to our reactions), we are speaking of a complex series of interacting sequences over time. Psychological research has long documented the existence of such interactions. What we think affects how we feel, what we feel affects how we think, what we think and feel affect how we behave, how we behave affects how we think and feel, and so on. Each time a spiraling sequence occurs, the sequence is stored in memory in strengthened form, making it more likely that the same or similar sequence will occur upon presentation of the same or similar event. In GAD (and indeed in all forms of psychopathology and perhaps in much of the daily behavior and experience of normal human beings), such spiraling sequences become stuck, rigid habits. As Foucault (1954/1987) states, "Illness suppresses complex, unstable, voluntary functions by emphasizing simple, stable, and compulsive functions" (p. 18).

This rigidity, or stuckness, has negative consequences. Kovac (2001) found rigidity to be negatively correlated with creativity, divergent thinking, and flexibility. Rigidity is also a characteristic of adult clients in general (Kalska, Punamäki, & Mäki-Pelli, 1999; MacLeod, 1991) and unipolar endogenous depression (Heerlein, Richter, Gonzalez, & Santander, 1998). On the other hand, other research has documented the benefits of increased flexibility. Flexible coping strategies predict better mental and physical health (Lazarus & Folkman, 1984; Perlin & Schooler, 1978). Mental flexibility is also associated with resiliency in children and correlates with playfulness (Snow, 1992), optimism and humor (Gelkopf & Kreitler, 1996), and lessened impact of trauma (Quota, El-Sarraj, & Punamäki, 2001). Because of these and other reasons we discuss later, emphasis in our GAD treatment is placed on increasing flexibility in our clients' reactions to their reactions.

Our view of psychopathology as involving multiple interacting systems and habitual, inflexible response patterns provides an interesting perspective on other schools of psychotherapy. Each school of therapy tends to place particular emphasis on a particular response system, considers that system to be rigid, and focuses intervention on that system. For CT, this involves nonadaptive cognition; for experiential therapy, it is denied or suppressed emotion; in psychoanalysis, "fixation" plays a key role; faulty interpersonal relations are central to interpersonal psychotherapy; environmental contingencies supporting nonadaptive overt behavior are critical to some behavioral views. In each case, it is assumed that changing the crucial response system will result in interactions throughout the remaining systems. For example, cognitive therapists believe that if one changes how clients are thinking, this will change how they feel and behave. Because psychological research has demonstrated that each system interacts with all others, each of these perspectives contains an element of relative truth; no theory or paradigm is preemptive (Feyerabend, 1993).

Our latest outcome study serves as a useful CBT example of change in the various interacting systems (Borkovec, Newman, Pincus, & Lytle, 2002). We contrasted CT alone, applied relaxation and self-control desensitization alone, and our CBT containing all of these elements. Considerable change occurred for all three groups, but no significant between-group effects were observed, largely because the component conditions were particularly effective. Because more therapy time had been devoted to each component in our study than in previous GAD investigations, we compared total amount of therapy time in those prior studies showing a superiority of CBT to its components versus those investigations wherein no difference occurred. Components were equivalent to CBT when lengthy treatment was provided (13.50 hours), and they were inferior to CBT with briefer therapy (9.25 hours). So if sufficient time is devoted in therapy to the modification of one response system, then it appears that changes in that system will eventually affect the other interacting systems.

Given these data, a route to increasing the effectiveness of a therapy, irrespective of what response system it is targeting, is to develop its techniques to maximize their impact on that one response system. Certainly, we would encourage such developments. However, the additional approach is to provide a client with interventions targeting many or all relevant response systems, while developing ways to maximize the effectiveness of each. We have taken the latter approach in our current pursuit of more efficacious treatments for GAD and hope that targeting multiple areas will create greater positive changes within the entire system.

THE DEVELOPMENT OF SPECIFIC INTERVENTIONS
FOR GENERALIZED ANXIETY DISORDER

Our development of techniques tailored to GAD evolved from initial applications of traditional CBT methods for teaching adaptive coping skills to adding an emphasis on teaching our clients how to live in the present moment in flexible ways, to eventually emphasizing whole-organism approach behavior in daily living through the cultivation of intrinsic values and motivations applied to each present moment. When an individual is living in perspectives such as the ones typical of our clients with GAD, attending to the present is not given high priority and would require considerable effort even if the client desired to do so. Constant threat perception yields hypervigilence for further threat cues and requires immediate actions to cope with the threat. Consequently, traditional CBT and its provision of coping skills to lessen anxiety may be an important first step for later work devoted to eventually increasing client focus on the present. Through a variety of techniques, we aim to replace automatic, anxiety-maintaining spirals (reactions to reactions) with more adaptive, flexible responses within each response system, using strategic choices repeatedly rehearsed, until the alternative responses have sufficient habit strength to provide greater choice and lessened determinism. Thus, therapy involves loosening up rigid habitual behavior and, ultimately, the creation of new meanings, not only with regard to the critical stress-producing aspects of life but also to life in general. Our brief descriptions of some of our techniques are organized in terms of the stuck habits among the various response systems involved in the maintenance of anxious meanings typical of our clients with GAD.

Stuck Awareness and Self-Monitoring

Self-monitoring has long been a foundational skill in behavior therapy for many adult psychological problems. Clients are asked to observe the environmental situations associated with their problems, the behaviors they emit, and the consequences, if any, that occur. With the later incorporation of CT techniques and recognition that internal events are involved in problematic functional relationships, self-monitoring was also directed to thoughts, images, feelings, and physiological reactions.

In our own treatment, self-monitoring is extremely important for three reasons. As in traditional CBT, we encourage our clients to pay attention to their inner and outer environments, and to observe the moment-to-moment interactions among their various response systems, and between those and their constantly changing external worlds. We are particularly interested in having our clients see causative relationships among these various elements and recognize that the characteristic ways in which they think, imagine, feel, and act have objective consequences for their internal and external worlds. This lays the groundwork for clients to achieve a more agentic position with regard to their characteristic response patterns. They become aware that anxiety is less an impingement from without and more a product of themselves that arises from within. They begin to see the possibility of real choice, because real choice is only won through the hard labor of gaining awareness of relevant personal processes over time.

However, in addition to providing functional analytic information to both the therapist and the client, self-monitoring provides opportunities for a special emphasis on learning to detect incipient changes in state as they happen. The goal is to catch anxiety spirals as early as possible, because the earlier the client catches a shift in an anxious or worrisome direction, the more effective will be the strategic choice and implementation of new coping strategies for moving his or her state away from that spiral. Practicing such monitoring occurs in-session, both by having the therapist alert the client to any observed changes in state and by actively generating anxiety or worry via traditional evocative methods (e.g., imagery recall of past events). Upon detection of incipient anxiety by either method, the therapist asks clients to identify what reactions they notice that indicate they are becoming anxious, and then asks them to identify what happened just before those noticed cues. Repeating the generation of anxious sequences through imagery recall allows a focus on the process and an awareness of internal events that emerge just before a clear recognition of incipient anxiety. Such repetition allows the client to make observations earlier and earlier in the sequence of anxious responding among the response systems.

Because so much of anxious process is habitual and outside of awareness, responsibility for noticing incipient anxiety spirals during a session initially falls to the therapist. Once clients are experiencing sufficient success, this control is gradually shifted over to them. The resulting increase in autonomy and responsibility likely engenders a more internal locus of control, which in turn engenders more novel actions. Self-monitoring and early cue detection are also practiced during daily living, and the therapist asks the client at the beginning of each session what new early cues were identified during the past week.

Self-monitoring also lays the foundation for one of the most critical goals in our treatment: a focus on the present. With so much time spent in thought and worry, clients with GAD have few attentional resources to devote to observing what is happening in their actual worlds. Asking clients to observe themselves and their environments objectively provides the opportunity to introduce the idea of living in the present moment and of paying attention to what actually exists, instead of the illusory world created in their thoughts and images.

While monitoring and observation in early sessions involve attending to external and internal events that directly relate to anxious experience, two further, sequential stages are later initiated. First, clients are asked to identify positive information and experiences during the day. Because of excessive negative filtering and confirmatory biases, it is important to direct their attention to, and encourage their processing of, positive features in their environment to create balance in their processing of information. Clients are asked to cultivate accuracy in all observations and judgments (rather than a Pollyannaish naivete) and to open their awareness to all information available in each present moment in order to facilitate choice and to foster emancipation from automatic responses. Empirical research supports the use of self-monitoring in this manner. Lord, Lepper, and Preston (1984) found that confirmatory biases in hypothesis testing can be overcome simply by instructing individuals to consider actively the possibility that the opposite could be correct. Neuberg (1989) found that merely giving subjects instructions to make accurate judgments motivated them to overrule expectations by gathering information in a more complete and rigorous manner. Tetlock (1985; Tetlock & Kim, 1987) found that making subjects feel accountable for their impressions or judgments (as they would feel when they give weekly descriptions of their past week's behavior during each therapy session) results in more effortful decision making and greater attention to situational constraints.

Stuck Physiological Functioning and Relaxation

Unlike persons with other anxiety disorders, clients with GAD do not typically show sympathetic activation when they are worrying or are confronted with challenges or threats. Instead, they display a reduction in cardiovascular variability and deficient parasympathetic tone (Hoehn-Saric, McLeod, & Zimmerli, 1989; Thayer, Friedman, & Borkovec, 1996). Such physiological rigidity makes sense given the psychological circumstance that they create. With frequent detection of threat but no place to run and no one to fight, sympathetic activation is not adaptive, so it is suppressed. Demonstrative of the interacting response systems, reduced vagal tone in children has been linked both to nonadaptive attentional deployment (providing a possible basis for threat-biased attention and interpretive biases consistently found in GAD; Mathews & MacLeod, 2002) and to later poor interpersonal behavior (Beauchaine, 2001). Moreover, both worry and its lack of autonomic variability are associated with significant health risks (Brosschot & Thayer, in press; Thayer & Lane, in press), and medical health care utilization is particularly high among people diagnosed with GAD (Roy-Byrne, 1996).

Given these data, relaxation is a very useful strategy for clients with GAD. Initially, we used only progressive muscle relaxation (Bernstein & Borkovec, 1973), and it has remained in our therapy because excessive muscle tension is one of the few physiological systems tonically elevated and particularly reactive in GAD (Hoehn-Saric et al., 1989). We later incorporated two significant additions: training in multiple relaxation techniques, and emphasis on applied relaxation training. For the former, we teach slowed, paced, diaphragmatic breathing in the first session. This relaxation method is easy to demonstrate, and the majority of clients notice nearly immediate benefits from even brief deployment. In the second session, full progressive muscle relaxation training is initiated and is completed over the course of the protocol sessions. Also in early sessions, we introduce clients to, and practice, pleasant relaxing imagery and meditational methods. Clients are encouraged to play and experiment with the various methods in order to discover which work best under which internal and external environmental circumstances, and to shift to an alternate technique if the first selected one is not effective in a particular situation. They practice their relaxation techniques twice a day to strengthen their ability to elicit rapid and deep relaxation responses. Training in multiple techniques reflects our emphasis on learning flexible coping responses and on creating increased choice. Moreover, research indicates that if relaxation-induced anxiety (common among diffusely anxious individuals) occurs with one technique, it is unlikely to occur with another (Heide & Borkovec, 1983).

Truly effective use of these methods comes, however, from applied relaxation training (Öst, 1987). Clients use their relaxation coping strategies to interrupt incipient anxiety or worry spirals during the session and in daily life upon self-monitoring detection of early cues throughout the day. In addition, they elicit calm and tranquil states frequently throughout the day in order to cultivate a relaxed lifestyle in general. As clients come to sessions reporting successes in both coping applications and the cultivation of relaxed lifestyles, therapy sessions start with elicitation of relaxation and a request that they maintain an awareness of this background tranquility throughout the session (and from now on, in daily living). The very earliest cue for intervention will now be an absence of this tranquility. Finally, and described in greater detail later, we encourage them increasingly to open up to, and positively approach, the present-moment environment after each relaxation reinduction and to attend to the information that this reality contains. As in the Pink Floyd song, we ask our clients to "Tear down the wall."

Just as self-monitoring was an introduction to attending to the present moment, so relaxation training is an introduction to creating and attending to a *pleasant* present moment. After relaxation inductions, we point out to our clients that they in fact produced that state, that they are capable of producing it anytime (although frequent practice is required to develop the habit of doing so), and that a goal of this procedure is learning to attend to things that are positive and pleasurable, with their relaxed states being an early example.

At the technical level, progressive relaxation involves tensing muscle groups and then letting go of the tension, while concentrating on the resulting sensations. As training progresses, we discuss the general metaphor of "letting go" beyond this physical example. We discuss the importance of learning to notice and then to let go of reactions to reactions involving negative thoughts, images, feelings, and any considerations of the future itself as soon as these events are detected. "Letting go" is described as mere observation of these internal reactions and of nonreaction to them, of detachment rather than attachment. In this sense, "letting go" overlaps with the variety of "acceptance" methods described elsewhere in this volume.

Beneficial effects of relaxation are well documented (Bernstein, Borkovec, & Hazlett-Stevens, 2000; Lehrer & Woolfolk, 1993; Lichstein, 1988) and have a particular relevance for clients with GAD. Relaxation facilitates behavioral change by diminishing the response priority of well-learned behaviors and increasing the response priority of weaker behaviors (Naka-mura & Broen, 1965). Thus, it can potentially loosen up rigid response patterns. It also facilitates imagery (Anderson & Borkovec, 1980) and so increases the effectiveness of imagery rehearsals (to be described in a later section). Relaxation directs the client's attention away from excessive focus on abstract conceptual activity. It also has been found to facilitate the emotional processing of phobic images (Borkovec & Sides, 1979). Finally, relaxation increases awareness. By definition, the act of achieving relaxation requires present-focused awareness to the feelings of muscular tension and relaxation; the relaxation response is rewarding only if awareness is sufficiently maintained to assess accurately the status of one's body.

Stuck Affect and Emotional Processing

Daily life of persons with GAD is filled with negative emotional experience, which is true even when persons with GAD relax in a laboratory (Borkovec & Inz, 1990). Although anxiety predominates, depression is a frequent accompaniment. Clients often have comorbid or past mood disorders (Brown & Barlow, 1992). Interestingly, the induction of worry in the laboratory will elicit about 60% anxious mood and 40% depressed mood, even in unselected normal individuals (Andrews & Borkovec, 1988).

Clients with GAD are also high in alexithymia (i.e., difficulty in identifying and describing emotional experience). Spending so much time worrying, they may simply have fewer attentional resources for noticing their emotions and their daily emotional variations. It is also possible that the muting effect of worry on somatic fear responses (Borkovec & Hu, 1990), and thus on the emotional processing of fear-related material, may generalize to other emotional experiences as well. Finally, clients with GAD may find emotions in general to be aversive (Turk, Heimberg, Luterek, Mennin, & Fresco, in press), similar to Hayes's (Hayes, Wilson, Gifford, Follette, & Strosahl, 1996) notion of experiential avoidance and further elaborated in Roemer and Orsillo's (2002) article on the potential integration of cognitive-behavioral and mindfulness/acceptance-based therapies.

Clearly, little joy exists in their phenomenological lives due to the anxiety and depression elicited by their illusory worlds of negative thought. This type of living in the future (and at times in the past) is in contrast with the emotional lives of most young children who experience (and readily show in their behavior) intense positive and negative emotions in response to immediate environmental events. Once the environment changes, they are synchronously moved in other behavioral and emotional directions appropriate to the environmental change. Adults often try to hold on to good events beyond their environmentally present reality and try to get rid of bad events. As a consequence, authentic emotion is often missing, and the intensity of real emotion is often lessened and/or inappropriate to changed environmental conditions. Individuals with GAD have the added burden of creating constant negative lives in their minds, therefore missing aspects of present-moment environments that contain emotionally significant experience and information: "When I was a child, I caught a fleeting glimpse, out of the corner of my eye. I turned to look, but it was gone. I cannot put my finger on it now. The child is grown, the dream is gone. I've become comfortably numb" (Pink Floyd, *The Wall*).

Our therapy approach contains three elements to address these affective features. As mentioned earlier, self-monitoring eventually includes paying attention to and experiencing all emotions (positive and negative) and their connections to present-moment events. Second, we now add interpersonal/emotional processing therapy (described later) to traditional CBT. The emotional processing element uses experiential techniques to deepen authentic, in-the-moment, primary affect. From a behavioral perspective, this provides repeated exposures to emotion to hypothetically lessen fear and avoidance of affect. From an experiential perspective, emotional deepening accesses denied or suppressed affects to facilitate their identification and processing. Third, as therapy progresses, increasing emphasis (described later) is placed on developing cognitive perspectives that cultivate approach to daily life and joy in its engagement.

Stuck Behavior

Unlike other anxiety disorders, behavioral avoidance of circumscribed environmental stimuli is not as salient for clients with GAD. They do, however, show subtle behavioral avoidances to a large variety of situations (Butler, Cullington, Hibbert, Klimes, & Gelder, 1987). More importantly, they display rigid interpersonal behavior that fails to adjust to changing interpersonal circumstances (Pincus & Borkovec, 1994).

Because so many circumstances are associated with GAD worries and anxieties, we have always used a coping, rather than mastery, approach. Clients use their applied relaxation skills early in therapy in response to any incipient anxiety or worrying, as well as before, during, and after stressful daily events. These responses are strengthened in-session through self-control desensitization (see Goldfried, 1971), wherein imagery of stressful or worrisome situations elicits incipient anxiety cues to which clients practice responding with their relaxation skills. Such repeated rehearsals help to build habit strength (i.e., to create greater choice) in the newly learned skills and to establish internal and external stimuli as daily reminders to deploy coping resources upon early detection of stress or worry. Finally, whenever opportunities for approach to feared situations do present themselves, we encourage exposures to those situations, combining clients' relaxation coping skills with whole-organism approach behaviors and the cultivation of intrinsic values (described later) during such approach.

As mentioned previously, our current package includes interpersonal/ emotional processing techniques. Based partly on work by Safran and Segal (1990), Michelle Newman (see Newman, Castonguay, Borkovec, & Molnar, 2004) expanded this integrative cognitive, interpersonal, and experiential approach and adapted it to our clients with GAD, based on what was known about their intrapersonal and interpersonal functioning. The interpersonal element is designed to identify the client's interpersonal needs and fears, to determine how the client is behaving to get those needs satisfied, and the ways that these behaviors are not succeeding, and to teach new and more flexible interpersonal behaviors. Emotional deepening methods contribute to the interpersonal goals by facilitating the identification of authentic emotions related to interpersonal relationships and, based on those, the emergence of authentic behavioral expressions (e.g., assertive responses and other forms of adaptive communication and ways of relating). In the process of functional analyses of interpersonal behaviors, use is made not only of clients' descriptions of their interpersonal patterns and how people react to those behaviors but also of the interpersonal behaviors that emerge between the client and the therapist. For example, the therapist will let the client know what kind of emotional impact his or her behavior is having in the moment and what behavioral tendencies those behaviors tend to pull from the therapist. Thus, the therapeutic relationship becomes a microcosm of the client's interpersonal realities, and feedback provides important information to the client for learning about actual, natural contingencies associated with the client's interpersonal actions and contains the possibility for corrective emotional experiences, similar to some of the features of the therapeutic relationship discussed by others in this volume.

Stuck Cognition

Traditional CT involves (1) identifying what clients are thinking, how they are perceiving, interpreting, and predicting, and what core beliefs they hold; (2) assessing the accuracy of these cognitions through a search for evidence for their truth value; (3) creating more accurate ways of seeing things and believing; and (4) testing these new views in daily life. We utilize this traditional and well-known approach with our clients with GAD, but given what we know about their idiosyncratic cognitive processes, we emphasize a number of additional features.

Rigidity in GAD is most pervasive in clients' cognitive activity. Their habitual engagement in worrisome thinking about the future precludes attending to other aspects of their immediate environments; they are thinking too much. GAD is also associated with persistent attentional biases to threat cues, often outside of awareness (MacLeod & Rutherford, 2004). Moreover, they display rigid interpretive biases, interpreting ambiguous information in threatening ways and perceiving higher than normal subjective risk that bad things will happen (MacLeod & Rutherford, 2004). Their streams of consciousness during worry show a lack of flexible thinking (Molina, Borkovec, Peasely, & Person, 1998), and they score high on measures of nonadaptive beliefs (e.g., the Dysfunctional Attitudes Scale; Behar & Borkovec, 2002), reflecting inaccurate and inflexible views of their worlds. Images in their mental life are often negatively valenced (Borkovec & Inz, 1990) and revolve around catastrophes that might happen. Because mental activities such as worry can be performed anytime, chronic worriers also associate worrisome activity with numerous environments, which results in a spread of worry throughout the day and a lack of stimulus control. Indeed, clients with GAD show classical acquisition of threat-detection responses to neutral stimuli (e.g., a colored square on a computer monitor) that have been paired with threatening words (e.g., *criticism*) used as unconditional stimuli in evaluative conditioning procedures (Thayer, Friedman, Borkovec, Johnsen, & Molina, 2000).

From this evidence, our cognitive interventions usefully focuses on modifying these characteristic inflexible habits, targeting clients' negatively biased attention, interpretations, predictions, expectations, and images, and establishing more adaptive stimulus control of worrisome activity. Below we describe our various therapeutic methods for addressing these cognitive domains. Our initial goal in therapy is to loosen up cognitive activity and provide alternatives to inaccurate and nonadaptive ways of perceiving the world via relatively more accurate, flexible, and adaptive ways of perceiving and interpreting. This "loosening up" includes, but is not limited to, a belief that emancipation occurs through the recognition of the ways in which the client is determined or "stuck" in nonadaptive, inflexible, or automatic cognitions. To influence automatic cognitive processes, a client requires awareness of the existence of such processes, an intention to override them, and sufficient attentional resources to do so (Bargh, 1994). These facets of change are continually facilitated during our treatment sessions. Once threat perceptions that would otherwise sabotage attempts to focus on the present moment are significantly lessened through cognitive change interventions, the goals of being able to stop thought altogether, get out of the head, and live increasingly in the present become more realistically achievable.

Open and Multiple Perspectives

Despite the value of the typical CT for generating more accurate views of the world, we do not want our clients to become rigid in their newfound beliefs. Replacing a habitual perspective with a more adaptive one would not be ideal if that new view also became inflexible and unresponsive to new information. As in traditional CT, we emphasize that any perspective must remain open to empirical testing, that no perspective is absolutely true, and that a particular perspective's accuracy, relevance, or usefulness may vary over changing times and changing environments. Most importantly, we emphasize the generation of multiple perspectives. This usually begins with discussions of neutral situations, wherein the client's habitual, defensive ways of thinking are not as likely to occur. The question "How many ways are there to see this?" is applied to things such as the forms that can be perceived in clouds, events in situational comedies from the viewpoints of different characters, simple objects in the therapy office, and Gestalt figures that contain more than one perceptual possibility. Once the client becomes familiar with the notion of multiple perspectives with these innocuous examples, the therapist moves to anxiety-producing or worry-relevant material. As in typical problem-solving approaches, the initial phase is a brainstorming period whose goal is to identify several views of the same situation, without evaluating their accuracy or usefulness.

Of particular note is our emphasis on the use of humorous views and play to facilitate multiple perspective taking. Humor not only adds an element of pleasantness and lightness to the process but also entails relatively large shifts away from habitual meanings, toward novel interpretations and responses (Kreitler, Dreshsler, & Kreitler, 1988). Thus, shifting and often incongruous perspectives involved in a humorous engagement facilitate the breaking of fixed and concretized habits and the use of novel approaches. Humor comprehension and appreciation are also positively associated with mental flexibility and the use of problem-solving strategies (Gelkopf & Kreitler, 1996). Moreover, Gelkopf and Kreitler (1996) regard the use of in-session humor as being akin to Beck's concept of "distancing," or the process of regarding thoughts objectively (1976, p. 243). Use of humor for shifting perspectives also facilitates cognitive reframing in which the conceptual and/or emotional context of a problem is changed to reconstruct its meaning in a more adaptive way (Walrond-Skinner, 1986).

In addition, the creation of multiple perspectives also involves an element of play. Play appears to be a central component of effective education (etymologically in Greek, *paidai* denotes "the harmless play of children," and *paideia* means "education"), and it is significant that the period in which mammals engage in the most play is also the time during which they are most likely to learn (Kolb, 2000). Moreover, Lowenfeld (1935/1991) delineated four ultimate purposes of play, all of which are desirable from a GAD therapeutic standpoint. Play (1) makes a connection with the immediate environment, (2) creates a bridge between conscious and emotional experience, (3) facilitates the experiencing of inner emotions, and (4) brings joy, relaxation, and amusement to one's life. Empirically determined benefits include increases in general flexibility and novelty of responses (Dansky

& Silverman, 1973; Singer & Singer, 1990); concentration and positive affect (Shmukler & Naveh, 1984–1985); creativity, divergent thinking, and originality (Feitelson, 1972; Smilansky, 1986); and cardiovascular flexibility (Hutt, 1981).

Once several perspectives are identified for a given situation, customary CT methods for assessing accuracy, advantages and disadvantages, and impact on anxiety and depression are applied, resulting in a set of multiple perspectives of varying degrees of estimated accuracy. Several of these will be seen as nearly equal in accuracy and so will provide flexible alternatives for the targeted situation. As with multiple relaxation techniques, our clients try out their multiple perspectives within situations during daily living, remaining playful and experimental with their cognitions, and loose and flexible in their approach to their lives. As Kuhn implies (1962/1996), it may be the case that, like Gestalt figures, we cannot view the world simultaneously through different paradigms/perspectives. However, this does not preclude the possibility that one can alternate between various perspectives from an evaluative position. Such alterations increase the probability of matching perspectives to existing circumstances in an appropriate and adaptive manner.

Rehearsal of Perspectives

Examples of dramatic insights leading to widespread changes occur in CT (e.g., Borkovec, Hazlett-Stevens, & Diaz, 1999), but it is more common that new perspectives have weak habit strength, old ones have been habitual for a long time, and rehearsal of new views is very important for increasing choice in ways of seeing. Thus, clients are asked to shift perspectives to newly developed views as soon as they detect anxiety or worry during their daily living, in addition to applying their relaxation and "letting go" skills. As cognitive products are identified in CT, these are incorporated into the self-control desensitization procedure: In the anxiety-generating scenes and at incipient anxiety detection, clients not only relax (and imagine themselves relaxing in the imagined situation) but they also imagine changing their perspectives. Repeated rehearsals of coping responses provide opportunities for creating increased habit strength and establishing environmental cues as reminders to shift perspectives.

Worry Outcome Diary

Clients with GAD do not process all of the information available in their moment-to-moment experience, and they especially do not process information that contradicts their habitual views. Although examining past evidence is useful in evaluating the accuracy of perspectives, it is important to have clients cultivate the skill of paying attention to reality in the present moment and of processing events that reflect accurately on the way things are. A useful device involves the Worry Outcome Diary. Clients write down each worry identified during the day and what outcome they fear will happen. Each evening, they review entries from past days to see whether actual outcomes have occurred. If so, they rate on a 5-point scale whether the outcome turned out better than expected, as bad as expected, or worse than expected. For things that turn out badly, they similarly rate how well they coped with the outcome. They are then asked to process any favorable outcome information by reliving in imagery the actual outcome as it related to the expectation and to draw conclusions from this real-life information relevant to their way of making predictions or having expectations. Diaries are reviewed with the therapist, who reinforces the new information and points out that the client is creating his or her first objective history of evidence about the way things actually are. Empirical data from our own laboratory demonstrates that the worried-about outcomes rarely happen, and even if they do, clients handle the situation much better than they predict that they will (Borkovec et al., 1999). Clients in turn gain an alternative perspective on the world and take steps toward creating new narratives for themselves. This may be similar to Teasdale's (1996) admonition that therapists should target holistic meanings rather than attempting to modify individual sentences of meaning. While the Worry Outcome Diary does focus on individual and concrete present worries, the dialectic of generating hypotheses, collecting data, and comparing the actual results to expectations provides a holistic meaning that goes beyond the modification of individual worry sentences.

Imagery as Reality and Imagination of Most Likely Outcomes

Imagery is reality in certain important senses. First, imagery is incipient action (efferent command into physiology, behavior, and affect; Lang, 1985). When we imagine something, we engage in internal behavior toward that something. If action is meaning, then imagery is a source of meaning. Second, the behavior of imagination is sufficiently powerful that imaginal rehearsal of skilled behaviors (as in a sporting activity) can increase the quality of performance, just as actual practice does, although possibly not to the same extent (Murphy, 1994). Third, emotional images elicit the same pattern of physiological response that actual events do (Lang, Levin, Miller, & Kozak, 1983). Finally, if people are asked to imagine a set of events happening and are later asked whether such events did indeed happen, then people will believe that those events happened to a greater degree than if they had not been asked to imagine those events (e.g., Garry, Manning, Loftus, & Sherman, 1996).

These points have several implication for our clients with GAD who are frequently experiencing catastrophic images. These images strengthen threatening meanings, and negative emotional reactions are experienced as if these catastrophes are actually happening. A further implication to the recall findings is that if one imagines bad events during worry, then these images are stored in memory with an ambiguous flag as to whether or not they happened in reality. So clients with GAD are constantly acquiring functional evidence that such bad things do indeed occur, even though they have not. This phenomenon is the likely basis for comments by clients that, although logical analysis and evidence indicate the inaccuracy of a non-adaptive perspective, it still *feels* true. Logic and intellectual recognition of evidence (as part of the abstract system) do not connect as strongly with efferent command as does imagery. Thus, inaccurate expectations contained in worry feel true, because our clients have experienced such events numerous times in their imaginal life; they have the evidence for the truth value of these events at an affective level.

Strong empirical evidence thus exists for the useful role of imagery in treatment, and we have incorporated it in our self-control desensitization method as a vehicle for rehearsing and strengthening adaptive reactions to incipient anxiety cues. Moreover, the imagery–recall research has prompted a further tactic: Desensitization segments end with repeated rehearsals of images of the most likely outcomes for a worrisome situation based on probability and evidence derived from CT segments of the session. Furthermore, the client is encouraged to substitute (and vividly imagine) the "most likely outcome," or several likely outcomes, upon early detection of worry. The goal is to reduce the frequency and duration of catastrophic images and to increase images that relate to what will actually happen. "Most likely" images facilitate moving the anxiety spiral in adaptive emotional directions, become more well established as an availability heuristic, and reinforce the feeling of the truth of cognitive products intellectually derived from preceding CT.

Stimulus Control and Worry-Free Zones

Because we can worry anywhere, many environmental cues become associated with it and so come to set the occasion for its occurrence. Two decades ago, we developed a stimulus control procedure for reducing worry. The technique antedated our eventual CBT approach but anticipated our emphasis on early cue detection and living in the present. Derived from Bootzin's (Bootzin & Epstein, 2000) stimulus control treatment for insomnia, our application involves five instructed steps for reducing worry: (1) Establish a half-hour worry period at the same time each day and in the same distinctive place; (2) monitor the worrying and learn to detect its initiation as soon as possible; (3) postpone any detected worrying until the worry period; (4) focus attention back to the present moment; and (5) use the worry period to worry about the concerns or to problem-solve about those concerns. Although telling worriers to stop worrying is not effective, they do find it much easier to postpone worries if time for them exists later. The method was found effective with chronic worriers (Borkovec, Wilkinson, Folensbee, & Lerman, 1983) and incorporated with changes into our eventual CBT. Although clients can worry during their worry period, emphasis is placed on problem solving and the application of the CT methods to generate cognitive coping responses for use when clients notice a worry. For problem solving, they distinguish between worries and feared outcomes over which they have some control (e.g., savings plan for children's college education) and those over which they have little or no control (e.g., global warming). In the worry period, clients work on behavioral strategies for increasing the likelihood of positive outcomes, but they implement actions based on those strategies as soon as possible, at which time that particular worry shifts to worries over which they have no further control. The latter are addressed by applying their usual CT methods in order to generate useful perspective shifts whenever that worry emerges.

One of our therapists, Mary Boutselis, created a related, often easier and more useful approach. Clients create a brief "worry-free" zone in their daily lives (e.g., whenever driving, when awakening and until after breakfast, or whenever in their living room). When they detect incipient worry in this zone, they let go of the worry and postpone it to any time outside of that zone. When clients report success within this first zone, additional zones are added, so that, over time, an increasing number of times and situations become free of worry.

Expectancy-Free Living

Once clients are reporting success with perspective shifts and are making more accurate predictions, we encourage one more step that is logically deducible from empirical literature on the pervasiveness of confirmatory biases. Because our preexisting perspectives influence what and how we see, present-moment reality is not easy to access. The therapeutic implication is that the greatest degree of adaptation, of new learning, and of access to reality occurs if we are able to let go of preexisting beliefs, predictions, and expectations, and simply pay attention to the reality that is in front of us. The ideal would involve our clients' movement from their habitual, negative expectations to relatively more accurate expectations, to eventually no expectations at all. Thus, the ultimate goal of CT, like the ultimate goal of self-monitoring and relaxation therapy, is living in the present moment.

Being completely free of preexisting perspectives is likely impossible, but we encourage our clients to practice letting go of these as much and as often as they can, and merely to pay attention to the actual events transpiring before their eyes. Early in therapy, this has to do with anxious and worrisome cognitions, but increasingly we ask clients to adopt the same approach to their experience of the entire day. Because evidence from the Worry Outcome Diary confirms that most things turn out well and that they cope quite well with whatever happens, clients learn that they can trust themselves and the world more than they have previously done, and that openness to present-moment reality can generate a lighter and freer life, where greater potential for joy and adaptive learning about themselves and their worlds exists.

Additional Components

In addition to the interventions targeting specific "stuck" systems, our work contains integrative components that cut across several domains and build on these more specific elements.

CT in a Relaxed State

We often have clients generate a deeply relaxed state just prior to conducting CT, especially that portion of therapy involving the generation of alternative perspectives. Increased parasympathetic tone provides for more flexible attentional deployment, and reduction of anxious states via relaxation facilitates more flexible and more accurate thinking in general. A pilot data study supports this: After choosing their two most pressing worries, half of the participants relaxed via slowed diaphragmatic breathing, whereas participants in the other half worried about one of their topics. They then wrote down as many possible outcomes to the second worry as they could think of. People who worried first generated mostly negative outcomes, whereas people who relaxed first listed mostly positive outcomes.

Focus on the Task at Hand, Whole-Organism Approach, and Intrinsic Values

Once in the present, there is the question of what to do in that moment. Simply paying attention to what actually exists is foundational to this approach. First, we emphasize (and practice in sessions) paying attention to sensations in all five modalities and the simplest level of perception as a method of getting out of the head and of decreasing reactions to these reactions by not judging, categorizing, or engaging in other associations and by merely observing the way things are. Second, if the present has a task, we encourage our clients to focus attention solely on that task, with minimal thought about future outcomes once engagement in the task has begun. Most importantly, we work to create intrinsic meanings and motivations for any present moment, whether that present contains a task or not. The purpose of cultivating intrinsic behaviors relates to what we previously meant by "whole-organism approach."

Whole-organism approach can be explained by an example. Consider the specific case of phobias. Traditional methods use exposure to feared stimuli, while motoric avoidance is prevented. The problem is that clients often engage in other defensive reactions during exposures even though they may be in the physical presence of the phobic situation and are in some limited sense behaviorally "approaching" it. We can close our eyes during exposures, engage in distraction, or shift to freezing responses as the evolutionarily significant backup response when escape or avoidance is prevented. Any of these reactions to reactions maintain the anxious meaning of the situation despite exposure to it. Indeed, Grayson, Foa, and Steketee (1982) demonstrated the deleterious effect of distraction during exposure with obsessive–compulsive disorder, while Borkovec (1974) showed the maintaining effects of imagined avoidance to imaginal phobic presentations. So whenever approach to feared situations becomes part of treatment, we work with our clients to develop ways in which they can engage in approach that involves all of their interacting systems, including cognitive and affective systems. A simple example that Borkovec uses involves phobias of bees. When asked to allow the bee to fly around without engaging in avoidance, people will usually freeze, with their eyes anxiously watching for the bee. Instead, they are asked to hold their hand out to the bee, as if inviting it to land on their hand, and to feel this action as a positive approach response, knowing cognitively that little chance exists that the bee would actually land, much less sting. Other perspectives based on the client's values and associated with positive affect (e.g., bees as makers of honey, as complex social animals, as one of nature's creatures) are encouraged to maximize positive approach feelings and cognitions during exposure.

Recent work supports the idea that values, sense of self, and intrinsic motivation may be critical in modifying long-held beliefs such as those typical of clients with GAD. Sherman and Cohen (2002) explain resistance to disconfirmatory evidence and biased interpretations of ambiguous stimuli as arising from a fundamental motivation to protect the integrity of the self. If self-worth and self-value are only affirmed by one view (e.g., any particular, dominant GAD perspective), people tend to defensive and resistant to novel, disconfirmatory evidence. So individuals need an alternative source of self-identity. Such alternatives are not always easy to locate when one is absorbed in worry and anxiety. A focus on values and intrinsic motivation is therefore very useful; making such values manifest leads to alternative self-affirmations. Moreover, any daily activity or experience can be enhanced by bringing intrinsic values to that present moment as a way of creating whole-organism approach. Goals and values markedly affect what information is attended to and how information is processed (Bargh & Chartrand, 1999). Although being Zorba, the Greek, might be idyllic, eliminating all preconceptions from one's processing of and engagement with present-moment reality is difficult, as mentioned before. While it is useful to cultivate increasingly objective observation, it is also additionally helpful to increase one's flexibility in the conceptions that are brought to the moment by enriching existing perspectives and by creating multiple perspectives that reflect one's most important or cherished values.

Social anxiety provides a good example of both attention to the task and the use of perspectives based on values. If we are socially anxious, focusing on ourselves during a conversation increases our anxiety, whereas focusing on the task at hand (i.e., conversation content) lessens anxiety (Przeworski, 2002). In addition, focusing on the conversation increases the likelihood that we will learn new and important things from its content or about the other person, things that might be useful or even critical to our lives someday. We can trust ourselves to emit the most adaptive behaviors we have learned so far, because we are paying attention to content rather than anything else, and this attentional focus maximizes the probability that those emitted behaviors will be adaptive, where adequate stimuli elicit adequate responses. This does not mean that our behavior will always be successful; we do make mistakes with others. However, as long as we continue to pay attention, we can continue to learn from our mistakes and thus maximize our survival in the long run.

Having focused on the present, we can also bring intrinsic values into the process of this conversation. Many conversations have explicit or implicit extrinsic goals (e.g., making a good impression, getting a job offer, creating a friendship, convincing someone to fund our proposal, or providing corrective feedback to change a student's behavior). Excessive focus on extrinsic goals during a task can result in anxiety over whether they will be achieved and depression over the prospect that they will not. Anxiety and depression decrease the quality of complex performances. Focus on the task precludes these emotions, thus maximizing the quality of performance. In turn, greater quality of performance increases the likelihood of achieving the goal. So we have to let go of the extrinsic outcome to maximize the chance of getting it, and focusing on the task at hand is one way to do this. Having additional intrinsic goals has the same effect but also provides opportunities to cultivate joy in the task or in the moment of the task. Although we may be talking to the other person for the sake of an extrinsic outcome, we can also maintain an awareness of other intrinsic values that we wish to bring to this conversation. We are attempting not to use people as means but as ends in themselves. For example, we might consciously bear in mind that we wish to affirm other human beings whenever we are with them, to make them feel good about themselves, or to convey caring.

The anthropologist, Carlos Casteneda, provided an interesting example. His teacher, Don Juan, asked that they meet in a town square. When Carlos arrived, he found Don Juan sitting in the square wearing a suit instead of his customary jeans. He laughed at Don Juan for being a hypocrite, for claiming in the past that one should never fear other's judgments, and here he was dressed up for the local people. Don Juan's reply described his distinction between internal and external consideration. Internal consideration involves dressing up for fear of others' opinions; external consideration involves dressing up out of respect. A striking implication of this particular example is that a socially anxious person could actually perform the very same behavior that in the past was designed to avoid disapproval, yet do it from an entirely different (non-anxiety-provoking) perspective. A significant feature to engaging in intrinsically valued behavior is that it is rewarding, pleasant, and potentially joyful in and of itself, has no direct reference to any extrinsic outcome, does not relate to the future, and it forms an effective basis for enhancing how one feels about oneself.

Additional examples can be given. Doing the dishes while worrying about other things that need to be done or being angry at having to do this chore can be contrasted with paying attention to the task (the warmth of the water, reflections in the soaped dish, movement of one's hands and arms through time and space) or doing the task out of love for one's family. Writing a grant proposal to obtain funding and more publications can be contrasted with a focus on getting on top of one's literature, obtaining new knowledge, writing beautiful sentences rich in meaning, or creating elegant designs and methodologies in pursuit of empirical pieces of the theoretical puzzle which, when discovered and placed into the mosaic of knowledge, change the entire mosaic. The important point is that we need to know our clients well enough to become familiar with their philosophical, religious, spiritual, or just daily life values that reflect what is truly important to them, and near and dear to their hearts. These qualities can provide the basis for creating an affective and cognitive approach, in addition to a behavioral approach, that can potentially bring happiness into each present moment. Moreover, unlike external goals, looseness and flexibility are inherent to values. Whereas goals possess fixed end points and the path to their attainment is specifiable in advance, values are more open, intrinsic, and flexible in their application and outcomes (Martin, Kleindorfer, & Brashers, 1987). Such an emphasis on value and autonomy is important for change: People generally gain more long-lasting changes if they attribute changes to themselves rather than to external environments (Mikulas, 2002).

Therapist Modeling of Flexibility

It is important that our therapists display the same flexibility that our clients are to learn. They become models for changes that we are trying to facilitate by these techniques. If we try to produce change in a client who is unwilling or unable to change in a particular way, or using a particular method, both clients and therapists become frustrated or fearful of failure in one another's (or supervisor's, or one's own) eyes. These states are not conducive to change, to the processing of new information, to being flexible in behavior, or to facilitating the critical therapeutic alliance (Constantino, Castonguay, & Schut, 2001). So our therapists make use of the large number of techniques available to them to move around in the session, addressing one system (e.g., via applied relaxation), then another (e.g., imagery rehearsals), then yet another (e.g., one further step in a CT sequence), and they make such shifts when the client does not seem to be understanding an application or is resistant to it, or does not feel that it is beneficial in that moment. Our CT, for example, does not attempt to take the client linearly from point A to point Z, whether or not clients wish to go there or can follow us there. Rather, the CT is designed to loosen up ways of seeing, to create multiple perspectives, and to give the client a sense of success along the way. Empirical support for one example of the importance of this approach comes from Castonguay, Goldfried, Wiser, Raue, and Hayes (1996) who demonstrated that when clients resist CT, the therapist's most common response is to increase adherence to the CT protocol, which results in a rupture in the working alliance and predicts poor outcome. An effective flexible alternative is to stop the CT and address the rupture with experiential repair techniques before proceeding (Safran & Muran, 2000).

It is useful to conceive of the therapist's modeling of flexibility, as well as the variety of other states created for the client, through the application of our various techniques in terms of altered states and their contribution to creating greater freedom within determinism. Internal and external environments in which we customarily live have developed functional properties as setting events and conditional stimuli that predispose habitual responding due to our learning histories. Many literatures in psychology have documented the potency of these environments in generating habitual ways of being (e.g., mood-dependent learning, state-dependent learning, drug-dependent learning, and decades of research in general learning theory and behavior therapy). The more novel the environment in which we find ourselves, the less strong the deterministic stimulus control of our behavior in that moment and the greater the degree of choice we have with regard to ways of responding at any of the levels of our information-processing systems. Therapy itself is a novel environment; clients are presented with numerous unfamiliar conditions. Whether these conditions involve the provision of an unconditional acceptance, exposure to feared situations without avoidance, therapist confrontation about nonadaptive interpersonal behaviors outside of client awareness, the experiencing of avoided emotions, or the creation of a deeply relaxed state, the client is exposed to relatively novel internal and external conditions that thereby provide an opportunity for greater choice. Although old habits are primed to occur, therapists can facilitate the enactment of new choices in these moments of relatively greater freedom.

EMPIRICAL SUPPORT FOR OUR THERAPY

Similar to earlier reviews (Borkovec & Whisman, 1996; Chambless & Gillis, 1993), a recent review of the outcome literature has clearly indicated that CBT is effective for GAD (Borkovec & Ruscio, 2001). The latter review covered 13 controlled trials involving this therapy, 11 of which provided information allowing the calculation of effect sizes. CBT generated the largest within-group effect sizes at both posttherapy (2.48) and long-term follow-up (2.44) compared to nonspecific or alternate treatments (2.09 and 2.00, respectively), component control conditions (1.72 and 1.71, respectively), and waiting-list no-treatment (0.01 at posttherapy; no follow-up available). Moderate to large between-group effect sizes also favored CBT (0.71 and 0.31 for posttherapy and follow-up compared to nonspecific or alternate treatments; 0.26 and 0.54, respectively, for component conditions; and 1.09 for posttherapy for no-treatment). Examination of each of the 13 studies determined that CBT generated significantly greater improvement than nonspecific or alternate treatments in 9 of 11 comparisons at posttherapy and 7 of 9 comparisons at follow-up, greater change than components in 2 of 10 posttherapy and 3 of 7 follow-up assessments (although findings of differences were due to duration of treatment, as described earlier in the Borkovec et al. [2002] report), and more favorable outcome than all no-treatment conditions at posttherapy. These studies included client samples whose subjects averaged 39 years of age, 7 years of chronicity, and 11 sessions of therapy. Among all of the conditions in these studies, CBT also had the lowest dropout rate (8%), and the changes it produced at the end of therapy routinely maintained at follow-up. CBT is thus a well-established, empirically supported treatment for GAD (Chambless & Ollendick, 2001).

Two additional controlled investigations (besides Borkovec et al. [2002] reviewed earlier) have since been published. First, Öst and Breitholtz (2000) found CT and behavior therapy equivalent in outcome, with within-group effect sizes matching average effect sizes for prior component conditions. Second, Ladouceur and colleagues (2000) determined that a CBT package (teaching acceptance of uncertainty in life and adaptive problem-solving orientations, and using exposure to catastrophic images underlying worrisome concerns and correction of erroneous beliefs about worry) was superior to no treatment. Absence of information precluded effect size calculations; absence of a nonspecific control condition limited conclusions about specific causal ingredients, and absence of component conditions prevented identification of active ingredients contained in this multicomponent package. However, it is the first controlled study to include an explicit type of acceptance therapy for GAD.

In addition to controlled trials, two open trials have been reported. Although further research employing control conditions is required before conclusions can be drawn, both studies employed interventions relevant to the theme of the conference upon which this volume is based. Kabat-Zinn and colleagues (1992) found mindfulness meditation effective with a mixed group of clients with panic disorder and GAD, and Crits-Christoff, Connolly, Azarian, Crits-Christoff, and Shappell (1996) found that supportive–expressive therapy focused on changing interpersonal relationships generated significant pre- to posttherapy improvements. Unfortunately, absence of effect size information in both investigations prevents a comparison of their outcomes to other GAD therapy studies.

It is also useful to examine our own series of five completed clinical trials to determine whether our evolving therapy is producing greater gains as our new directions have been incorporated. Our first investigations (Borkovec & Mathews, 1988; Borkovec et al., 1987) involved solely traditional CBT. The next study (Borkovec & Costello, 1993) incorporated our various ways of teaching clients to focus on the present moment. The fourth investigation (Borkovec et al., 2002) continued that emphasis and added the creation of intrinsic values. Our fifth study (Newman, Castonguay, & Borkovec, 2002) continued the emphasis on these elements and added interpersonal and emotional deepening techniques. Average within-group effect sizes over these investigations at posttherapy were 1.84, 2.60, 2.69, 2.80, and 3.29. Our first study did not obtain systematic follow-up data, but the effect sizes for the other consecutive studies were 2.64, 3.04, 2.45, and 3.19. We may simply be getting better at what we do in general, but the data are also consistent with the hypothesis that each new direction that we have taken has resulted in increments in clinical effectiveness. We are currently conducting a randomized clinical trial contrasting our CBT with and without the interpersonal and experiential components. This additive design will provide a direct experimental test of whether the interpersonal and experiential elements are causatively linked to incremented improvements over and above what our CBT is able to produce.

EPILOGUE

The purpose of this book is to describe "new" developments within behavioral and cognitive therapy. The claim that something new is happening raises some interesting issues.

First, something new in therapeutic interventions is definitely needed. A recent meta-analysis demonstrated that, with the single exception of specific phobias, no significant increase in effect sizes has occurred over the decades of outcome research on each of the other anxiety disorders (Öst, 2002). Although the principles of operant and classical conditioning have been successfully applied to an increasing number of psychological problems (see Chambless & Ollendick's [2001] for a review of "empirically supported treatments"), no further increments in effectiveness have occurred within most of the anxiety disorders since their original applications.

Second, "new" within the field of behavior therapy would, strictly speaking, mean "the application of additional empirical knowledge and principles." Since the early days of behavior therapy, there have been no further applications of any other psychological principles that have led to new interventions that are as dramatically effective as the applications of those original principles. In a sense, the commitment of early behavior therapy to use the best known principles of human behavior in the development of psychological interventions has not been fulfilled over the past four decades. Although we have described the evolution (and not revolution) of our own therapy approach for GAD in terms of its grounding in psychological knowledge, our specific techniques, and those presented in other chapters in this volume, vary in the degree to which each rests upon solid empirical foundations. Those techniques with grounding in psychological principles might be new in terms of their content but do not represent anything new within the fundamental spirit of behavior therapy. Those techniques with little or no basis in empirically derived principles might be "new" in a second, broader sense of the term, but they would not be a part of behavior therapy. Rather, they would more correctly be portrayed as integrations of behavior therapy methods with techniques based on other nonempirical sources of presumed knowledge.

There are many sources of potential knowledge (e.g., philosophy, theology, natural sciences, social sciences, personal observation, clinical observation), each with its own advantages and disadvantages, and its own specific rules of evidence for the truth–value of its conclusions. We rightfully become particularly excited when two or more such sources agree in their conclusions about a particular phenomenon. This would represent a kind of interrater reliability about a piece of knowledge, encouraging its further pursuit because of the likelihood that something very important has been identified by two or more separate paths. There appear to be two levels of such interrater reliability present in the content of this volume. First, it is striking how similar the perspectives are among the contributors to this volume, all with a professional history within behavior therapy, but with each person largely operating independently and drawing from differing resources in eventually coming to the same place (e.g., the potential importance of the therapeutic relationship, of mindfulness, of life in the present moment, and of bringing values to bear on life in that moment). How and why this has occurred in this cohort of behavior therapists at this particular moment in time is unclear and would require historical analysis of the *zeitgeist* to explain it fully. But such an analysis would likely touch upon the second level of reliability. Potential insights about human behavior from humanistic traditions within clinical psychology (e.g., Carl Rogers) and from outside of Western psychology (e.g., Buddhism) became particularly popular with a generation growing up in the 1960s and 1970s, a time when alternatives to prevailing worldviews were being sought. Many of the authors in this volume are from that generation. We were thus exposed simultaneously to this cultural experience on the one hand, and to the emergence of behavior therapy and its rigorous scientifically based approach to psychotherapy on the other. When these traditions seem to be overlapping in what they tell us about the nature of human beings, there is additional incentive to pursue them further. We see such overlap frequently throughout this volume, so there is good reason for some excitement.

But third, there are two emotion-related issues. First, growing up in early behavior therapy has given us an enormous respect for the contributions of its founding parents. All sources of knowledge build upon the insights of earlier generations. Out of respect for those great thinkers, we should be very cautious in proclaiming a "new movement." Indeed, until the new therapy methods described in this volume are shown by research to significantly increment therapeutic change beyond that degree of change already documented for basic behavioral therapy, such a movement contains only a hope anyway, and not much reality. And "movements" have a tendency to have certain by-products that are not optimal for the continuing discovery of knowledge. They may inadvertently result in an overly enthusiastic zeal that contributes to beliefs that affect the things to which we selectively attend, and how we interpret the things to which we attend, thus increasing the likelihood of confirmatory bias instead of seeing what is real.

Our hope is that we will continue to ground our methods and their development in empirical science, that we will experimentally evaluate the potential causal contributions of any technical additions that we make to our therapies, and that we will remain humble about the course upon which we have embarked.

ACKNOWLEDGMENT

Preparation of this chapter was supported in part by National Institute of Mental Health Grant No. MH-58593 to T. D. Borkovec.

REFERENCES

Anderson, M. P., & Borkovec, T. D. (1980). Imagery processing and fear reduction during repeated exposure to two types of phobic imagery. *Behaviour Research and Therapy, 18,* 537–540.

Andrews, V. H., & Borkovec, T. D. (1988). The differential effects of induction of worry, somatic anxiety, and depression on emotional experience. *Journal of Behavior Therapy and Experimental Psychiatry, 19,* 21–26.

Bargh, J. A. (1994). The four horsemen of automaticity: Awareness, intention, efficiency, and control in social cognition. In R. S. Wyer & T. K. Srull (Eds.), *Handbook of social cognition* (2nd ed., pp. 1–40). Hillsdale, NJ: Erlbaum.

Bargh, J. A., & Chartrand, T. L. (1999). The unbearable automaticity of being. *American Psychologist, 54*(7), 462–479.

Baumeister, R. F., Bratslavsky, E., Muraven, M., & Tice, D. M. (1998). Ego depletion: Is the active self a limited resource? *Journal of Personality and Social Psychology, 74,* 1252–1265.

Baumeister, R. F., & Sommer, K. L. (1997). Consciousness, free choice, and automaticity. In R. S. Wyer, Jr. (Ed.), *Advances in social cognition* (Vol. X, pp. 75–81). Mahwah, NJ: Erlbaum.

Beauchaine, T. (2001). Vagal tone, development, and Gray's motivational theory: Toward an integrated model of autonomic nervous system functioning in psychopathology. *Development and Psychopathology, 13,* 183–214.

Beck, A. T. (1976). *Cognitive therapy and the emotional disorders.* New York: New American Library.

Behar, E., & Borkovec, T. D. (2002, November). *Cognitive-behavioral therapy for generalized anxiety disorder: Changes in dysfunctional attitudes.* Poster presented at the 35th annual meeting of the Association for the Advancement of Behavior Therapy, Reno, NV.

Bernstein, D. A., & Borkovec, T. D. (1973). *Progressive relaxation training.* Champaign, IL: Research Press.

Bernstein, D. A., Borkovec, T. D., & Hazlett-Stevens, H. (2000). *New directions in progressive relaxation training: A guidebook for helping professionals.* Westport, CT: Praeger.

Bernstein, R. J. (1983). *Beyond objectivism and relativism.* Philadelphia: University of Pennsylvania Press.

Bootzin, R. R., & Epstein, D. R. (2000). Stimulus control instructions. In K. L. Lichstein & C. M. Morin (Eds.), *Treatment of late-life insomnia* (pp. 167–184). Thousand Oaks, CA: Sage.

Borkovec, T. D. (1974). Heart-rate process during systematic desensitization and implosive therapy for analogue anxiety. *Behavior Therapy, 5,* 636–641.

Borkovec, T. D., Abel, J. L., & Newman, H. (1995). The effects of therapy on comorbid conditions in generalized anxiety disorder. *Journal of Consulting and Clinical Psychology, 63,* 479–483.

Borkovec, T. D., Alcaine, O. M., & Behar, E. (2004). Avoidance theory of worry and generalized anxiety disorder. In R. G. Heimberg, C. L. Turk, & D. S. Mennin (Eds.), *Generalized anxiety disorder: Advances in research and practice* (pp. 77–108). New York: Guilford Press.

Borkovec, T. D., & Costello, E. (1993). Efficacy of applied relaxation and cognitive behavioral therapy in the treatment of generalized anxiety disorder. *Journal of Consulting and Clinical Psychology, 61,* 611–619.

Borkovec, T. D., Hazlett-Stevens, H., & Diaz, M. L. (1999). The role of positive beliefs about worry in generalized anxiety disorder and its treatment. *Clinical Psychology and Psychotherapy, 6,* 126–138.

Borkovec, T. D., & Hu, S. (1990). The effect of worry on cardiovascular response to phobic imagery. *Behaviour Research and Therapy, 28,* 69–73.

Borkovec, T. D., & Inz, J. (1990). The nature of worry in generalized anxiety disorder: A predominance of thought activity. *Behaviour Research and Therapy, 28,* 153–158.

Borkovec, T. D., & Mathews, A. M. (1988). Treatment of nonphobic anxiety disorders: A comparison of nondirective, cognitive, and coping desensitization therapy. *Journal of Consulting and Clinical Psychology, 56,* 877–884.

Borkovec, T. D., Mathews, A. M., Chambers, A., Ebrahimi, S., Lytle, R., & Nelson, R.

(1987). The effects of relaxation training with cognitive therapy or nondirective therapy and the role of relaxation-induced anxiety in the treatment of generalized anxiety.
Journal of Consulting and Clinical Psychology, 25, 883–888.

Borkovec, T. D., Newman, M. G., Pincus, A., & Lytle, R. (2002). A component analysis of
cognitive behavioral therapy for generalized anxiety disorder and the role of interpersonal problems. *Journal of Consulting and Clinical Psychology, 70*, 288–298.

Borkovec, T. D., Robinson, E., Pruzinsky, T., & DePree, J. A. (1983). Preliminary exploration of worry: Some characteristics and processes. *Behaviour Research and Therapy,
21*, 9–16.

Borkovec, T. D., & Ruscio, A. (2001). Psychotherapy for generalized anxiety disorder.
Journal of Clinical Psychiatry, 62, 37–45.

Borkovec, T. D., & Sides, J. K. (1979). The contribution of relaxation ad expectancy to fear
reduction via graded, imaginal exposure to feared stimuli. *Behaviour Research and
Therapy, 17*, 529–540.

Borkovec, T. D., & Whisman, M. A. (1996). Psychological treatment for generalized anxiety disorder. In M. R. Mavissakalian & R. F. Prien (Eds.), *Long-term treatments of
anxiety disorders* (pp. 171–199). Washington, DC: American Psychiatric Association.

Borkovec, T. D., Wilkinson, L., Folensbee, R., & Lerman, C. (1983). Stimulus control applications to the treatment of worry. *Behaviour Research and Therapy, 21*, 247–251.

Brosschot, J. F., & Thayer, J. F. (in press). Worry, perseverative thinking and health. In L.
Temoshok (Ed.), *The expression and non-expression of emotion in health and disease.* Mahwah, NJ: Erlbaum.

Brown, T. A., & Barlow, D. H. (1992). Comorbidity among anxiety disorders: Implications
for treatment and DSM-IV. *Journal of Consulting and Clinical Psychology, 60*, 835–
844.

Brown, T. A., Barlow, D. H., & Liebowitz, M. R. (1994). The empirical basis of generalized
anxiety disorder. *American Journal of Psychiatry, 151*, 1272–1280.

Bruner, J. S., & Postman, L. (1949). On the perception of incongruity: a paradigm. *Journal
of Personality, 18*, 206–223.

Butler, B., Cullington, A., Hibbert, G., Klimes, I., & Gelder, M. (1987). Anxiety management for persistent generalized anxiety. *British Journal of Psychiatry, 151*, 535–542.

Castonguay, L. G., Goldfried, M. R., Wiser, S., Raue, P. J., & Hayes, A. M. (1996). Predicting outcome in cognitive therapy for depression: A comparison of unique and
common factors. *Journal of Consulting and Clinical Psychology, 64*, 497–504.

Chambless, D. L., & Gillis, M. M. (1993). Cognitive therapy of anxiety disorders. *Journal
of Consulting and Clinical Psychology, 61*, 248–260.

Chambliss, D. L., & Ollendick, T. H. (2001). Empirically supported psychological interventions: Controversies and evidence. *Annual Review of Psychology, 52*, 685–716.

Clark, D. A., & Steer, R. A. (1996). Empirical status of the cognitive model of anxiety and
depression. In P. M. Salkovskis (Ed.) *Frontiers of cognitive therapy: The state of the
art and beyond* (pp. 75–96). New York: Guilford Press.

Constantino, M. J., Castonguay, L. G., & Schut, A. J. (2001). The working alliance: A flag-
ship for the scientific-practitioner model in psychotherapy. In G. S. Tryon (Ed.),
Counseling based on process research (pp. 81–131). New York: Allyn & Bacon.

Crits-Christoff, P., Connolly, M. B., Azarian, K., Crits-Christoff, K., & Shappell, S. (1996).
An open trial of brief supportive-expressive psychotherapy in the treatment of generalized anxiety disorder. *Psychotherapy, 33*, 418–431.

Dansky, J. L., & Silverman, I. W. (1973). Effects of play on associative fluency in pre-school
aged children. *Developmental Psychology, 9*, 38–43.

Fehr, F. S., & Stern, J. A. (1970). Peripheral physiological variables and emotion: The
James–Lange theory revisited. *Psychological Bulletin, 74*, 411–424.

Feitelson, D. (1972). Developing imaginative play in pre-school children as a possible approach to fostering creativity. *Early Childhood Development and Care, 1,* 181–195.

Feyerabend, P. K. (1993). *Against method* (3rd ed.). London: Verso.

Floyd, Pink. (1979). Comfortably numb. On *The wall* [Album]. New York: Capitol/EMI Records.

Foucault, M. (1987). *Mental illness and psychology* (A. Sheridan, Trans.). Berkeley: University of California Press. (Original work published 1954)

Gadamer, H. G. (1975). *Truth and method* (J. Weinsheimer & D. G. Marshall, Trans.). New York: Continuum. (Original work published 1960)

Garry, M., Manning, C. G., Loftus, E. F., & Sherman, S. J. (1996). Imagination inflation: Imagining a childhood event inflates confidence that it occurred. *Psychonomic Bulletin and Review, 3,* 208–214.

Gelkopf, M., & Kreitler, S. (1996). Is humor only fun, an alternative cure or magic?: The cognitive therapeutic potential of humor. *Journal of Cognitive Psychotherapy: An International Quarterly, 10,* 235–254.

Goldfried, M. R. (1971). Systematic desensitization as training in self-control. *Journal of Consulting and Clinical Psychology, 37,* 228–234.

Grayson, J. B., Foa, E. B., & Steketee, G. (1982). Habituation during exposure treatment: Distraction vs. attention-focusing. *Behaviour Research and Therapy, 20,* 323–328.

Hayes, S. C., Wilson, K. W., Gifford, E. V., Follette, V. M., & Strosahl, K. (1996). Emotional avoidance and behavioral disorders: A functional dimensional approach to diagnosis and treatment. *Journal of Consulting and Clinical Psychology, 64,* 1152–1168.

Heerlein, A., Richter, P., Gonzalez, M., & Santander, J. (1998). Personality patterns and outcomes in depressive and bipolar disorders. *Psychopathology, 31,* 15–22.

Heide, F. J., & Borkovec, T. D. (1983). Relaxation-induced anxiety: Paradoxical anxiety enhancement due to relaxation training. *Journal of Consulting and Clinical Psychology, 51,* 171–182.

Hoehn-Saric, R., McLeod, D. R., & Zimmerli, W. D. (1989). Somatic manifestations in women with generalized anxiety disorder: Physiological responses to psychological stress. *Archives of General Psychiatry, 46,* 1113–1119.

Hutt, (1981). Toward a taxonomy and conceptual model of play. In H. Day (Ed.), *Advances in motivation and aesthetics.* New York: Plenum Press.

Kabat-Zinn, J., Massion, A. O., Kristeller, J., Peterson, L. G., Fletcher, K. E., Pbert, L., et al. (1992). Effectiveness of a meditation-based stress reduction program in the treatment of anxiety disorders. *American Journal of Psychiatry, 149,* 936–943.

Kalska, H., Punamäki, R. L., & Mäki-Pelli, M. (1999). Memory performance and metamemory among depressive patients. *Applied Neuropsychology, 6,* 96–107.

Kant, I. (1996). *Critique of pure reason* (W. S. Pluhar, Trans.). Indianapolis, IN: Hackett. (Original work published 1781)

Kierkegaard, S. A. (1990). *Eighteen upbuilding discourses* (H. V. Hong & E. H. Hong, Trans.). Princeton, NJ: Princeton University Press. (Original work published 1843)

Kolb, A. Y. (2000). *Play: An interdisciplinary integration of research.* Unpublished doctoral dissertation, Case Western Reserve University, Cleveland, OH.

Kovac, T. (2001). Rigidity assessment: A possible way to identify a creative personality. *Studia Psychologica, 43,* 125–129.

Kreitler, S., Drechsler, I., & Kreitler, H. (1988). How to kill jokes cognitively?: The meaning structure of jokes. *Semiotica, 68,* 297–319.

Kuhn, T. S. (1996). *The structure of scientific revolutions* (3rd ed.). Chicago: University of Chicago Press. (Original work published 1962)

Ladouceur, R., Dugas, M. J., Freeston, M. H., Leger, E., Gagnon, F., & Thibodeau, N.

(2000). Efficacy of a cognitive-behavioral treatment for generalized anxiety disorder: Evaluation in a controlled clinical trial. *Journal of Consulting and Clinical Psychology, 68,* 957–964.

Lang, P. J. (1985). The cognitive psychophysiology of emotion: Fear and anxiety. In A. H. Tuma & J. D. Maser (Eds.), *Anxiety and the anxiety disorders* (pp. 131–170). Hillsdale, NJ: Erlbaum.

Lang, P. J., Levin, D. N., Miller, G. A., & Kozak, M. J. (1983). Fear behavior, fear imagery, and the psychophysiology of emotion: The problem of affective response integration. *Journal of Abnormal Psychology, 92,* 276–306.

Lazarus, R. S., & Folkman, S. (1984). *Stress, appraisal, and coping.* New York: Springer.

Lehrer, P. M., & Woolfolk, R. L. (1993). *Principles and practice of stress management* (2nd ed.). New York: Guilford Press.

Lichstein, K. L. (1988). *Clinical relaxation strategies.* New York: Wiley.

Lord, C. G., Lepper, M. R., & Preston, E. (1984). Considering the opposite: A corrective strategy for social judgment. *Journal of Personality and Social Psychology, 47,* 1231–1243.

Lowenfeld, M. (1991). *Play in childhood.* New York: Cambridge University Press. (Original work published 1935)

MacLeod, C., & Rutherfored, E. (2004). Information-processing approaches: Assessing the selective functioning of attention, interpretation, and memory in GAD patients. In R. G. Heimberg, C. L. Turk & D. S. Mennin (Eds.), *Generalized anxiety disorder: Advances in research and practice* (pp. 109–142). New York: Guilford Press.

MacLeod, C. M. (1991). Half a century of research on the Stroop effect: An integrative review. *Psychological Bulletin, 109,* 163–203.

Mathews, A., & MacLeod, C. (2002). Induced processing biases have causal effects on anxiety. *Cognition and Emotion, 16,* 310–315.

Martin, J. E., Kleindorfer, G. B., & Brashers, W. R. (1987). The theory of bounded rationality and the problem of legitimation. *Journal for the Theory of Social Behavior, 17,* 63–82.

Mikulas, W. L. (2002). *The integrative helper: Convergence of Eastern and Western traditions.* Pacific Grove, CA: Brooks/Cole.

Molina, S., Borkovec, T. D., Peasely, C., & Person, D. (1998). Content analysis of worrisome streams of consciousness in anxious and dysphoric participants. *Cognitive Therapy and Research, 22,* 109–123.

Mowrer, O. H. (1947). On the dual nature of learning: A re-interpretation of "conditioning" and "problem-solving." *Harvard Educational Review, 17,* 102–148.

Murphy, S. (1994). Imagery interventions in sport. *Medicine and Science in Sports and Exercise, 26,* 334–345.

Nakamura, C. Y., & Broen, W. E. (1965). Facilitation of competing responses as a function of "subnormal" drive conditions. *Journal of Experimental Psychology, 69,* 180–185.

Neuberg, S. L. (1989). The goal of forming accurate impressions during social interactions: Attenuating the impact of negative expectancies. *Journal of Personality and Social Psychology, 56,* 374–386.

Newman, M. G., Castonguay, L. G., & Borkovec, T. D. (2002, June). *Integrating cognitive behavioral and interpersonal/emotional processing treatments for generalized anxiety disorder: Preliminary outcome findings.* Symposium presentation at the annual meeting of the Society for Psychotherapy Research, Santa Barbara, CA.

Newman, M. G., Castonguay, L. G., Borkovec, T. D., & Molnar, C. (2004). Integrative psychotherapy. In R. G. Heimberg, C. L. Turk, & D. S. Mennin (Eds.), *Generalized anxiety disorder: Advances in research and practice* (pp. 320–350). New York: Guilford Press.

Öst, L. (1987). Applied relaxation: Description of a coping technique and review of controlled studies. *Behaviour Research and Therapy, 25,* 397–409.

Öst, L.-G. (2002, July). *CBT for anxiety disorders: What progress have we made after 35 years of randomized clinical trials?* Keynote address, British Association for Behavioural and Cognitive Psychotherapy, Warwick, UK.

Öst, L.-G., & Breitholtz, E. (2000). Applied relaxation vs. cognitive therapy in the treatment of generalized anxiety disorder. *Behaviour Research and Therapy, 38,* 777–790.

Palmer, S. E. (1999). *Vision science: Photons to phenomenology.* Cambridge, MA: MIT Press.

Perlin, L. I., & Schooler, C. (1978). The structure of coping. *Journal of Health and Social Behavior, 19,* 2–21.

Pincus, A. L., & Borkovec, T. D. (1994, June). *Interpersonal problems in generalized anxiety disorder: Preliminary clustering of patients' interpersonal dysfunction.* Paper presented at the annual meeting of the American Psychological Society, New York.

Przeworski, A. (2002, May). *Effects of focus of attention and anxiety levels in high and low socially anxious individuals.* Unpublished master's thesis, Pennsylvania State University, University Park, PA.

Quota, S., El-Sarraj, E., & Punamäki, R. (2001). Mental flexibility as resiliency factor among children exposed to political violence. *International Journal of Psychology, 36,* 1–7.

Roemer, L., & Orsillo, S. M. (2002). Expanding our conceptualization of and treatment for generalized anxiety disorder: Integrating mindfulness/acceptance-based approaches with existing cognitive-behavioral models. *Clinical Psychology: Science and Practice, 9,* 54–68.

Roy-Byrne, P. P. (1996). Generalized anxiety and mixed anxiety–depression: Association with disability and health care utilization. *Journal of Clinical Psychiatry, 57*(Suppl. 7), 86–91.

Safran, J., & Segal, Z. V. (1990). *Interpersonal process in cognitive therapy.* New York: Basic Books.

Safran, J. D., & Muran, J. C. (2000). *Negotiating the therapeutic alliance: A relational treatment guide.* New York: Guilford Press.

Singer, D. G., & Singer, J. L. (1990). *The house of make believe.* Cambridge, MA: Harvard University Press.

Sherman, D. K., & Cohen, G. L. (2002). Accepting threatening information: Self-affirmation and the reduction of defensive biases. *Current Directions in Clinical Science, 11,* 119–123.

Shmukler, D., & Naveh, I. (1984–1985). Structured vs. unstructured play training with economically disadvantaged preschoolers. *Imagination, Cognition and Personality, 4,* 293–304.

Smilansky, S. (1986). *The effects of sociodramatic play on disadvantaged preschool children.* New York: Wiley.

Snow, J. H. (1992). Mental flexibility and planning skills in children and adolescencts with learning disabilities. *Journal of Learning Disabilities, 25,* 265–270.

Snyder, M. (1984). When belief creates reality. *Advances in Experimental Social Psychology, 18,* 247–305.

Swann, W. B., & Read, S. J. (1981). Acquiring self-knowledge: The search for feedback that fits. *Journal of Personality and Social Psychology, 41*(6), 1119–1128.

Teasedale, J. D. (1996). Clinically relevant theory: Integrating clinical insight with cognitive science. In P. M. Salkovskis (Ed.) *Frontiers of cognitive therapy: The state of the art and beyond* (pp. 26–47). New York: Guilford Press.

Tetlock, P. E. (1985). Accountability: A social check on the fundamental attribution error. *Social Psychological Quarterly, 48,* 227–236.

Tetlock, P. E., & Kim, J. I. (1987). Accountability and judgment processes in a personality prediction task. *Journal of Personality and Social Psychology, 53,* 700–709.

Thayer, J. F., Friedman, B. H., & Borkovec, T. D. (1996). Autonomic characteristics of generalized anxiety disorder and worry. *Biological Psychiatry, 39,* 255–266.

Thayer, J. F., Friedman, B. H., Borkovec, T. D., Johnsen, B. H., & Molina, S. (2000). Phasic heart period reactions to cued threat and non-threat stimuli in generalized anxiety disorder. *Psychophysiology, 37,* 361–368.

Thayer, J. F., & Lane, R. D. (in press). Perseverative thinking and health: Neurovisceral concomitants. *Psychology and Health.*

Turk, C. L., Heimberg, R. G., Luterek, J. A., Mennin, D. S., & Fresco, D. M. (in press). Delineating emotion regulation deficits in generalized anxiety disorder: A comparison with social anxiety. *Cognitive Therapy and Research.*

Walrond-Skinner, S. (1986). *A dictionary of psychotherapy.* London: Routledge & Kegan Paul.

11

Acceptance and Change in the Treatment of Eating Disorders

The Evolution of Manual-Based Cognitive-Behavioral Therapy

G. Terence Wilson

The primary focus of this chapter is bulimia nervosa (BN), which has been more intensively researched than other eating disorders. However, the clinical principles and procedures discussed here are directly applicable to anorexia nervosa (AN) and many of the atypical eating disorders (eating disorders not otherwise specified; American Psychiatric Association, 1994). The most notable of the latter category is binge eating disorder (BED).

MANUAL-BASED TREATMENT OF BULIMIA NERVOSA

BN is characterized by recurrent binge eating (defined as the uncontrolled consumption of a large amount of food), recurrent compensatory behavior designed to influence body shape and weight (e.g., self-induced vomiting, laxative misuse, severe dieting, fasting, or excessive exercise), and dysfunctional self-evaluation that is unduly determined by body shape and weight. Comorbid psychiatric disorders are common, especially depression and personality disorders (American Psychiatric Association, 1994).

Treatment Efficacy

Manual-based cognitive-behavioral therapy (CBT) is currently the treatment of choice for BN. (This treatment will be referred to as CBT-BN in the remainder of the chapter.) As the evidence has been extensively reviewed elsewhere (Whittal, Agras, & Gould, 1999; Wilson & Fairburn, 2002), it suffices here to highlight some of the main findings:

1. CBT-BN typically eliminates binge eating and purging in roughly 40–50% of all cases. Dysfunctional dieting is reliably decreased, and patients' body images are improved. In addition, there is usually a reduction in the level of general psychiatric symptoms and an improvement in self-esteem and social functioning. Therapeutic improvement is reasonably well maintained at 1-year follow-up.
2. CBT-BN has been shown to be more effective than antidepressant medication, especially in producing a complete cessation of binge eating and purging as opposed to percentage reduction in these behaviors. This is a telling comparison, because antidepressant medication is reliably more effective than pill placebo, at least in the short term.
3. A combination of CBT-BN and antidepressant medication is significantly more effective than medication alone. The data do not show that the combined treatment is reliably more effective in addressing specific eating disorder psychopathology than CBT-BN alone.
4. CBT-BN has proved superior to other psychological treatments with which it has been compared.
5. CBT-BN is quick acting, achieving much of its ultimate therapeutic effect within the first 4–6 weeks of treatment.

Treatment Limitations

The well-documented efficacy of CBT-BN is the good news, and it represents a substantial achievement. The bad news is that many patients show only an incomplete response to CBT-BN, and some completely fail to respond. We need a more effective intervention.

It obviously would be helpful if we could identify those patients for whom CBT-BN is not the treatment of choice. However, the available literature shows that reliable predictors of response to any treatment—psychological or pharmacological—have yet to be identified (Agras et al., 2000; Wilson & Fairburn, 2002). Certainly no empirically based guidance is available to clinicians that would enable them to match patients with one form of treatment or another.

One of the advantages of manual-based CBT-BN is that it has a rapid effect, as noted earlier. We know that BN patients who fail to respond by

6–8 weeks are unlikely to improve with the continuation of current CBT-BN (Agras et al., 2000; Wilson, Fairburn, Agras, Walsh, & Kraemer, 2002). The pragmatic approach, therefore, would be to identify and concentrate on these early nonresponders. But how then do we treat these patients?

One option would be to provide some alternative form of psychological therapy. However, there is still no evidence to suggest that a different type of psychotherapy would be effective when CBT-BN is not, the clinical popularity of this notion notwithstanding. A second option would be to use pharmacotherapy. Initial research has shown promising results in this regard. In a small pilot study, fluoxetine was significantly more effective than pill placebo in the treatment of nonresponders to CBT-BN (Walsh et al., 2000). Even if this proves to be a robust finding, there will still be questions about the long-term efficacy of antidepressant medication for BN (Wilson & Fairburn, 2002). The third, and in my view the most logical option, is to develop a more flexible and effective form of CBT.

ENHANCING THE EFFICACY OF MANUAL-BASED COGNITIVE-BEHAVIORAL THERAPY

Current manual-based CBT-BN is based on a cognitive-behavioral model of the maintenance of the disorder (Fairburn, Marcus, & Wilson, 1993). According to this model, dysfunctional overconcern with body shape and weight is the primary psychopathology of BN and related eating disorders. Fairburn (1997) has argued that the other clinical features of BN derive directly from this "core" psychopathology. As shown in Figure 11.1, these extreme concerns drive maladaptive attempts to control body shape and weight, including dysfunctional dieting (or even fasting), excessive exercise, and purging behaviors such as vomiting or laxative misuse. Dieting, in turn, leads to periodic loss of control over eating (binge eating) because of both biological (e.g., a state of energy deficit) and psychological pressures. The latter include adherence to arbitrary, rigid, and self-imposed dietary rules, the perceived violation of which triggers loss of control (Fairburn, 1997; Fairburn, Marcus, et al., 1993). Overconcern with shape and weight is also responsible for various forms of body avoidance and checking.

The Fairburn cognitive-behavioral model enjoys considerable empirical support. The role of dietary restraint in triggering and maintaining binge eating has been confirmed in laboratory research (Polivy & Herman, 1993), prospective studies of risk factors for BN (Patton, Selzer, Coffey, Carlin, & Wolfe, 1999), and a prospective study of the natural course of BN (Fairburn, Stice, et al., 2003). Manual-based CBT-BN was designed to modify dietary restraint and has proved effective in doing so. Reduction of dietary restraint has been shown to mediate, at least in part, the efficacy of

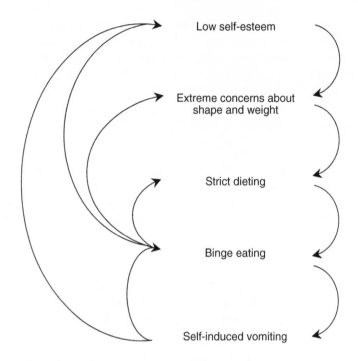

FIGURE 11.1. Cognitive-behavioral model of the maintenance of bulimia nervosa.

CBT-BN in eliminating binge eating and purging (Wilson, Fairburn, et al., 2002).

There is persuasive evidence that dysfunctional concern with body shape and weight plays a causal role in the development and maintenance of BN. Overconcern with shape and weight has been shown to be a risk factor for the development of BN (e.g., Patton et al., 1999). Stice (2001) showed that internalization of current societal ideals of physical beauty ("thin-ideal internalization") predicts body dissatisfaction that in turn drives dieting and generates negative affect that results in binge eating and purging. Studies using structural equation modeling have also yielded findings consistent with the model (Byrne & McLean, 2002; Spangler, 2002). Moreover, failure to reduce shape and weight concerns has been associated with risk of relapse (Fairburn, Jones, Peveler, Hope, & O'Connor, 1993).

CBT-BN was designed to modify dysfunctional concern with body shape and weight, but the evidence that it succeeds is far less strong than in the case of dietary restraint. For example, a large, multisite study showed that CBT-BN was significantly more effective than interpersonal psychotherapy (IPT) in reducing and eliminating binge eating, purging, and dietary restraint (Agras, Walsh, Fairburn, Wilson, & Kraemer, 2000). However, there were no differences in the reduction of body dissatisfaction and the importance of shape and weight. Given the causal significance of concerns about body shape and weight, an obvious goal would be to develop more effective methods for its treatment.

Treating Dysfunctional Overconcern with Body Shape and Weight

Current CBT-BN directly addresses body dissatisfaction and overconcern about the importance of body shape and weight via behavioral interventions and cognitive restructuring (Fairburn, Marcus, & Wilson, 1993).

The behavioral strategies consist of ensuring that patients cease avoiding body exposure (e.g., wearing form-fitting clothes or taking part in activities such as swimming) on the one hand, or limiting frequent body checking on the other. The cognitive restructuring focuses primarily on helping patients to challenge the accuracy or validity of specific beliefs about their physical appearance. For example, a patient who reports that she "feels fat" despite having a lower than average body weight would be encouraged to evaluate the evidence for and against this particular belief, with a view toward changing (disconfirming) the belief. In addition, patients would also be asked to evaluate the implications of holding a belief about the importance of being thin.

In an analysis of treatments for modifying dysfunctional attitudes about body shape and weight, Rosen (1996) suggested that the interventions in the Fairburn, Marcus, and Wilson (1993) manual might be too brief and recommended ways to strengthen this component of CBT-BN. In addition, the explicit targeting of body dissatisfaction occurs toward the end of treatment. As a result, there is often insufficient time to devote to these procedures in difficult patients whose progress through the earlier components of the sequenced course of CBT-BN has been prolonged or unsuccessful. It can be argued that enhancing the efficacy of CBT-BN will require more effective strategies for addressing dysfunctional attitudes about body shape and weight. Sufficient time would have to be devoted to these strategies to ensure that they are implemented optimally.

Behavioral Strategies

What is needed in an enhanced CBT approach to treating BN is a more intensive focus on implementing exposure and response prevention regarding body image (Fairburn, Cooper, & Shafran, 2003; Reas, Whisenhunt, Netemeyer, & Williamson, 2002; Rosen, 1997). Treatment should comprise a detailed analysis of idiosyncratic avoidance patterns and checking behaviors, as is now commonplace in effective CBT for anxiety disorders. Avoidance and checking behaviors should be a specific focus of assessment and self-monitoring.

Cognitive Strategies

Challenging the validity of a maladaptive belief is effective when that belief can be disconfirmed, often on the basis of behavioral experiments collabor- atively devised by patient and therapist. Thus, in the treatment of BN, patients learn that many of their rules about what and when to eat are without merit and are clearly dysfunctional. They discover, for example, that consumption of a particular "forbidden food" need not result in loss of control and subsequent weight gain. But challenging the validity of a be- lief is less useful in addressing issues of shape and weight. A functional ap- proach is better suited to this task.

A Functional Focus

In this approach, the emphasis is on the implications of holding dysfunc- tional core beliefs about shape and weight (e.g., "I must be thin in order to be happy and successful"). Vitousek, Watson, and Wilson (1998) have pointed out that "a focus on functionality is indicated when clients' be- liefs are highly valued [or] culturally shared . . . so that *evidence about their validity is unavailable or irrelevant*. In these instances, a shift in focus to the utility of beliefs and associated behaviors may penetrate bar- riers that arguments about their correctness cannot breach" (p. 408, emphasis added).

   A functional analysis helps patients to examine the pros and cons of sticking to their dysfunctional beliefs and behaviors (see Wilson, Fairburn, & Agras, 1997, for details). Fennell (1999) has described an expanded form of this exploration of pros and cons that lends itself particularly well to addressing problematic shape and weight concerns. Consistent with the Fennell approach, Vitousek and colleagues (1998) recommend that thera- pists deliberately begin by asking patients to spell out the advantages of their core beliefs about shape and weight. This is a useful means of commu- nicating a sympathetic understanding of the patients' problems, and of vali- dating their experience and struggles with weight and shape issues in a social context that emphasizes the value of thinness (Linehan, 1994). Patients with AN, in particular, often have a history of having been warned that unless they change, they will suffer serious medical problems and even die. However, as Linehan (1996) notes, "An unremitting focus on change can increase perceptions of unpredictability and loss of control, increasing anxiety or anger so that the processing of new information is shut-off" (p. 18).

Validation of the patient's experience, as Linehan (1996) has argued, increases self-acceptance and thereby facilitates a willingness to explore attempts at change. Accordingly, this functional focus on the consequences of specific beliefs and behaviors is a powerful means of addressing problems with commitment to treatment and resistance to change (Vitousek et al., 1998). It can be used to address problems with commitment to change at any stage in the therapy and may have to be repeated at different points in the treatment process (Wilson et al., 1997). Developing and then maintaining motivation to change is a continuing task.

Consider, for example, a patient with BN, with a body mass index (BMI) of 21, whose fiercely held goal is to eat nothing during the day and then as little as possible at an evening meal. She is adamant that eating anything more would be "unacceptable." Obviously, it is impossible to proceed with the task of having her eat three meals plus two planned snacks, and all of the other interventions as prescribed in CBT-BN, until she is willing to try to change. Using the Socratic method, the CBT therapist must patiently but persistently focus the patient on the consequences of her choice and the need to explore alternative options. The therapist blends empathy (validation) with firmness in emphasizing the need for change (Wilson et al., 1997).

The notion of "readiness for change," drawn from Miller and Rollnick's (1991) description of motivational enhancement therapy as a means of overcoming resistance to change in alcohol-dependent patients has become increasingly popular in the treatment of eating disorders (Geller, 2002; Treasure et al., 1999). Overcoming ambivalence about change and enhancing commitment to therapy using strategies such as the functional focus summarized earlier have always been an integral part of CBT (Marlatt, 1985; Vitousek et al., 1998; Wilson et al., 1997). This explains the results of a study that assessed the predictive value of a pretreatment measure of readiness to change in patients with BN treated with either manual-based CBT-BN or IPT (Wolk & Devlin, 2001). Readiness for change was linked to posttreatment outcome in IPT but not CBT-BN. Since CBT in general directly targets motivation to change with demonstrably effective strategies, pretreatment patient variables are less likely to have predictive value. However, in less effective treatments that do not directly focus on motivation to change, pretreatment patient characteristics would tend to assume greater significance.

Acceptance and Change

A significant development within CBT in the 1990s was the focus on balancing the traditional emphasis on behavior change with the value of acceptance, and the importance of the relationship between the two (Hayes, Jacobson, Follette, & Dougher, 1994). Perhaps the most prominent example of this innovative approach was Linehan's (1993) dialectical behavior therapy (DBT) for borderline personality disorder. Elsewhere (1996a) I have suggested that the same dialectic—a comparable balance between acceptance and change—is central to the treatment of eating disorders.

Patients with eating disorders tend to define their self-worth in terms of their body shape and weight, at least in part because physical appearance may seem more controllable than many other aspects of life. Yet body shape and weight are relatively immutable, and it is more realistic for these patients to make other changes in their lives. Thus, they become invested in changing what cannot be changed, and avoid making other important life changes. The preoccupation with shape and weight often serves to mask important psychological and interpersonal problems. The patient's dilemma is captured in the Serenity Prayer: "God give me the serenity to accept the things I cannot change, the courage to change the things I can, and the wisdom to know the difference." Once patients make nutritionally sound and psychologically adaptive lifestyle changes, they need to accept the resulting shape and weight of their bodies.

The thrust of the functional focus within CBT-BN, as described earlier, is to help patients accept that extreme weight control measures, such as unhealthy dieting, purging, and excessive exercise, do not work. These extreme and unhealthy attempts to influence weight do not accomplish patients' goals of achieving an ideal body shape and weight, and they undermine self-esteem. It is also important to balance the maladaptive consequences of trying to change what cannot be changed, or changed without serious personal cost, as in dysfunctional diet-driven eating disorders, with a more positive focus on other fulfilling aspects of life. McClintock and Evans (2002) have shown that low self-acceptance mediates the impact of fear of negative evaluation and poor social support on disordered eating and low body self-esteem in a nonclinical sample of women. Acceptance is an active process of self-affirmation rather than the passive giving up of constructive and realistic efforts at change (Linehan, 1994).

Acceptance in this sense is especially difficult for patients with eating disorders. Major obstacles to acceptance include social and cultural pressures regarding body weight, low self-esteem, and perfectionism (Wilson, 1996a). Clinical observations have long linked perfectionism to eating disorders, especially AN, and recent findings have confirmed the association (Shafran, Cooper, & Fairburn, 2002; Wonderlich, 2002). In their cognitive-behavioral analysis of perfectionism, Shafran and colleagues (2002) view it as a form of dysfunctional self-evaluation characterized by rigid and dichotomous thinking in which self-worth is defined in terms of meeting demanding personal standards despite adverse consequences. They argue that this self-evaluative system is essentially the same as the core psychopathology of AN and BN. In contrast to the rigidity of perfectionism, acceptance involves balance, flexibility, and the ability to tolerate ambiguity.

Mindfulness and Acceptance

Innovative and potentially more powerful strategies than conventional CBT-BN methods for addressing dysfunctional shape and weight concerns have been proposed. A number of clinicians have recommended the use of systematic body exposure, in which patients are asked to observe themselves in a full-length mirror as a means of modifying negative body image (e.g., Rosen, 1997; Tuschen-Caffier, Pook, & Frank, 2001). This technique is based on the well-established principle of exposure. Patients react with anxiety and aversion to their body image, as if it were a phobic stimulus (Laberg, Wilson, Eldredge, & Nordby, 1991; Tuschen-Caffier, Vogele, Bracht, & Hilbert, 2003). Systematic exposure should reduce this anxiety and the body avoidance it generates.

More recently, Wilson (1999, 2002b) has described a mindfulness-based adaptation of mirror exposure. In brief, the patient stands in front of a full-length mirror and describes her entire body from head to toe. She is asked to focus on a holistic view of her body, not just the "hot spots" that cause distress. Following Linehan's (1993) mindfulness training, the patient is instructed to *observe* her body, to *describe* it, to be *nonjudgmental*, and to *stay in the present*. The goal of this intervention is to help the patient shift from an automatic (and dysfunctional) mind-set to a more controlled one, in which she does not dwell on the past, worry about the future, try to "problem-solve," or avoid any unpleasant aspect of the situation (Segal, Williams, & Teasdale, 2002; Teasdale, 1997).

A mindfulness-based approach to accepting body shape and weight makes persuasive clinical and theoretical sense. Linehan (1993) and Teasdale (1997) describe three ways of processing emotion-related material: "mindless emoting" (being immersed in affective responding with little self-awareness); "intellectualizing/doing" (trying to "do something" to cope or change the situation); and "mindful experiencing/being" (the nonevaluative awareness of self). In mirror exposure, patients with BN typically start by engaging in one of the first two modes of emotional processing. They have great difficulty not automatically emoting and harshly judging their bodies in very negative terms. Patients' selective attention on real and perceived imperfections serves to maintain their dysfunctional concerns about shape and weight. Patients also often envision ways they could change their bodies. Veale and Riley (2001) coined the phrase "mental cosmetic surgery" in describing the reactions of patients with body dysmorphic disorder to mirror exposure, and this applies to patients with BN as well. This lack of self-acceptance generates frustration and negative affect, trapping patients in a continuing cycle of distress. Mindful experiencing of shape and weight, which promotes self-acceptance and attenuates maladaptive rumination, offers a way out of this cycle of negative self-evaluation.

Mindfulness-based mirror exposure can also serve as a prototypical situation for training patients to cope with negative affect in general. As noted below, mood intolerance can contribute directly to the development and maintenance of BN (Fairburn, Cooper, & Shafran, 2003). The presence of negative affect in both BN and BED is associated with more severe eating disorder psychopathology and predicts a poorer clinical outcome (Stice & Agras, 1999; Stice et al., 2001). Moreover, mindfulness is a key element of DBT for borderline personality disorder (Linehan, 1993), which is commonly associated with BN and BED.

As yet, there is little empirical support for the specific efficacy of mirror exposure. In a study of inpatients with AN, Key et al. (2002) compared a standard body image treatment with one that also included mirror exposure. Whereas the standard treatment had no effect, the addition of mirror exposure produced significant and sustained reduction in body dissatisfaction, body anxiety, and avoidance behaviors. In this study, mirror exposure was conducted within the framework of systematic desensitization. To date, there is no controlled research on mindfulness-based training in the treatment of negative body image.

DBT for Binge Eating Disorder

Mindfulness is a principal component of Linehan's (1993) DBT for borderline personality disorder. Telch and her colleagues have adapted DBT for the treatment of BED (Telch, Agras, & Linehan, 2001; Wiser & Telch, 1999). A primary goal of this treatment is to teach patients how to use mindfulness and emotional regulation skills to cope with negative affect, without resorting to binge eating or other maladaptive coping responses. Preliminary findings, which are promising, show that DBT is significantly more effective than a delayed-treatment control group, at least in the short term (Telch et al., 2001). Kristeller and Hallett (1999) have similarly reported positive preliminary results for a mindfulness-based treatment of BED. A preliminary report of the adaptation of DBT to BN has similarly yielded promising results (Safer, Telch, & Agras, 2001).

Mindfulness and CBT: Some Comments

This chapter on eating disorders is part of a volume devoted to the understanding and application of mindfulness and acceptance. A fundamental question is how different is this focus on mindfulness and acceptance from current CBT? Is it part of the continuing evolution of CBT, or some discontinuous change (what some years ago might have been called a "paradigm shift")?

Answering this question will obviously require the relevant empirical research. Proponents of treatments derived from these new concepts face the challenge of not only demonstrating that they are effective but that they also improve upon the effectiveness of existing CBT methods. This applies to mindfulness-based mirror exposure, as noted earlier. I am also proposing a broad view of effectiveness that goes beyond efficacy. Efficiency and disseminability are important criteria. The treatment of depression provides an instructive example. It appears that behavioral activation might be as effective as cognitive therapy (Jacobson, Martell, & Dimidjian, 2001), and it might be more broadly disseminable (Hollon, 2001). As a brief, well-defined, and arguably disseminable intervention, mindfulness-based cognitive therapy for depression has considerable clinical appeal (Segal et al., 2001).

The view taken in this chapter is that mindfulness and acceptance supplement and can enhance the existing principles and procedures of CBT. Thus, a functional focus is vital for changing some dysfunctional beliefs, whereas disconfirming the validity of other beliefs through behavioral experiments is appropriate for others. Mindfulness-based interventions are well-suited to problems of emotional regulation, but they complement rather than supplement CBT-BN. This is a conservative approach, with a relatively high empirical threshold for departing from current evidence-based methods that are treatments of choice for a number of clinical disorders such as CBT-BN.

A more radical view is that the emphasis on concepts such as mindfulness and acceptance represents a more far-reaching development that departs significantly from current CBT—one that entails different theory, generates different methods, and provides potentially greater clinical effectiveness (e.g., Hayes, Strosahl, & Wilson, 1999).

It may be useful to examine two areas in which the application of mindfulness and acceptance is well-developed. Mindfulness-based cognitive therapy for depression is very different procedurally from Beck's cognitive therapy (Beck, Rush, Shaw, & Emery, 1979). It would seem to be a different therapy. But it can be argued that the theory that informs this approach is more consistent with current models of information and emotional processing than cognitive therapy, and might even explain the success of cognitive therapy (e.g., Teasdale, 1997). In this sense, it fits naturally with the evolution of CBT, a hallmark of which is supposed to be the application to clinical problems of the findings of psychological science.

The application of mindfulness to the treatment of eating disorders, as summarized earlier, derives from Linehan's (1993) DBT. The latter is a creative clinical blend of traditional behavior therapy and the philosophy of mindfulness and acceptance. DBT is different from traditional CBT. But does it represent a "paradigm shift," or is it part of the continuing development of CBT? Pending more experimental analysis and treatment outcome data, arguments could be made on both sides of this issue.

It might be useful to consider the strategies of mindfulness and acceptance within a broader framework of the ongoing action within CBT. Concerns that the advent of manual-based treatment would result in stagnation have been completely misplaced (Wilson, 2002a). Innovation in CBT is alive and well. The treatment of depression, again, provides a good example. The efficacy of cognitive therapy is well documented. However, not only has the mindfulness-based adaptation been shown to be effective in reducing risk for relapse, but so also has behavioral activation treatment (Hollon, 2001; Jacobson et al., 2001). There might be some link between the latter two approaches given their basic functional focus, but they are fundamentally different—cognitive versus behavioral—procedures. The efficacy of these different treatments challenges our understanding of why these therapies work. Are there common change mechanisms that can be addressed through different procedures? Or are different change mechanisms responsible for the effects of these different treatment methods?

EXPANDING AND INDIVIDUALIZING TREATMENT: THE EVOLUTION OF MANUAL-BASED THERAPY

Thus far, I have summarized innovative and potentially more powerful methods for treating dysfunctional body shape and weight concerns as a means of improving the efficacy of current manual-based CBT-BN. Fairburn, Cooper, and Shafran (2003) have advocated a more radical approach to enhancing treatment efficacy. They have developed an expanded cognitive-behavioral model of the maintenance of BN that highlights the important role of factors beyond the core psychopathological mechanisms of overconcern with body shape and weight, and dietary restraint. Furthermore, they have detailed a broader range of treatment techniques that can be administered in a more flexible and individualized treatment approach than current CBT-BN. In so doing, they have formulated a more sophisticated form of manual-based treatment that may well provide a model for the future development of manual-based CBT in general.

Individualizing Treatment

A continuing misconception about all manual-based CBT is that it precludes individualization of treatment. In fact, CBT-BN allows the therapist to individualize treatment in several different ways, which include formulating a treatment plan for the individual patient within the overall treatment model; ongoing, session-to-session assessment based on self-monitoring that helps determine the timing and nature of treatment; identifying specific dysfunctional beliefs, specific triggers for binge eating, and idiosyncratic body checking and avoidance behaviors; using multiple techniques, some of which may be better suited to some patients than to others; and addressing comorbid disorders, when necessary (Wilson, 1998, 2002a).

Nonetheless, more needs to be done in crafting manual-based treatments that can address the specific needs of individual patients. A major limitation of manual-based treatment is that selection of manual-based therapies is currently dictated in large part by categorical DSM-IV diagnoses. Thus, there is one CBT protocol specifically for BN (CBT-BN), another for BED, and so on. The unsatisfactory nature of this scheme for matching treatments to individual patients' problems is widely recognized. Considerable heterogeneity exists across individuals within DSM-IV diagnostic categories. The mechanisms that maintain the specific disorder will vary across individuals; therefore, the same treatment will not be equally effective for all members of a diagnostic category. Matching interventions to DSM-IV diagnoses as the sole basis for treatment selection is fundamentally at odds with the "functional analysis" of the individual patient, which has been a core conceptual and clinical feature of behavior therapy from its earliest days. We need to move beyond the atheoretical, heterogeneous categories of DSM-IV to more refined matches of specific treatments with particular problems in individual patients.

The challenge in emphasizing a greater individualization of treatment is to balance this clinically appealing flexibility with the well-documented strengths of the structured focus of manual-based treatment. The problems of clinical judgment have been amply documented (Dawes, 1994), and they provide a compelling reason for the use of manual-based treatment (Wilson, 1996b). Ultimately, valid matching of specific treatments to particular patients will hinge on an improved understanding of (1) the mechanisms that maintain the clinical disorder in question, and (2) the mechanisms whereby specific treatments work. The challenge for the next generation of treatment manuals was succinctly summarized by Hayes (1998, p. 33): "What the health delivery system needs is a very small set of generally applicable manuals with information about how to modify them to fit particular problems and patient subgroups. . . . [This] requires a theoretical understanding of the process that technology manipulates."

Enhanced Manual-Based Treatment for Eating Disorders

Fairburn, Cooper, and Shafran (2003) have developed an innovative and enhanced manual-based treatment not only for BN but also for eating disorders in general. They have broadened the cognitive-behavioral model of the mechanisms that maintain BN and other eating disorders. The mechanisms they have added to those outlined in Figure 11.1 are core low self-esteem, clinical perfectionism, mood intolerance, and interpersonal difficulties.

There are sound conceptual and empirical grounds for incorporating these mechanisms into the model. One goal of the enhanced treatment is to identify specific patient profiles, so that treatment can be tailored accordingly, using new therapy modules that address the expanded range of maintaining mechanisms.

In a radical departure from the current use of manual-based treatments, Fairburn, Cooper, and Shafran (2003) declare that "diagnosis is not of relevance to treatment" in this new approach. Rather, they propose a "transdiagnostic" theory and treatment of all eating disorders. Their fundamental rationale is that all the eating disorders share common maintaining mechanisms. Furthermore, Fairburn and colleagues (2003) underscore the necessarily "idiographic nature" of "personalized treatment formulations" in implementing this new framework. The latter emphasis, of course, represents a return to the philosophy of the "functional analysis" that has always been part of behavior therapy.

In their new transdiagnostic treatment approach for manual-based treatment, Fairburn, Cooper, and Shafran (2003) also address another common criticism of manual-based treatment. It is often argued that clinical practice in the "real world" is self-correcting—if one method is unsuccessful, another is adopted. In contrast, it is alleged that manual-based treatment proceeds in an unchanging, lockstep fashion. Yet there is scant evidence to indicate that routine clinical practice is self-correcting; if anything, the data indicate that therapists tend to stick with the treatment they started regardless of outcome (Wilson, 1998).

Fairburn, Cooper, and Shafran (2003) do not leave accountability and constant monitoring of patient progress to therapist discretion. They build into their treatment a "self-correcting" feature. Stage 1 involves eight sessions of core CBT treatment, with a primary focus on behavioral change. The next one to three sessions are devoted to methodically evaluating progress. In the case of problems, the focus is on identifying barriers to change and assessing the role of additional maintaining mechanisms, with a view toward formulating a revised, personalized treatment plan. This structure provides an instructive example of reliance on clinical research findings rather than intuitive therapist judgment in individualizing treatment. As noted earlier in this chapter, early treatment response is the most potent predictor of outcome in BN.

More than any other existing approach, this innovative approach seeks to balance the strengths of evidence-based treatment protocols with clinical flexibility and individualization (Wilson, 2002a). The approach is designed to treat eating disorders, but it is plausible to assume that it could be applied to the full range of "anxiety disorders" and other related groups of clinical disorders. Empirical research on these clinical and conceptual innovations is already well under way.

ACKNOWLEDGMENT

I am grateful to Tanya Schlam for her helpful comments on this chapter.

REFERENCES

Agras, W. S., Crow, S. J., Halmi, K. A., Mitchell, J. E., Wilson, G. T., & Kraemer, H. C. (2000). Outcome predictors for the cognitive-behavioral treatment of bulimia nervosa: Data from a multisite study. *American Journal of Psychiatry, 57*, 459–466.

Agras, W. S., Walsh, B. T., Fairburn, C. G., Wilson, G. T., & Kraemer, H. C. (2000). A multicenter comparison of cognitive-behavioral therapy and interpersonal psychotherapy for bulimia nervosa. *Archives of General Psychiatry, 157*, 1302–1308.

American Psychiatric Association. (1994). *Diagnostic and statistical manual of mental disorders* (4th ed.). Washington, DC: Author.

Beck, A. T., Rush, A. J., Shaw, B. F., & Emery, G. (1979). *Cognitive therapy of depression.* New York: Guilford Press.

Byrne, S. M., & McLean, N. J. (2002). The cognitive-behavioural model of bulimia nervosa: A direct evaluation. *International Journal of Eating Disorders, 31*, 17–31.

Dawes, R. M. (1994). *House of cards.* New York: Free Press.

Fairburn, C. G. (1997). Eating disorders. In D. M. Clark & C. G. Fairburn (Eds.), *The science and practice of cognitive behaviour therapy* (pp. 209–242). Oxford, UK: Oxford University Press.

Fairburn, C. G., Cooper, Z., & Shafran, R. (2003). Cognitive behaviour therapy for eating disorders: A "transdiagnostic" theory and treatment. *Behaviour Research and Therapy, 41*, 509–529.

Fairburn, C. G., Jones, R., Peveler, R. C., Hope, R. A., & O'Connor, M. (1993). Psychotherapy and bulimia nervosa: The longer-term effects of interpersonal psychotherapy, behaviour therapy and cognitive behaviour therapy. *Archives of General Psychiatry, 50*, 419–428.

Fairburn, C. G., Marcus, M. D., & Wilson, G. T. (1993). Cognitive-behavioral therapy for binge eating and bulimia nervosa: A comprehensive treatment manual. In C. G. Fairburn & G. T. Wilson (Eds.), *Binge eating: Nature, assessment, and treatment* (pp. 361–404). New York: Guilford Press.

Fairburn, C. G., Stice, E., Cooper, Z., Doll, H., Norman, P. A., & O'Connor, M. E. (2003). Understanding persistence in bulimia nervosa: A five-year naturalistic study. *Journal of Consulting and Clinical Psychology, 71*, 103–109.

Fennell, M. (1999). *Overcoming low self-esteem.* London: Robinson.

Geller, J. (2002). Estimating readiness for change in anorexia nervosa: Comparing clients, clinicians, and research assessors. *International Journal of Eating Disorders, 31*, 251–260.

Hayes, S. C. (1998). Market-driven treatment development. *Behavior Therapist, 21*, 32–33.

Hayes, S. C., Jacobson, N. S., Follette, V. M., & Dougher, M. J. (Eds.). (1994). *Acceptance and change: Content and context in psychotherapy.* Reno, NV: Context Press.

Hayes, S. C., Strosahl, K. D., & Wilson, K. G. (1999). *Acceptance and commitment therapy: An experiential approach to behavior change.* New York: Guilford Press.

Hollon, S. (2001). Behavioral activation treatment for depression: A commentary. *Clinical Psychology: Science and Practice, 8*, 271–274.

Jacobson, N. S., Martell, C. R., & Dimidjian, S. (2001). Behavioral activation treatment for depression: Returning to contextual roots. *Clinical Psychology: Science and Practice, 8,* 255–270.

Key, A., George, D., Beattie, K., Stammers, K., Lacey, H., & Waller, G. (2002). Body image treatment within an inpatient program for anorexia nervosa: The role of mirror exposure in the desensitization process. *International Journal of Eating Disorders, 31,* 185–190.

Kristeller, J. L., & Hallett, C. B. (1999). An exploratory study of a meditation-based intervention for binge eating disorder. *Journal of Health Psychology, 4,* 357–363.

Laberg, J., Wilson, G. T., Eldredge, K., & Nordby, H. (1991). Effect of mood on heart rate reactivity in bulimia nervosa. *International Journal of Eating Disorders, 10,* 169–178.

Linehan, M. M. (1993). *Skills training manual for treating borderline personality disorder.* New York: Guilford Press.

Linehan, M. M. (1994). Acceptance and change: The central dialectic in psychotherapy. In S. C. Hayes, N. S. Jacobson, V. Follette, & M. J. Dougher (Eds.), *Acceptance and change: Content and context in psychotherapy* (pp. 73–86). Reno, NV: Context Press.

Linehan, M. M. (1996). Validation and psychotherapy. In A. Bohart & L. S. Greenberg (Eds.), *Empathy and psychotherapy: New directions in theory, research, and practice* (pp. 1–21). Washington, DC: American Psychological Association.

Marlatt, G. A. (1985). Cognitive assessment and intervention procedures for relapse prevention. In G. A. Marlatt & J. R. Gordon (Eds.), *Relapse prevention: Maintenance strategies in the treatment of addictive behaviors* (pp. 201–279). New York: Guilford Press.

McClintock, J. M., & Evans, W. I. M. (2002). The underlying psychopathology of eating disorders and social phobia: A structural equation analysis. *Eating Behaviors, 2,* 247–262.

Miller, W. R., & Rollnick, S. (1991). *Motivational interviewing: Preparing people to change addictive behavior.* New York: Guilford Press.

Patton, G. C., Selzer, R., Coffey, C., Carlin, B., & Wolfe, R. (1999). Onset of adolescent eating disorders: Population-based cohort study over 3 years. *British Medical Journal, 318,* 765–768,

Polivy, J., & Herman, C. P. (1993). Etiology of binge eating: Psychological mechanisms. In C. G. Fairburn & G. T. Wilson (Eds.), *Binge eating: Nature, assessment, and treatment* (pp. 173–205). New York: Guilford Press.

Reas, D. L., Whisenhunt, B. L., Netemeyer, R., & Williamson, D. A. (2002). Development of the Body Checking Questionnaire: A self-report measure of body-checking behaviors. *International Journal of Eating Disorders, 31,* 324–331.

Rosen, J. C. (1996). Body image assessment and treatment in controlled studies of eating disorders. *International Journal of Eating Disorders, 20,* 331–344.

Rosen, J. C. (1997). Cognitive-behavioral body image therapy. In D. M. Garner & P. E. Garfinkel (Eds.), *Handbook of treatment for eating disorders* (2nd ed., pp. 188–201). New York: Guilford Press.

Safer, D. L., Telch, C. F., & Agras, W. S. (2001). Dialectical behavior therapy for bulimia nervosa. *American Journal of Psychiatry, 158,* 632–634.

Segal, Z. V., Williams, J. M. G., & Teasdale, J. D. (2001). *Mindfulness-based cognitive therapy for depression: A new approach to preventing relapse.* New York: Guilford Press.

Shafran, R., Cooper, Z., & Fairburn, C. G. (2002). Clinical perfectionism: A cognitive-behavioural analysis. *Behaviour Research and Therapy, 40,* 773–791.

Spangler, D. L. (2002). Testing the cognitive model of eating disorders: The role of dysfunctional beliefs about appearance. *Behavior Therapy, 33,* 87–105.

Stice, E. (2001). A prospective test of the dual pathway model of bulimic pathology: Mediating effects of dieting and negative affect. *Journal of Abnormal Psychology, 110*, 124–135.

Stice, E., & Agras, W. S. (1999). Subtyping bulimics along dietary restraint and negative affect dimensions. *Journal of Clinical and Consulting Psychology, 67*, 460–469.

Stice, E., Agras, W. S., Telch, C. F., Halmi, K., Mitchell, J., & Wilson, G. T. (2001). subytping binge eating disordered women along dietary restraint and negative affect dimensions. *International Journal of Eating Disorders, 30*, 11–27.

Teasdale, J. D. (1997). The relationship between cognition and emotion: The mind-in-place in mood disorders. In D. M. Clark & C. G. Fairburn (Eds.), *Science and practice of cognitive behaviour therapy* (pp. 67–94). New York: Oxford University Press.

Telch, C. F., Agras, S. W., & Linehan, M. M. (2001). Dialectical behavior therapy for binge eating disorder. *Journal of Consulting and Clinical Psychology, 69*, 1061–1065.

Treasure, J. L., Katzman, M., Schmidt, U., Troop, N., Todd, G., & de Silva, P. (1999). Engagement and outcome in the treatment of bulimia nervosa. *Behaviour Research and Therapy, 37*, 405–418.

Tuschen-Caffier, B., Pook, M., & Frank, M. (2001). Evaluation of manual-based cognitive-behavioral therapy for bulimia nervosa in a service setting. *Behaviour Research and Therapy, 39*, 299–308.

Tuschen-Caffier, B., Vogele, C., Bracht, S., & Hilbert, A. (2003). Psychological responses to body shape exposure in patients with bulimia nervosa. *Behaviour Research and Therapy, 41*, 573–586.

Veale, D., & Riley, S. (2001). Mirror, mirror on the wall, who is the ugliest of them all?: The psychopathology of mirror gazing in body dysmorphic disorder. *Behaviour Research and Therapy, 39*, 1381–1393.

Vitousek, K., Watson, S., & Wilson, G. T. (1998). Enhancing motivation for change in treatment-resistant eating disorders. *Clinical Psychology Review, 18*, 391–420.

Walsh, B. T., Agras, W. S., Devlin, M. J., Fairburn, C. G., Wilson, G. T., Kahn, C., et al. (2000). Fluoxetine in bulimia nervosa following poor response to psychotherapy. *American Journal of Psychiatry, 157*, 1332–1333.

Whittal, M. L., Agras, W. S., & Gould, R. A. (1999). Bulimia nervosa: A meta-analysis of psychosocial and pharmacological treatments. *Behavior Therapy, 30*, 117–135.

Wilson, G. T. (1996a). Acceptance and change in the treatment of eating disorders and obesity. *Behavior Therapy, 27*, 417–439.

Wilson, G. T. (1996b). Treatment of bulimia nervosa: When CBT fails. *Behaviour Research and Therapy, 34*, 197–212.

Wilson, G. T. (1998). Manual-based treatment and clinical practice. *Clinical Psychology: Science and Practice, 5*, 363–375.

Wilson, G. T. (1999). Cognitive behavior therapy for eating disorders: Progress and problems. *Behaviour Research and Therapy, 37*, 579–596.

Wilson, G. T. (2002a). *The evolution of cognitive behavior therapy: Manual-based treatment and beyond.* Keynote address, 30th Anniversary Annual Conference, British Association for Behavioural and Cognitive Psychotherapies, Warwick, UK.

Wilson, G. T. (2002b). *Mirror exposure treatment for bulimia nervosa.* Unpublished manual, Rutgers University, Piscataway, NJ.

Wilson, G. T., & Fairburn, C. G. (2002). Eating disorders. In P. E. Nathan & J. M. Gorman (Eds.), *Treatments that work* (2nd ed., pp. 559–592). New York: Oxford University Press.

Wilson, G. T., Fairburn, C. G., & Agras, W. S. (1997). Cognitive-behavioral therapy for bulimia nervosa. In D. M. Garner & P. Garfinkel (Eds.), *Handbook of treatment for eating disorders* (2nd ed., pp. 67–93). New York: Guilford Press.

Wilson, G. T., Fairburn, C. G., Agras, W. S., Walsh, B. T., & Kraemer, H. (2002). Cognitive behavior therapy for bulimia nervosa: Time course and mechanisms of change. *Journal of Consulting and Clinical Psychology, 70*, 267–274.

Wiser, S., & Telch, C. F. (1999). Dialectical behavior therapy for binge-eating disorder. *Journal of Clinical Psychology, 55*, 755–768.

Wolk, S. L., & Devlin, M. J. (2001). Stage of change as a predictor of response to psychotherapy for bulimia nervosa. *International Journal of Eating Disorders, 30*, 96–100.

Wonderlich, S. A. (2002). Personality and eating disorders. In C. G. Fairburn & K. D. Brownell (Eds.), *Eating disorders and obesity: A comprehensive handbook* (2nd ed., pp. 204–209). New York: Guilford Press.

12

Vipassana Meditation as a Treatment for Alcohol and Drug Use Disorders

G. Alan Marlatt, Katie Witkiewitz, Tiara M. Dillworth,
Sarah W. Bowen, George A. Parks, Laura Marie Macpherson,
Heather S. Lonczak, Mary E. Larimer, Tracy Simpson,
Arthur W. Blume, *and* Rick Crutcher

The excessive use of alcohol and other substances represents a significant public health problem worldwide (World Health Organization, 1999). The United Nations Office for Drug Control and Crime Prevention (UNODCCP; 2002) recently reported that approximately 185 million people worldwide are current drug users, and the demand for treatment is on the rise in countries around the world. In the United States, epidemiological data suggest that nearly 20% of the population will experience a substance use disorder (abuse or dependence) at some point in their lives (Grant, 1997). Yet approximately 90% of those Americans in need of treatment are not receiving any care (Grant et al., 1994). The poor utilization of available treatments indicates an urgent need for brief, low cost, and accessible interventions to serve those individuals with alcohol and drug use disorders (Marlatt & Witkiewitz, 2002).

Interventions derived from two general approaches, cognitive-behavioral therapy (CBT) and the 12-step disease model treatment approach (as exemplified by the Minnesota Model), have been the most widely disseminated and empirically tested substance abuse treatments. Cognitive-behavioral approaches to substance use have received considerable attention in the research literature, with many studies demonstrating the efficacy and effectiveness of CBT for a variety of addictive disorders in diverse populations (Carroll, 1996; Kadden, 2001; McCrady & Ziedonis, 2001). Based on the premise that maladaptive drinking and drug use are learned behaviors, CBT is an intervention that attempts to identify contextual, social, affective, and cognitive precipitants of pathological substance use. Once the possible causes of maladaptive behavior are identified, the treatment focuses on altering and/or reducing the influence of high-risk precipitants to substance use (e.g., negative affect, stress, peer pressure). CBT-type interventions (e.g., coping skills training, relapse prevention, cue exposure, behavioral marital therapy) incorporate the identification and modification of deficits in coping skills (e.g., inability to resist use in the presence of substance-related cues), the bolstering of self-efficacy (e.g., encouraging any steps toward positive behavior change), and the reduction of positive outcome expectancies (e.g., challenging a person's belief that he or she must be drinking to feel relaxed).

The Minnesota Model of alcohol treatment is based on a conceptualization of alcohol abuse and dependence as a chronic, progressive disease that affects a person physically, mentally, and spiritually (Spicer, 1993). The foundation of the model is based on the 12 steps of Alcoholics Anonymous (AA), which is the most well-known and widely available mutual support group worldwide (Room, 1998). The 12 steps are primarily focused on fellowship and the importance of finding "God" or a "higher power," prayer and spiritual awakening, and the reliance on the higher power for coping with the disease of alcoholism. Recent research has demonstrated that AA affiliation following treatment is related to an increase in self-efficacy, motivation, and coping behavior (Morganstern, Labouvie, McCrady, Kahler, & Frey, 1997), and there is growing empirical support for the effectiveness of posttreatment AA affiliation (McKellar, Stewart, & Humphreys, 2003; Miller, 1998; Morganstern et al., 1997).

The cognitive-behavioral and Minnesota models of substance abuse treatment differ in both theory and practice, with cognitive-behavioral approaches focused both on skills training and cognitive and behavioral antecedents to substance use (e.g., self-efficacy, expectancies, negative affect), and the Minnesota Model focused on spiritual awakening and acceptance of one's disease. Despite these differences, the data suggest considerable overlap in the outcomes (Moos, Finney, Ouimette, & Suchinsky, 1999; Project MATCH Research Group, 1998) and mechanisms of change (Morganstern et al., 1997) for both treatments. There are also major drawbacks in both approaches. CBT is not as widely available as AA and NA (Narcotics Anonymous), and it is more cost-prohibitive. The theocentric focus of AA and NA is not preferred by many treatment seekers, particularly those belonging to Eastern religions (e.g., Buddhism, Hinduism) or those who do not subscribe to any religion (e.g., atheists, agnostics). Also, data suggest that one of the barriers to seeking formal addiction treatment is the stigma and embarrassment associated with the labels of "addict" or "alcoholic" (Sobell, Ellingstad, & Sobell, 2000).

From a consumer choice perspective (Marlatt & Witkiewitz, 2002), the development of less theistic, more tolerant, nonstigmatizing, widely available, and affordable alternatives to the current substance abuse treatment systems is warranted. In this chapter, we provide an introduction to an alternative spirituality-based treatment, Vipassana meditation. This form of treatment may fill the treatment gap for those who would benefit from a spirituality-based approach but do not wish to participate in AA. First, we review the concepts of spirituality, meditation, and mindfulness, followed by an overview of the process of Vipassana meditation. The link between spirituality, mindfulness, and addiction is discussed, with a particular emphasis on the cognitive, behavioral, and neurobiological mechanisms that may be affected by mindfulness. Second, we then describe preliminary data from two empirical studies investigating the psychological functioning and substance use of incarcerated and nonincarcerated participants following a 10-day Vipassana course.

SPIRITUALITY

Broadly defined, spirituality has been characterized as a "search for the sacred" with particular emphasis on transcending the boundaries of human material existence (Miller, 1998). Spirituality has been operationally defined as a latent construct with multidimensional properties representing aspects of beliefs, motivation (goals and values), mystical or transcendent experiences, and behaviors related to these beliefs, motivations, or experiences. Most religions are organized systems designed to support and encourage the attainment of a spiritual life, shared by a community of believers and practitioners. Thus, spirituality can be thought of as overlapping but not synonymous with any particular religious orientation or value system. While the specific beliefs, moral codes, and spiritual practices of religions vary, there are common themes, such as transcending human suffering and the development of greater conscious awareness.

Addictive behaviors, such as alcohol abuse and dependence, viewed from a spiritual perspective might be understood as misguided attempts to solve the problems of human existence by artificially altering one's state of consciousness with psychoactive substances that temporarily mimic authentic spiritual transformation (by altering senses, thoughts, and behavior), but which ultimately decrease spiritual capacity, resulting in both

physical and mental disorders (Miller, 1998). From this perspective, authentic spiritual beliefs and practices are natural and healthy ways to
prevent, and effectively treat, substance use disorders. Traditionally, the
spiritual approach to recovery and alcohol treatment has been most associated with the 12-step Minnesota Model of substance abuse treatment
(Cook, 1988a, 1988b). However, there is evidence that other spiritual interventions, including meditation and mindfulness training, are associated
with reduced alcohol and substance use (Breslin, Zack, & McMain, 2002).

MINDFULNESS: EASTERN AND WESTERN APPROACHES

Mindfulness is based on the ability to focus on the present moment, with
full participation in that experience and an attitude of nonjudgmental acceptance. It is an important construct in both Western psychology (Langer,
1989; Teasdale, Segal, & Williams, 1995) and various Eastern spiritual traditions (Goldstein & Kornfield, 1987; Marlatt & Kristeller, 1998). Both
perspectives offer theoretical models of how mindfulness may be a useful
cognitive skill in the alleviation of personal suffering and behavioral problems, including addiction to alcohol and other drugs.

From a Western psychology perspective, Langer (1989) has defined
"mindfulness" as a cognitive skill, and has extended this theory to the
study of addiction etiology and treatment (Margolis & Langer, 1990).
From this perspective, addiction is a mindless state in which one is bound
by rigid cognitive dichotomies (e.g., using or not using) and a reliance on
alcohol or drugs as the only available means of escaping stress and anxiety.
Similarly, substance-induced altered states may enhance thought suppression, which may provide further avoidance of anxious thoughts (Wegner &
Zanakos, 1994).

Mindfulness has also been described as a metacognitive state of detached awareness (Teasdale et al., 1995). Introduced by Flavell (1979),
metacognition is most typically understood as knowledge, or cognition
about cognition (Flavell, 1981). Metacognitive processing not only consists
of acquiring knowledge regarding one's cognitions but also involves regulatory processes such as planning, monitoring, and evaluating (Schraw,
1998). In a clinical context, regulatory processes might involve removal of
the effect of maladaptive thoughts on processing, modification of responses
to anxiety-provoking stimuli, and development of metacognitive plans for
controlling thought processes (Wells, 2002). Notably, while cognitive therapy has traditionally prescribed the modification of maladaptive thoughts,
a mindfulness stance would espouse a detached acceptance of thoughts
(Teasdale, 1999). Thus, a mindfulness perspective would encourage a person experiencing a craving or some other form of anxiety to change the
metacognitive beliefs regarding the aversive cognitions rather than the ac-

tual cognitions themselves (Teasdale, 1999). In his application of meta-cognitive theory to the treatment of substance use, Toneatto (1999), who conceptualizes cravings as metacognitions, outlines the following three-step approach to the treatment of cravings: (1) the description of particular craving statements; (2) the identification of perceived consequences of such cravings; and (3) the elucidation of perceived effects of the psychoactive substance on such cognitive events. This therapeutic approach addresses the functions of a substance rather than simply the cravings themselves (Toneatto, 1999).

The goal of mindfulness training is not to challenge or change the content of thoughts (as in Beck's [1976] cognitive therapy for depression), but to develop a different attitude or relationship to thoughts, feelings, and sensations. Mindfulness meditation is similar to the traditional behavioral technique of self-monitoring (Thoreson & Mahoney, 1974) or, in this case, "thought monitoring." Mindfulness involves bringing one's complete attention to the present experience on a moment-to-moment basis (Marlatt & Kristeller, 1998), and embracing an attitude of acceptance.

Eastern approaches to mindfulness focus on facilitating spiritual awakening (Goldstein & Kornfield, 1987). To be fully mindful in the present moment is to be aware of the full range of experiences that exist in the here and now. Rather than judging experiences as good or bad, mindfulness accepts all experiences (thoughts, emotions, sensations, and events) as simply "what is" in the present moment. Kumar (2002) describes mindfulness as a "nonjudgmental, present-centered awareness ... directed toward all thoughts, feelings, and sensations that occur during [meditation] practice" (p. 42). Vipassana is a Sanskrit word that means "seeing things the way they are," as in the state of mindfulness meditation.

Mindfulness Meditation

Meditation is one medium used to practice and develop mindfulness. Meditation has been described as both a practical method of attaining deep relaxation and a spiritual path toward the attainment of enlightenment (Marlatt & Kristeller, 1998). From the perspective of Western psychology, meditation also has been described as a method of enhancing awareness or mindfulness of ongoing behavior and cognitions (self-monitoring of thoughts, feelings, and actions). From a behavioral point of view, meditation has been described as a form of "global desensitization," in which meditative practice acts as a form of counterconditioning similar to Wolpe's systematic desensitization as a treatment for fear and anxiety (Goleman, 1971; Goleman & Schwartz, 1984). Anxiety is extinguished during meditation, because the relaxation state replaces the negative reinforcement (tension reduction) previously associated with avoidance or escape from the feared stimulus.

Meditation is often recommended as a practice that can be learned and applied as a general stress-reduction procedure to deal with a variety of related health problems, including pain management, hypertension, and muscular disorders (Marlatt & Kristeller, 1998). The practice can elicit a hypometabolic state of mental and physical relaxation that has been documented to reduce tension and mitigate reactions to stress (Benson, 1975).

Meditation has also been described as a spiritual practice and is recommended as such by many religious disciplines, particularly those associated with Eastern spiritual approaches, such as Buddhism, Hinduism, and Sufism. There are a variety of different types of meditation with somewhat different interpretations and methods, but underlying each is a focus on transcendence, including acceptance of self and compassion for others. Meditation practices can be used to develop mindfulness at physical, psychological, and spiritual levels (Marlatt & Kristeller, 1998).

The first empirical studies on meditation and substance abuse came from practitioners of the transcendental meditation (TM) technique (Benson, 1975; Marcus, 1974). Practitioners of TM meditate for two 20-minute daily sitting periods and silently repeat a "mantra" (a relaxing Sanskrit word, e.g., *sherim*) as the focus for concentrative meditation. As of 1994, there have been over 30 studies investigating the effectiveness of TM as a treatment for alcohol and drug problems (Alexander, Robinson, & Rainforth, 1994), with all of these studies demonstrating some positive effect of TM in reducing alcohol and drug use (see Alexander et al., 1994, for a review). Over 25 years ago, Marlatt and Marques (1977) began using meditation for high-risk drinkers as an intervention with anecdotal success. The acceptance and clinical effectiveness of the intervention led Marlatt, Pagano, Rose, and Marques (1984) to conduct a randomized trial of three relaxation techniques (a mantra-based meditation similar to TM, deep muscle relaxation, and daily quiet recreational reading) in heavy drinking college students. All three groups reported significant reductions in alcohol consumption, and those in the TM group reported the most consistent reductions in alcohol use compared to no-treatment control group participants. In a second randomized trial with college students, meditation and aerobic exercise were equally effective in reducing daily alcohol consumption, and both groups reduced their drinking significantly more than a no-treatment control group (Murphy, Pagano, & Marlatt, 1986).

Vipassana Meditation

Initially used in the prison system in India, Vipassana meditation has shown promising support as an intervention for alcohol and other substance abuse in incarcerated populations (Kishore, Verma, & Dhar, 1996; Parks et al., 2003). Results with inmate populations have demonstrated effectiveness in reducing recidivism and psychopathological symptoms, and increasing more positive behaviors, such as cooperation with prison authorities (Kishore et al., 1996). In noninmate populations, the practice of Vipassana has been shown to be effective in reducing impulsiveness and increasing tolerance of common stressors (Emavardhana & Tori, 1997).

Vipassana means "seeing things the way they really are," or mindful awareness of what is happening in the present moment. Distinct from the common use of "mindfulness" in the psychological literature, Vipassana meditation seeks to teach the practitioner how to transcend the cognitive understanding of physical and mental events in the moment and reach a direct, perceptive experience of events as impermanent *(anicca)*. There is extensive documentation, drawn from the Buddhist Pali Canon, showing that continuous, concentrated focus on the sensations, with a direct understanding of their impermanent nature, was the practice that led the Buddha to his state of complete, awakened enlightenment (Vipassana Research Institute, 1990). Specifically related to the problem of addiction to alcohol and drug use, this practice of Vipassana addresses the root cause of craving. Goenka says, "The discovery of the Buddha that the real cause of [craving] lies in [sensations] is the unparalleled gift of the Buddha to humanity. With this one discovery he gave us the key to open the door of liberation within ourselves" (p. 4).

Vipassana meditation been made available to individuals around the world by the revered Vipassana master, S. N. Goenka (Hart, 1987). Goenka has presented Vipassana in the form of a 10-day meditation course, offered in over 100 meditation centers in 56 countries. It is taught and explained by Goenka in thoroughly modern and secular terminology that makes it accessible to practitioners of any religion or no religion. The course consists of daily practice of meditation, with a focus on attending to one's breath (for the first 3 days) and awareness of any bodily sensation during meditation "body scans" (for the final week of the 10-day course).

The course is taught in a standardized manner by assistant teachers who have been certified by Goenka and his staff, and includes a videotaped series of hour-long discourses (or "Dhamma Talks") delivered by Goenka each evening. These talks cover basic Buddhist principles, including the "Four Noble Truths" associated with the cause and cure of human suffering: (1) Suffering (distress, pain, anxiety, depression, addiction, etc.) is basic to all human experience; (2) suffering is caused by ego-based attachment to pleasure (craving) and avoidance of pain (aversion); (3) there is a "way out" of suffering; and (4) the "Eight-Fold Path" leads to enlightenment and the cessation of suffering.

The practice of Vipassana addresses the root cause of craving. In Buddha's first discourse, he says, "Having experienced as they really are, the arising of sensations, their passing away, the relishing of them, the danger in them, and the release from them, the Enlightened one . . . is fully liberated, being free from all attachment" (Rhys, 1910, p. 36). One learns through experience that suffering is impermanent and that there is an inter-dependence of thoughts, emotions, and experiences, such that one's experi-ences and actions are connected to all other experiences and actions. This aspect of the teaching highlights that the identification of "the self" as a separate autonomous being is an illusion and may exacerbate or cause most human problems, including addiction (Marlatt, 2002).

MECHANISMS OF CHANGE IN MINDFULNESS PRACTICE

The demonstration of an empirical relationship between meditation prac-tice and reduced alcohol and/or drug use leads us to ask the question, "*How* does mindfulness elicit change?" Exposure and desensitization, thought monitoring, relaxation, and acceptance have all been suggested as potential "active ingredients" of mindfulness training (Breslin et al., 2002; Hayes, Strosahl, & Wilson, 1999; Linehan, 1993; Marlatt, 2002). During mindfulness practice, the exposure to negative thoughts, emotions, and sen-sations (e.g., physical urges), in conjunction with inaction, may encourage desensitization and the acceptance of unwanted emotions or thoughts. This response prevention would help to extinguish operant responding that was learned via the negative reinforcement of escaping negative affective states through substance use. Monitoring one's reactions to thoughts and sensa-tions without acting on them requires acceptance of negative affect, includ-ing unwanted thoughts and temptations.

Meditation is highly regarded for its effects on mental states, but there is increasing evidence that meditation may also influence physiological re-activity. Recent neurobiological and psychophysiological studies have dem-onstrated changes in neurotransmitter levels (Infante et al., 2001; Kjaer et al., 2002), brain wave activity (Dunn, Hartigan, & Mikulas, 1999; Far-goso, Grinberg, Perez, Ortiz, & Loyo, 1999), activation of neural struc-tures (Lazar et al., 2000), and cerebral blood flow (Newberg et al., 2001). Kjaer and colleagues (2002) found increased dopamine release during med-itation, which was strongly associated with a reduced desire for action. Using functional magnetic resonance imaging, Lazar and colleagues (2000) concluded that meditation practice leads to the activation of neural struc-tures (dorsolateral prefrontal and parietal cortices, hippocampal regions, temporal lobe, anterior cingulated cortex, striatum, and pre- and post-central gyri) that are involved in attention and the functioning of the auto-nomic nervous system. Many of the findings from these studies suggest that meditation results in neurological changes that are associated with in-creased levels of alertness, relaxation, attentional control, and reduced readiness for action.

The neurobiological findings support the hypothesis that meditation enhances awareness and the cultivation of alternatives to mindless, compulsive behavior (Marlatt, 2002). As stated by Groves and Farmer (1994), "In the context of addictions, mindfulness might mean becoming aware of triggers for craving . . . and choosing to do something else which might ameliorate or prevent craving, so weakening the habitual response" (p. 189). Craving responses that are common in addiction create a complex system composed of environmental cues and rigid cognitive responding (subject experience of craving), increased outcome expectancies for the desired effects of the substance (positive reinforcement) and/or increased motivation for engaging in the addictive behavior to provide a reduction in negative affect or withdrawal symptoms (negative reinforcement). Mindfulness meditation may disrupt this system by providing heightened awareness and acceptance of the initial craving response, without judging, analyzing, or reacting. By interrupting this system, meditation may act as a form of counterconditioning, in which a state of metacognitive awareness and relaxation replaces the positive and negative reinforcement previously associated with engaging in the addictive behavior. In this sense, mindfulness may serve as a "positive addiction" (Glasser, 1976). Therefore, mindfulness is more than just a coping strategy for dealing with urges and temptations; it could also be a gratifying replacement or substitute for addictive behavior.

It is important to note that the success seen with mindfulness can be attributed to similar components found in CBT and AA. For example, the surrender and acceptance of one's powerlessness are pervasive themes in the 12 steps of AA (Alchoholics Anonymous, 1976). In Buddhist teachings, the acceptance of one's thoughts, feelings, and sufferings is also fundamental. Both AA and mindfulness orientations also include a focus on ego-transcendence and aspirations toward spiritual enlightenment (Alexander, 1997).

Although CBT focuses on changing thoughts, the first step in this process is becoming aware of cognitions, such as cravings or self-doubt, and realizing how an initial reaction to those thoughts can lead to physically or mentally harmful behaviors. Similarly, through the development of awareness and the understanding that reaction is unnecessary, mindfulness helps to enhance coping skills, improve self-efficacy, and lower the desire to use substances for the alleviation of negative affective states. Thus, AA, CBT, and mindfulness each share several common ingredients and have been of great benefit to many individuals struggling with substance use/abuse. Our aim is not to dismiss the value of these approaches, but rather to offer a promising alternative to those for whom CBT or AA may not represent the best fit for their needs or belief systems.

Recently, the Addictive Behaviors Research Center at the University of Washington conducted two studies on the use of Vipassana meditation as a stand-alone treatment for alcohol and drug problems. In the first study, we recruited inmates, many of whom were heavy substance abusers prior to incarceration, from a minimum security county jail (North Rehabilitation Facility, Seattle) to participate in a research study while attending a 10-day Vipassana meditation course. We assessed the participants immediately before and after the course, and 3 months following release from the facility. In the second study, we invited individuals who attended Vipassana meditation courses in Michigan, California, Massachusetts, and Washington to complete assessments immediately before and after the course, and 3 and 6 months following course completion. Although follow-up data are still being collected, in the next section, we provide a summary of the designs of these studies and some preliminary findings. In Study 1, the incarcerated sample, we have collected precourse, postcourse, and 3-month follow-up assessments, and in Study 2, the nonincarcerated sample, we have complete data for the pre- and postcourse assessments.

STUDY 1: INCARCERATED SAMPLE

Design

Vipassana meditation, taught by teachers from the Northwest Vipassana Center, Dhamma Kunja, was one of many treatment programs offered to inmates at the North Rehabilitation Facility (NRF). The first study used a quasi-experimental design consisting of two groups, Vipassana meditation course completers and a case-matched comparison group that did not volunteer for the meditation course. This design was chosen over the more rigorous random assignment to condition for two reasons. First, Vipassana course recruitment was not a research requirement and was solely under the control of NRF officials and the Vipassana teachers. Second, the number of Vipassana volunteers was too low to have enough statistical power to randomly assign participants who desired the course to one of the two conditions.

Interested NRF residents attended a four-session orientation held before the course and watched videos about Vipassana meditation with correctional populations, including one filmed in India's largest prison and another about a previously held NRF women's course (Menahemi & Ariel, 1997). After completing the group orientation session, each potential Vipassana student was individually interviewed by the teacher to ascertain his or her motivation for taking the course and to screen out those who were not good candidates (i.e., individuals unable to sit for extended periods, unwilling to comply with the code of conduct, or suffering from severe psychiatric illnesses) to complete the meditation training. The Vipassana courses were offered five times per year at regular intervals throughout the 2 years of the study, yielding nine Vipassana courses over the study time period. In the tradition of Vipassana practice, men and women participated in separate courses.

Vipassana Meditation Course Condition

As the 10-day Vipassana training began, residents were housed in a wing separate from the rest of the inmate population and instructed to maintain silence throughout the training, unless given permission by the instructors to speak (i.e. during didactics with instructors, issues related to logistics such as meals, etc.). No outside contact was allowed during the course. Participants had two vegetarian meals daily and one snack of fruit and tea. A typical daily schedule for the course is described as follows:

4:00 A.M.	Wake up
4:30–6:30 A.M.	Silent meditation
6:30–8:00 A.M.	Breakfast and personal time (shower, sleep, walk, etc.)
8:00–11:00 A.M.	Silent meditation/instruction
11:00–1:00 P.M.	Lunch, personal time, and meetings with instructor
1:00–5:00 P.M.	Silent meditation/instruction
5:00–6:00 P.M.	Tea/fruit
6:00–7:00 P.M.	Silent meditation/instruction
7:00–8:00 P.M.	Discourse (video narrated by S. N. Goenka)
8:00–9:00 P.M.	Silent meditation/instruction
9:00–10:00 P.M.	Return to residence or question–answer period with instructor
10:00 P.M.	Lights out

During the first 3 days of the Vipassana training, students focus on meditation breathing techniques designed to calm and focus the mind. By day 4, participants focus on meditative observations of both physical and mental sensations without reacting emotionally. With practice, participants become increasingly capable of observing thoughts, feelings, and sensations without experiencing cravings, fears, or aversion.

Control Group

The control participants received services as usual in the NRF facility during the intervention period but did not choose to participate in the Vipassana meditation course. There were a rich array of rehabilitation programs available for NRF inmates, and the majority of inmates participated in one or more of these interventions, including chemical dependency treatment, alcohol and other drug education, mental health services, parenting training, adult basic education and General Educational Development (GED) testing, acupuncture, housing, case management, and vocational programs. More than 50% of the general population at NRF participated in some form of substance abuse treatment.

Methods

Participants and Recruitment

Participants included 306 male and female inmates ranging in age from 19 to 58 ($M = 37.71$, $SD = 8.11$). All residents at NRF incarcerated during the the nine separate 10-day Vipassana meditation courses were eligible for recruitment. The low proportion of female participants (19%) was representative of the typical gender breakdown at NRF, with women comprising between 14% and 20% of the inmate population.

The majority of NRF inmates have significant alcohol and substance abuse problems, as well as learning disabilities and mental illness. Participants were incarcerated for a wide range of offenses. However, NRF does not accept inmates who have been convicted for violent felony charges or sex offenses, or who have a high-risk escape profile. The 88 participants (Vipassana = 29, control = 59) who completed 3-month follow-up assessments had an average of 12.33 ($SD = 12.28$) previous bookings, including driving under the influence (DUI), assault, theft, prostitution, and traffic violations. The majority (61.2%) identified as European American, and 14.1% identified as African American, 9.4% as Latino, 8.2% as Native Americans, 2.4% as Alaskan Native, 1.2% as Asian/Pacific Islander, and 3.5% as multiethnic or other. Approximately 20% of the sample had a middle school education or less. Sixty-three percent had a high school education, 13% graduated from college, and 5% had some level of postgraduate education. Thirty-one percent of the sample had been unemployed prior to incarceration, 12% were receiving public assistance or supplementary security income (SSI), 22% had been employed part time, and 36% had been employed full time. Twenty-eight percent endorsed no formal religion at the time of the baseline assessment. Over 50% identified as Christian (24% Protestant, 20% Catholic, 7% no denomination specified), 14% as other (not specified), and 3% as agnostic. Buddhist, Jewish, and "multiple religions" were each chosen by 1% of the sample.

In the 90 days prior to incarceration, the majority of residents in the sample reported using alcohol (81%) and marijuana (53%). Almost 57% had used crack or powder cocaine, 25% had used amphetamines, 18% had used heroin, and 12%, other opiates or analgesics. Additionally, 10% had used hallucinogens and 5% had abused methadone. On average, those who consumed alcohol drank 52.87 ($SD = 33.88$) out of the last 90 days. Their peak day of drinking in the last 90 days averaged 8.31 ($SD = 8.75$) drinks. There were no significant differences (alpha = .05) between the Vipassana and control groups on any demographic, alcohol and drug, or psychosocial measures based on independent sample t tests and chi-square analyses.

In order to evaluate any systematic attrition biases, participants who completed assessments at all three time points ($N = 88$) were compared to those who, for various reasons, did not complete the study ($N = 218$). Inadequate record keeping prevented us from determining the reasons for some participants (N = 88) not completing the study and other participants (N = 95) being declared ineligible for participation past the baseline assessment. The known reasons for not completing the study include release from NRF prior to postcourse evaluation (N = 22), refusal to continue (N = 9), reincarceration at another facility (N = 3), and escape from NRF (N = 1). Independent sample t tests showed no significant differences (alpha = .05) between those who completed the study and those who dropped on baseline measures of age, gender, ethnicity, psychiatric symptoms, frequency of alcohol use, or level of education.

Procedures

All inmates residing at NRF within 1 week prior to an upcoming Vipassana course were offered the opportunity to participate in a study on the effects of Vipassana meditation and other rehabilitation programs on alcohol and drug use, alcohol and drug-related consequences, psychological functioning, spirituality, and criminal behavior. It was made clear to the inmates that participation in the Vipassana meditation course did not require volunteering for the research study, and that being in the research study did not require taking the Vipassana meditation course.

Pre- and postcourse questionnaires were administered to groups of 6–12 inmates in classrooms at NRF, 2 to 3 days before and after each Vipassana meditation course. Participants were asked to provide locator information (e.g., phone numbers, address, collateral contact information, date of birth, employment) after the postcourse questionnaire in order to continue in the study after their release from NRF, and they were interviewed within 1 week following the course to verify contact information and schedule the 3-month follow-up. Follow-up questionnaires were administered 3 and 6 months after the inmates were released. Only participants who completed the first two questionnaires and provided locator information were eligible to complete the follow-up questionnaires.

Measures

Demographics, thought suppression (White Bear Suppression Inventory [WBSI]; Wegner & Zanakos, 1994), type and severity of any psychiatric symptoms experienced (Brief Symptom Inventory [BSI]; Derogatis & Melisaratos, 1983), and optimism (Life Orientation Test [LOT]; Scheier & Carver, 1985) were all assessed. Alcohol and drug questionnaires included measures of quantity and frequency (Daily Drinking Questionnaire [DDQ]; Collins, Parks, & Marlatt, 1985); the adverse consequences experienced due to use (Short Inventory of Problems [SIP]; Miller, Tonigan, & Longabaugh, 1995); Addiction Severity Index—Self-Report [ASI]; McLellan,

Luborsky, O'Brien, & Woody, 1980); alcohol dependency (Alcohol Use Disorders Identification Test [AUDIT]; Saunders, Aasland, Babor, de la Puente, & Grant, 1993; Alcohol Dependence Scale [ADS]; Skinner & Horn, 1984; Drug Abuse Screening Test [DAST]; Skinner, 1982); control and confidence that they can abstain from alcohol and drug in various circumstances (Drinking-Related Locus of Control Scale [DRIE]; Donovan & O'Leary, 1978); and motivation to change their addictive behaviors (Readiness to Change Questionnaire [RCQ]; Heather, Gold, & Rollnick, 1991).

Results

The following is a brief summary of preliminary results from the entire sample of Vipassana and control participants who completed the precourse and 3-month follow-up assessments. We have focused our attention on significant changes in alcohol and drug use, and substance-related cognitions between the 3 months prior to incarceration and the 3 months following release from NRF. When we have completed the follow-up assessments, we intend to use post hoc matching procedures (Rosenbaum & Rubin, 1985) to control for baseline differences between the Vipassana and control groups based on demographics (age, gender, and ethnicity) and substance use (frequency of alcohol and drug use).

For the preliminary analysis of these data, we were interested in two distinct effects: the relationship between precourse and 3 months within each group and the time-by-treatment interactions between groups. We hypothesized that the Vipassana participants would have better outcomes at 3 months than the control participants, but that, given the treatment orientation of NRF, the control participants would also improve from precourse to the 3-month assessment. To test these hypotheses, we first calculated the main univariate effects for time within each treatment group, then performed repeated-measures analyses to evaluate the time-by-treatment group interaction. Due to the large number of analyses and multiple dependent variables, we recognize a heightened risk for making Type I errors. To correct for this, we used a corrected alpha level (alpha = .01) for evaluating the main effects. We provide the actual p values for the time-by-treatment interactions.

Table 12.1 provides the means and standard deviations for each treatment group on several dependent measures at precourse and 3-month follow-up. Significant main effects within each treatment group are designated by an asterisk to the 3-month means and standard deviations. The F values, degrees of freedom, and p values for time-by-treatment interactions are provided in the last column of Table 12.1. Repeated-measures analyses indicated significant treatment-by-time interactions over the 3-month period, favoring the Vipassana group, on the physical and impulse control scales of the SIP (Miller et al., 1995), drug abuse severity (DAST; Skinner, 1982), av-

TABLE 12.1. North Rehabilitation Facility Results

| Measure | Vipassana | | Control | | $F(df)^b$ |
	Precourse	3-month	Precourse	3-month	
SIP					
Physical	4.07 (3.47)	1.43 (2.33)*	3.27 (0.41)	2.45 (0.41)	$F(1, 81) =$ 8.71, $p = .004$
Impulse control	4.00 (3.23)	1.93 (2.67)*	3.16 (2.83)	2.76 (0.41)	$F(1, 80) =$ 6.54, $p = .01$
AUDIT	1.78 (1.11)	1.18 (1.09)*	1.62 (1.11)	1.40 (1.06)	$F(1, 78) =$ 3.34, $p = .07$
ADS	14.24(12.46)	13.10(13.90)	13.74(10.41)	13.29(10.50)	$F(1, 61) =$ 0.16, $p = .69$
DAST	15.52 (8.77)	9.74 (7.58)*	15.02 (7.81)	13.71 (8.96)	$F(1, 73) =$ 6.76, $p = .01$
No. of drinks^a	54.85(56.54)	8.63(13.78)*	49.77(63.45)	29.60(46.53)	$F(1, 77) =$ 3.15, $p = .08$
Marijuana use^a	2.56 (3.09)	0.37 (0.93)*	2.14 (2.91)	1.20 (2.39)*	$F(1, 81) =$ 4.07, $p = .05$
Powder cocaine^a	1.26 (2.38)	0.11 (0.42)	0.58 (1.38)	0.56 (1.58)	$F(1, 82) =$ 5.58, $p = .02$
Crack cocaine^a	2.81 (3.37)	0.70 (1.90)*	2.23 (2.96)	1.56 (2.55)	$F(1, 82) =$ 4.50, $p = .04$
DRIE	6.32 (4.70)	3.40 (3.52)*	5.96 (4.63)	5.81 (5.10)	$F(1, 70) =$ 5.90, $p = .02$
LOT	17.76 (4.08)	20.72 (4.65)	19.67 (4.63)	19.04 (4.51)	$F(1, 77) =$ 12.43, $p = .001$
WBSI	53.04 (2.46)	2.98 (0.16)*	47.89(15.45)	46.75(16.44)	$F(1, 77) =$ 4.37, $p = .04$

^{a} Peak weekly use.

^{b} Time-by-treatment interaction.

*Main effect for treatment group, $p < .01$.

erage weekly drug use, including peak weekly marijuana and powder and crack cocaine use, drinking-related locus of control (DRIE; Donovan & O'Leary, 1978), optimism (LOT; Scheier & Carver, 1985), and thought suppression (WBSI; Wegner & Zanakos, 1994).

Reductions on the WBSI demonstrate decreased thought suppression among Vipassana participants, a finding that is consistent with the basic tenets of Vipassana meditation and could play an important role in the reduction of temptations and craving responses. However, these data are not conclusive, and further research should explore the relationship between craving, thought suppression, and mindfulness meditation.

STUDY 2: COMMUNITY SAMPLE

The second study assessed participants attending Vipassana meditation courses in four different states across the country. Three courses in Washington, two courses in California, and one each in Illinois and Massachusetts agreed to participate in the study. Due to a limited time frame and lack of resources, we conducted this as an observational study with follow-up program evaluation and no control group. This pilot study was designed to test the feasibility of conducting research at Vipassana centers nationwide, the characteristics and level of substance use among individuals who willingly attended the course, and the effectiveness of Vipassana training in a nonincarcerated population.

Methods

Participants and Recruitment

One hundred fifty-three participants were recruited from seven separate 10-day Vipassana meditation courses. Of these, 102 participants (male: $N = 51$; female: $N = 49$; missing gender information: $N = 2$) ranging in age from 19 to 76 ($M = 41.09$, $SD = 12.78$) completed both pre- and post-course questionnaires. The majority (74%) identified as European American; 14% identified as Asian/Pacific Islander, 4% as African American, and 6% as multiethnic or other (2% did not respond). Twenty-one percent had a high school education, 27% graduated from college, and 52% had some level of postgraduate education. Eighteen percent of the sample had been unemployed prior to the course, 4% were receiving public assistance or SSI, 32% had been employed part time, and 46% had been employed full time. Fifty-three percent identified themselves as having no formal religion at the time of the baseline assessment, 16% as Buddhist, 6% as Christian (5% Protestant, 1% Catholic), 5% as Hindu, 3% as atheist, 3% as agnostic, 2% as Jewish, and 10% identified as other (not specified).

In the 90 days prior to each course, the majority of participants had used alcohol (64%), Twenty-four percent had used marijuana, 9% had used hallucinogens, and 4% had used sedatives/hypnotics/tranquilizers. Powder cocaine and crack, amphetamines, and opiates/analgesics were each used by 1% of the sample. Those who used alcohol drank an average of 15.76 days ($SD = 13.04$) out of the last 90 days. Their peak day of drinking in the last 90 days averaged 8.03 ($SD = 9.21$) drinks.

Procedures

Participants were recruited on the first day of the course and completed a precourse assessment before the evening session began. Postcourse questionnaires were either completed on the last day of the course or given to participants to mail within a week of the course ending. Follow-up assessments were mailed 3 and 6 months after the course ended.

Measures

The measures that were administered to the NRF sample were also used in the community sample, with the addition of a Vipassana Meditation Questionnaire (Frazier, 2002) to assess opinions about meditation and to rate expectations of the course. At baseline, we assessed substance use, substance-related problems, locus of control and motivation, spirituality, and measures of psychosocial functioning. At the postcourse assessment we assessed drinking-related locus of control (DRIE; Donovan & O'Leary, 1978), optimism (LOT; Scheier & Carver, 1985), thought suppression (WBSI; Wegner & Zanakos, 1994), psychiatric symptoms (BSI; Derogatis & Melisaratos, 1983), readiness to change (RCQ; Heather et al., 1991), and self-regulation skills (Self-Regulation Questionnaire [SRQ]; Brown, Miller, & Lawendowski, 1999).

Results

Data from the 3- and 6-month follow-up assessments are still being collected; therefore, we focused on the acute psychosocial effects of the course by analyzing the differences between pre- and postcourse assessments. As shown in Table 12.2, preliminary paired samples t tests and chi-square analyses indicated significant improvements on motivation to change, depression, interpersonal skills, somatization, drinking-related locus of control, and self-regulation. There were no significant improvements on optimism or thought suppression. Alcohol and drug use were not assessed postcourse, because participants made a commitment not to use alcohol or other psychoactive substances during the course. Therefore, we are unable to report on any substance use outcomes in this sample. After 3- and 6-month follow-up assessments are collected, we will be report in future publications any changes on measures of psychosocial and substance use following participation in the course.

Discussion

Taken together, the preliminary findings from this ongoing series of studies provide support for the feasibility and clinical effectiveness of the Vipassana meditation course for reducing alcohol and drug use and related problems, psychiatric symptoms, and thought suppression, and for improving drinking-related cognitions, optimism, self-regulation, and readiness to change. The positive findings in the two diverse populations sampled for these investigations lend support for the generalizability of Vipassana as an intervention for substance use and psychiatric disorders for both incarcerated and nonincarcerated individuals. The widespread availability of Vipassana centers all over the world, and the tradition of these centers not charging fees for participation in Vipassana courses, provides further evidence for the applicability of Vipassana as a low-cost alternative to current systems of addiction treatment. Furthermore, cognitive-behavioral approaches and interventions based on the Minnesota Model are primarily focused on reducing substance use, whereas Vipassana appears to influence more

TABLE 12.2. Community Trial Results

Measure	Precourse M(SD)	Postcourse M(SD)	t
RCQ			
Precontemplation	3.36 (2.48)	3.31 (2.20)	$t(55) = 0.31, p = .76$
Contemplation	−3.99 (4.12)	−2.63 (4.08)*	$t(59) = −3.40, p = .001$
Action	−1.36 (4.57)	−0.67 (4.47)	$t(55) = −1.95, p = .06$
BSI			
Anxiety	2.27 (2.39)	2.18 (2.79)	$t(82) = 0.96, p = .34$
Depression	3.57 (3.82)	2.66 (3.23)*	$t(84) = 3.24, p = .002$
Hostility	2.21 (2.16)	1.74 (2.36)	$t(85) = 2.05, p = .04$
Interpersonal	3.20 (3.05)	2.38 (2.64)*	$t(85) = 3.16, p = .002$
OCD	4.38 (3.83)	4.03 (3.70)	$t(85) = 1.22, p = .23$
Paranoia	2.11 (2.64)	1.61 (2.39)	$t(83) = 2.46, p = .02$
Phobic anxiety	0.77 (1.45)	0.89 (2.16)	$t(85) = 0.90, p = .37$
Psychoticism	1.78 (2.30)	1.87 (2.74)	$t(82) = 0.30, p = .77$
Somatization	1.94 (2.62)	3.22 (2.84)*	$t(86) = −4.41, p = .0005$
DRIE	1.99 (2.15)	0.85 (1.29)*	$t(54) = 3.69, p = .001$
SRQ	194.09(19.87)	197.91(20.62)*	$t(78) = −2.82, p = .006$
LOT	21.87 (4.70)	21.64 (4.22)	$t(92) = 0.18, p = .86$
WBSI	42.76 (11.27)	42.60(11.25)	$t(96) = −0.12, p = .90$

*$p < .01$.

metacognitive processes, which may have broader and more long-term effects. To this end, we propose that one possible mechanism of cognitive change in Vipassana, and other mindfulness approaches to cognitive-behavioral treatment, may be described from a metacognitive perspective.

For example, in Study 1, the improvements in alcohol-related control orientations and expectations among those who participated in the Vipassana meditation group versus the control group might be, in part, a function of relatively greater metacognitive insight and regulatory skills. Such findings could have important treatment implications. If metacognitive skills operate as significant mechanisms mediating the effect of treatment on psychological outcomes, therapists could then provide additional metacognitive training to those functioning at a lower skills level. Consideration of treatment approaches for both addictive behaviors and psychiatric disorders such as depression and anxiety (e.g., Teasdale, 1999; Teasdale et al., 2000; Toneatto, 2002; Wells & Papageorgiou, 1998), within a metacognitive theoretical context, may be of enormous benefit for the identification and modification of thought processes that may significantly compromise well-being. More specifically, the use of meditation combined with exposure components of cognitive-behavioral treatments for co-occurring disorders may bolster traditional exposure techniques by providing clients with skills necessary to engage, rather than distract or avoid, in early treatment phases.

Craving, as a cognitive response, may be one thought process that is inherently tied to substance use and relapse. Many individuals who are trying to abstain from substances cite "craving," the desire to ingest a substance, as a major contributor to later substance use. Often related to positive outcome expectancies, the subjective experience of craving may be part of a complex system of environmental cues and cognitive or behavioral responding. Mindfulness meditation may interrupt this system by increasing awareness and acceptance of the initial experience of craving, replacing the "temptation" to use with a more positive, adaptive response to substance cues. Future research should test these hypotheses by measuring the influence of mindfulness meditation on reports of craving, metacognition, and the occurrence of substance use.

FUTURE DIRECTIONS

Two important questions that emerge from this review require additional study. First, as previously discussed, many questions remain concerning the identification of mechanisms of action that may underlie the effectiveness of mindfulness meditation in the treatment of addictive behavior problems. A variety of potential mechanisms or mediators have been proposed, both in terms of Western psychological theories and Eastern principles of spirituality and awakening. Western psychologists have focused on an array of processes, ranging from physiological relaxation and stress management to metacognitive variables (e.g., attentional control, enhanced awareness, and self-monitoring). From the perspectives of Eastern philosophy, such as those promoted by Buddhist practitioners of meditation, the focus is on spiritual practices that promote enlightenment and relief from suffering. Potential mechanisms include radical acceptance based on nonjudgmental awareness (Brach, 2003), letting go of "ego-attachment" and craving, recognition of addiction as a "false refuge," and a preoccupation with past and future events as compared to the "here and now" of mindful awareness (Marlatt, 2002). As additional measures are developed and refined to assess both Western and Eastern constructs and postulated mechanisms of action, future research studies will be able to address both how and why mindfulness meditation is effective in both the prevention and treatment of addiction.

The second question concerns the relative effectiveness of mindfulness meditation training when administered either as a specific Buddhist spiritual practice or as form of cognitive therapy that is targeted to a specific clinical problem, such as depression or addiction. The Vipassana meditation course is based on fundamental Buddhist practices that provide a pathway to eventual spiritual enlightenment and the realization of one's "Buddha nature." During the 10-day course, no specific instructions are given as to how to apply mindfulness skills to specific behavioral or psychological problems. Mindfulness skills are assumed to be effective in relieving suffering in a global sense, but it is left to the practitioner as to how he or she could apply these skills to deal with clinical symptoms or maladaptive behaviors. In a recent discussion of this issue, Teasdale, Segal, and Williams (2003) argued that a combination of mindfulness training coupled with a therapy program (individual or group format) designed to help clients apply meditation to their personal problems may be more effective than a more generic approach, such as the Vipassana course. The mindfulness-based cognitive therapy for relapse prevention in depression program described by Segal, Williams, and Teasdale (2002) is an example of a program that integrates Eastern and Western coping skills to prevent depression relapse.

The prevention of relapse in the treatment of substance use disorders, described initially in the text *Relapse Prevention* by Marlatt and Gordon (1985), has been a major focus of our work for the past 30 years. Through the evolution of relapse prevention (RP), as well as the evidence supporting mindfulness meditation as a treatment for addictive behavior (Benson, 1975; Marcus, 1974; Murphy et al., 1986) has led us to develop a revolutionary new treatment approach called mindfulness-based relapse prevention (MBRP), which combines mindfulness techniques and established RP principles and practices (Witkiewitz, Marlatt, & Walker, 2004). Traditional RP treatment begins with the assessment of potential risk factors and high-risk situations for relapse, such as low self-efficacy, ineffective coping responses, and stressful situations. RP then combines skills training with specific cognitive interventions and global self-management strategies designed to prevent or limit the occurrence of relapse episodes. The cornerstones of RP are identifying and modifying coping skills deficits and self-efficacy, educating about the abstinence violation effect, and challenging positive outcome expectancies.

Unlike traditional RP and cognitive-behavioral interventions, which are focused on challenging maladaptive thoughts and changing the content of thoughts (Kadden, 2001), MBRP focuses on changing one's relationship to thoughts. The goal of MBRP is to develop awareness of thoughts, feelings, and sensations (including urges or cravings) by developing mindfulness skills that can be applied in high-risk situations for relapse. Clients are taught specific RP strategies (enhancing self-efficacy and training in behavioral activation and coping, education about positive outcome expectancies, and the abstinence violation effect) to be used in conjunction with mindfulness practice. Clients can learn, through mindfulness techniques, that arising thoughts and cravings are just that; they are mental events that come and go. It is the attachment or aversion to the thoughts or sensations that causes suffering or discomfort that may potentially lead to relapse. The mindfulness techniques in MBRP teaches clients to recognize these thoughts and cravings, and accept them and let them pass, without necessarily reacting to them.

In future research, we plan to conduct a randomized clinical trial that would compare the traditional Vipassana meditation course with an MBRP program that combines meditation practice with RP (administered in a group therapy format) for individuals seeking help for their problems with alcohol. The results of this treatment outcome study should help shed light on this important remaining question.

AN INTEGRATION AND FORMULATION

Going beyond the application of mindfulness meditation in the treatment of addictive behaviors, can this practice, with its origins in Eastern spirituality, be integrated into contemporary CBT, most of which is based on Western psychological theory? Would such an integration be viewed as an evolution or a revolution in the developmental growth of CBT? We argue that both views are accurate. The integration of mindfulness as a practice to enhance awareness and acceptance is consistent with the evolution of cognitive therapy, the "C" of CBT. Because mindfulness operates at the metacognitive level and is not designed to modify or alter thought content (as is the case with traditional cognitive therapy, à la Beck), some would call this a revolutionary development, perhaps even the emergence of "radical cognitivism."

For those whose bent is more on the radical behavioral side of the fence, mindfulness meditation is consistent with viewing thoughts and ideas as "behavior of the mind" or "thoughts without a thinker" (Epstein, 1996). Buddhist psychology is congruent with radical behaviorism, in that it holds that egoistic determination (seeing the self or ego as the controlling agent or "cause" of behavioral outcomes) is an illusion. Mindfulness practice enhances awareness of the "big picture" of how the mind operates. As thoughts and feelings arise, mindfulness pulls the camera of awareness back for a long view, without attachment or holding the focus on any one object of attention. The meditator develops a deeper understanding of the multi-determinants and contextual source of thinking and ideas (behavior of the mind), and feeling and sensations (behavior of the body). In many ways, this has been a shared objective in behavioral analysis and therapy: Self-monitoring, behavioral analysis, and awareness of behavioral contingencies have all been central components of a behavioral approach.

The central controversy between the radical cognitive and radical behavioral approaches concerns the role or function of mindfulness itself. From the perspective of Buddhist psychology (Marlatt, 2002), mindfulness is a state of nonjudgmental awareness that permits the meditator to observe the ebb and flow of covert thoughts and feelings, without being caught up in ego-based attributions about past and present events or plans for future activities. Instead of being trapped in our usual story lines about the self as a causative agent, our awareness is focused on the present moment, with attention placed on the breath and ongoing bodily sensations. When unpleasant thoughts or feelings arise, attention is directed fully toward the experience, with no deliberate attempt to escape or avoid what is happening in the moment. This is, again, consistent with contemporary CBT practices such as exposure therapy or systematic desensitization. The enhancement of relaxation associated with meditation practice is also congruent with CBT stress-management programs that teach clients how to induce the "relaxation response" as an alternative to stress or anxiety. Relaxation is also linked to the practice of teaching clients how to accept and "let go" of potentially problematic thoughts and feelings rather than trying to exert additional control or willpower to change the experience (usually by avoidance or escape strategies).

From the perspective of radical cognitive theory, however, mindfulness provides the "skillful means" to enhance awareness of how the mind and body behave in any given time and place. Instead of racing along from thought to feeling to thought, under the conditioned control of the "automatic pilot," mindfulness permits the meditator to observe the connections between habitual behaviors and their associated thoughts (Segal et al., 2002). As meditation progresses, there is the increased opportunity to observe the gaps or spaces between the otherwise habitual stimulus–response connections. The process of meditation "slows down the action," so that the meditator has greater access to moments of "pausing" prior to reacting in the usual habitual manner (Brach, 2003). Such "pauses" represent choice points for engaging in alternative responses, such as focusing on the breath and the physical sensations one is experiencing in the present moment, before responding in a habitual manner. Mindfulness facilitates proactive awareness and a greater sense of freedom of choice, in contrast with a more habitual, reactive pattern of responding.

If mindfulness provides the capacity to rise above the mindless "automatic pilot" mode of consciousness, what is the mechanism of action involved in this transition? Take driving as an example. Many drivers operate on "automatic pilot" (complete with competing activities such as talking on their cellphones, eating snacks, smoking, etc.) until they encounter an emergency situation or unexpected road conditions that serve to "break the spell" and awaken the driver's acute awareness of the immediate situation. Mindful of the potential danger, the now alert driver engages in skillful maneuvers such as slowing down, changing lanes, or pulling over at the next rest stop to check the road map. As such, although mindfulness enhances navigational skills, it is not the "cause" of good driving behavior. Mindfulness is linked with heightened awareness of driving conditions, including increased attention to early warning signs and current road conditions. The past can be viewed through the rearview mirror, and the future is represented by the road ahead, both at the same moment in time. Drivers steer their cars and adjust the speed, but they are not the sole "cause" of events on the road. Whether the outcome is a safe trip or a car crash depends on multiple causative factors, including the state of the driver (awake or asleep, sober or intoxicated, mindful or distracted, etc.), the condition of the road and the driving environment (weather conditions, traffic, accidents, detours, etc.), and the state of the vehicle (seat belts, air bags, condition of the engine, fuel level, etc.). Only the driver is capable of mindfulness as an alternative to operating on automatic pilot (Berger, 1988).

If life is a journey, how do we help the driver stay on track and practice mindful navigation skills? Society recommends that adolescents attend driver's education in high school, prior to receiving their licenses. Students learn the rules of the road, traffic regulations, and the principles of safe and courteous driving. They may learn these skills in a driving simulator or with a driving instructor, who often has access to a separate steering wheel, gas pedal, and brake on the passenger side of the front seat of the training car. Mindfulness is also a skill that can be acquired in practice (such as attending an intensive Vipassana retreat), under the guidance of an experienced instructor. The instructor may have experience as a meditation teacher, a therapist, or be trained in both roles. In mindfulness training, the instructor/teacher/therapist serves as a guide, someone to help the student acquire the skills required for a safe journey. The bottom line remains the same: The driver is at the wheel.

REFERENCES

Alcoholics Anonymous. (1976). *Alcoholics Anonymous: The big book*. New York: Alcoholics Anonymous World Services.

Alexander, C. N., Robinson, P., & Rainforth, M. (1994). Treating and preventing alcohol, nicotine, and drug abuse through transcendental meditation: A review and statistical meta-analysis. *Alcoholism Treatment Quarterly, 11*(1/2), 13–87.

Alexander, W. (1997). *Cool water: Alcoholism, mindfulness, and ordinary recovery*. Boston: Shambhala.

Beck, A. (1976). *Cognitive therapy and the emotional disorders*. Oxford, UK: International Universities Press.

Benson, H. (1975). *The relaxation response*. New York: Morrow.

Berger, K.T. (1988). *Zen driving*. New York: Ballantine.

Brach, T. (2003). *Radical acceptance*. New York: Bantam.

Breslin, F. C., Zack, M., & McMain, S. (2002). An information-processing analysis of mindfulness: Implications for relapse prevention in the treatment of substance abuse. *Clinical Psychology: Science and Practice, 9*(3), 275–299.

Brown, J. M., Miller, W. R., & Lawendowski, L. A. (1999). The Self-Regulation Questionnaire. In L. VandeCreek & T. L. Jackson (Eds.), *Innovations in clinical practice: A source book* (Vol. 17, pp. 281–293). Sarasota, FL: Professional Resource Press/Professional Resource Exchange.

Carroll, K. M. (1996). Relapse prevention as a psychosocial treatment: A review of controlled clinical trials. *Experimental and Clinical Psychopharmacology, 4,* 46–54.

Collins, R. L., Parks, G. A., & Marlatt, G. A. (1985). Social determinants of alcohol consumption: The effects of social interaction and model status on the self-administration of alcohol. *Journal of Consulting and Clinical Psychology, 53*(2), 189–200.

Cook, C. C. H. (1988a). The Minnesota Model in the management of drug and alcohol dependency: Miracle method or myth?: Part I: The philosophy and the programme. *British Journal of Addiction, 83,* 625–634.

Cook, C. C. H. (1988b). The Minnesota Model in the management of drug and alcohol dependency: Miracle method or myth?: Part II: Evidence and conclusions. *British Journal of Addiction, 83,* 735–748.

Derogatis, L. R., & Melisaratos, N. (1983). The Brief Symptom Inventory: An introductory report. *Psychological Medicine, 13,* 595–605.

Donovan, D. M., & O'Leary, M. R. (1978). The Drinking-Related Locus of Control Scale: Reliability, factor structure and validity. *Journal of Studies on Alcohol, 39*(5), 759–784.

Dunn, B. R., Hartigan, J. A., & Mikulas, W. L. (1999). Concentration and mindfulness meditations: Unique forms of consciousness? *Applied Psychophysiology and Biofeedback, 24,* 147–165.

Emavardhana, T., & Tori, C. D. (1997). Changes in self-concept, ego defense mechanisms, and religiosity following seven-day Vipassana meditation retreats. *Journal for the Scientific Study of Religion, 36*(2), 194–206.

Epstein, M. (1996). *Thoughts without a thinker: Psychotherapy from a Buddhist perspective.* New York: Basic Books.

Fargoso, C. M., Grinberg, Z. J., Perez, M. A. G., Ortiz, C. A., & Loyo, J. R. (1999). Effects of meditation on brain electrical activity. *Revista Mexicana de Psicologia, 16*(1), 101–115.

Flavell, J. H. (1979). Metacognition and cognitive monitoring: A new area of cognitive-developmental inquiry. *American Psychologist, 34,* 906–911.

Flavell, J. H. (1981). Monitoring social cognitive enterprises: Something else that may develop in the area of social cognition. In J. H. Flavell & L. Ross (Eds.), *Social cognitive development* (pp. 272–287). London: Cambridge University Press.

Frazier, D. (2002). *Vipassana Meditation Questionnaire.* Unpublished manuscript.

Glasser, W. (1976). *Positive addiction.* Oxford, UK: Harper & Row.

Goldstein, J., & Kornfield, J. (1987). *Seeking the heart of wisdom: The path of insight meditation.* Boston: Shambhala.

Goleman, D. (1971). Meditation as meta-therapy. *Journal of Transpersonal Psychology, 3,* 1–25.

Goleman, D., & Schwartz, G. E. (1984). Meditation as an intervention in stress reactivity. In D. H. Shapiro, Jr. & R. N. Walsh (Eds.), *Meditation: Classic and contemporary perspectives* (pp. 77–88). New York: Aldine.

Grant, B. F. (1997). Prevalence and correlates of alcohol use and DSM-IV alcohol dependence in the United States: Results of the National Longitudinal Alcohol Epidemiologic Survey. *Journal on Studies of Alcohol, 58*(5), 464–473.

Grant, B. F., Harford, T. C., Dawson, D. A., Chou, P., Dufour, M., & Pickering, R. (1994). Prevalence of DSM-IV alcohol abuse and dependence: United States, 1992. *Alcohol Health and Research World, 18*(3), 243–248.

Groves, P., & Farmer, R. (1994). Buddhism and addictions. *Addiction Research, 2*(2),183–94.

Hart, W. (1987). *The art of living: Vipassana meditation as taught by S. N. Goenka.* San Francisco: HarperCollins.

Hayes, S. C., Strosahl, K. D., & Wilson, K. G. (1999). *Acceptance and commitment therapy: An experiential approach to behavior change.* New York: Guilford Press.

Heather, N., Gold, R., & Rollnick, S. (1991). *Readiness to Change Questionnaire: User's manual* (Technical Report No. 15). Kensington, Australia: National Drug and Alcohol Research Centre, University of New South Wales.

Infante, J. R., Torres-Avisbal, M., Pinel, P., Vallejo, J. A., Peran, F., Gonzalez, F., et al. (2001). Catecholamine levels in practitioners of the transcendental meditation technique. *Physiology and Behavior,* 72(1–2), 141–146.

Kadden, R. M. (2001). Behavioral and cognitive-behavioral treatment for alcoholism research opportunities. *Addictive Behaviors,* 26, 489–507.

Kishore, C., Verma, S. K., & Dhar, P. L. (1996). *Psychological effects of Vipassana on Tihar Jail inmates: Research report.* New Delhi: All India Institute of Medical Sciences.

Kjaer, T. W., Bertelsen, C., Piccini, P., Brooks, D., Alving, J., & Lou, H.C. (2002). Increased dopamine tone during meditation-induced change of consciousness. *Cognitive Brain Research,* 13, 255–259.

Kumar, S. M. (2002). An introduction to Buddhism for the cognitive-behavioral therapist. *Cognitive and Behavioral Practice,* 9, 40–43.

Langer, E. J. (1989). *Mindfulness.* Reading, MA: Addison-Wesley.

Lazar, S. W., Bush, G., Gollub, R. L., Fricchione, G. L., Khalsa, G., & Benson, H. (2000). Functional brain mapping or the relaxation response and meditation. *Neuroreport,* 11, 1581–1585.

Linehan, M. M. (1993). *Cognitive-behavioral treatment of borderline personality disorder.* New York: Guilford Press.

Marcus, J. B. (1974). Transcendental meditation: A new method of reducing drug abuse. *Drug Forum,* 3, 113–136.

Margolis, J., & Langer, E. (1990). An analysis of addictions from a mindful/mindless perspective. *Psychology of Addictive Behaviors,* 4(2), 107–115.

Marlatt, G. A. (2002). Buddhist psychology and the treatment of addictive behavior. *Cognitive and Behavioral Practice,* 9(1), 44–49.

Marlatt, G. A., & Gordon, J. R. (1985). *Relapse prevention: Maintenance strategies in the treatment of addictive behaviors.* New York: Guilford Press.

Marlatt, G. A., & Kristeller, J. (1998). Mindfulness and meditation. In W. R. Miller (Ed.), *Integrating spirituality in treatment: Resources for practitioners* (pp. 67–84). Washington, DC: American Psychological Association.

Marlatt, G. A., & Marques, J. K. (1977). Meditation, self-control, and alcohol use. In R. B. Stuart (Ed.), *Behavioral self-management: Strategies, techniques, and outcomes* (pp. 117–153). New York: Brunner/Mazel.

Marlatt, G. A., Pagano, R. R., Rose, R. M., & Marques, J. K. (1984). Effects of meditation and relaxation training upon alcohol use in male social drinkers. In D. H. Shapiro & R. N. Walsh (Eds.), *Meditation: Classic and contemporary perspectives* (pp. 105–120). New York: Aldine.

Marlatt, G. A., & Witkiewitz, K. (2002). Harm reduction approaches to alcohol use: Health promotion, prevention, and treatment. *Addictive Behaviors,* 27, 867–886.

McCrady, B. S., & Ziedonis, D. (2001). American Psychiatric Association practice guideline for substance use disorders. *Behavior Therapy,* 32, 309–336.

McKellar, J., Stewart, E., & Humphreys, K. (2003). Alcoholics Anonymous involvement and positive alcohol-related outcomes: Cause, consequence, or just a correlate?: A prospective 2-year study of 2,319 alcohol-dependent men. *Journal of Consulting and Clinical Psychology,* 71(2), 302–308.

McLellan, A. T., Luborsky, L., O'Brien, C. P., & Woody, G. E. (1980). An improved diagnostic instrument for substance abuse patients: The Addiction Severity Index. *Journal of Nervous and Mental Diseases,* 168, 26–33.

Menahemi, A., & Ariel, E. (Producers & Directors). (1997). *Doing time, doing Vipassana.* [Motion picture]. India: Karuna Films.

Miller, W. R. (1998). Researching the spiritual dimensions of alcohol and other drug problems. *Addictions, 93*(7), 979–990.

Miller, W. R., Tonigan, J. S., & Longabaugh, R. (1995). *The Drinker Inventory of Consequences (DrInC).* Project MATCH Monograph Series Vol. 4 (Margaret E. Mattson, Ed.). Rockville, MD: National Institute on Alcohol Abuse and Alcoholism.

Moos, R. H., Finney, J. W., Ouimette, P. C., & Suchinsky, R. T. (1999). A comparative evaluation of substance abuse treatment: I. Treatment orientation, amount of care, and 1-year outcomes. *Alcoholism: Clinical and Experimental Research, 23*(3), 529–536.

Morganstern, J., Labouvie, E., McCrady, B. S., Kahler, C. W., & Frey, R. M. (1997). Affiliation with Alcoholics Anonymous after treatment: A study of its therapeutic effects and mechanisms of action. *Journal of Consulting and Clinical Psychology, 65*(5), 768–777.

Murphy, T. J., Pagano, R. R., & Marlatt, G. A. (1986). Lifestyle modification with heavy alcohol drinkers: Effects of aerobic exercise and meditation. *Addictive Behaviors, 11,* 175–186.

Newberg, A., Alavi, A., Baime, M., Pourdehnad, M., Santanna, J., & d'Aquili, E. (2001). The measurement of regional cerebral blood flow during the complex cognitive task of meditation: A preliminary SPECT study. *Psychiatry Research: Neuroimaging, 106,* 113–122.

Parks, G. A., Marlatt, G. A., Bowen, S. W., Dillworth, T. M., Witkiewitz, K., Larimer, M., et al. (2003, July/August). The University of Washinton Vipassana Meditation Research Project at the North Rehabilitation Facility. *American Jails Magazine, 17,* 13–17.

Project MATCH Research Group. (1998). Matching patients with alcohol disorders to treatments: Clinical implications from Project MATCH. *Journal of Studies on Alcohol, 7,* 589–602.

Rhys Davids, T. W. (1910). *Dialogues of the Buddha II.* Oxford, UK: Pali Text Society.

Room, R. (1998). Mutual help movements for alcohol problems in an international perspective. *Addiction Research, 6*(2), 131–145.

Rosenbaum, P. R., & Rubin, D. B. (1985). Discussion of "On State Education Statistics": A difficulty with regression analyses of regional test score averages. *Journal of Educational Statistics, 10*(4), 326–333.

Saunders, J. B., Aasland, O. G., Babor, T. F., de la Puente, J. R., & Grant, M. (1993). Development of the Alcohol Use Disorders Screening Test (AUDIT): WHO collaborative project on early detection of persons with harmful alcohol consumption, II. *Addiction, 88,* 791–804.

Scheier, M. F., & Carver, C. S. (1985). Optimism, coping, and health: Assessment and implications of generalized outcomes expectancies. *Health Psychology, 4,* 219–247.

Schraw, G. (1998). Promoting general metacognitive awareness. *Instructional Science, 26*(1–2), 113–125.

Segal, Z., Williams, J. M. G., & Teasdale, J. D. (2002). *Mindfulness-based cognitive therapy for depression: A new approach to preventing relapse.* New York: Guilford Press.

Skinner, H. A. (1982). The Drug Abuse Screening Test. *Addictive Behaviors, 7*(4), 363–371.

Skinner, H. A., & Horn, J. L. (1984). *Alcohol Dependence Scale (ADS): User's guide.* Toronto: Addiction Research Foundation.

Sobell, L. C., Ellingstad, T. P., & Sobell, M. B. (2000). Natural recovery from alcohol and drug problems: Methodological review of the research with suggestions for future directions. *Addiction, 95,* 749–764.

Spicer, J. (1993). *The Minnesota Model: The evolution of the multidisciplinary approach to addiction recover.* Minneapolis, MN: Hazelden.

Thoreson, C. G., & Mahoney, M. H. (1974). *Behavioral self-control*. New York: Holt, Rinehart & Winston.

Teasdale, J. D. (1999). Metacognition, mindfulness and the modification of mood disorders. *Clinical Psychology and Psychotherapy, 6*, 146–155.

Teasdale, J. D., Segal, Z., & Williams, J. M. G. (1995). How does cognitive therapy prevent depressive relapse and why should control (mindfulness) training help? *Behaviour Research and Therapy, 33*, 25–39.

Teasdale, J. D., Segal, Z. V., & Williams, J. M. G. (2003). Mindfulness training and problem formulation. *Clinical Psychology: Science and Practice, 10*, 157–160.

Teasdale, J. D., Segal, Z. V., Williams, J. M. G., Ridgeway, V. A., Soulsby, J. M., & Lau, M. A. (2000). Prevention of relapse/recurrence in major depression by mindfulness-based cognitive therapy. *Journal of Consulting and Clinical Psychology, 68*, 615–623.

Toneatto, T. (1999). A metacognitive analysis of craving: Implications for treatment. *Journal of Clinical Psychology, 55*(5), 527–537.

Toneatto, T. (2002). A metacognitive therapy for anxiety disorders: Buddhist psychology applied. *Cognitive and Behavioral Practice, 9*, 72–78.

United Nations Office for Drug Control and Crime Prevention. (2002). *Global illicit drug trends 2002*. New York: United Nations.

Vipassana Research Institute. (1990). *The importance of Vedana and Sampajañña: A seminar, February 1990, Dhamma Giri, Igatpuri*. Igatpuri, India: Author.

Wegner, D. M., & Zanakos, S. (1994). Chronic thought suppression. *Journal of Personality, 62*, 615–640.

Wells, A. (2002). GAD, metacognition and mindfulness: An information processing analysis. *Clinical Psychology: Science and Practice, 9*(1), 95–100.

Wells, A., & Papageorgiou, C. (1998). Relationships between worry, obsessive–compulsive symptoms and meta-cognitive beliefs. *Behavior Research and Therapy, 36*, 899–913.

Witkiewitz, K., Marlatt, G. A., & Walker, D. E. (in press). Mindfulness-based relapse prevention for alcohol and substance use disorders: The meditative tortoise wins the race. *Journal of Cognitive Psychotherapy*.

World Health Association. (1999). *Global status report on alcohol*. Geneva: WHO, Substance Abuse Department, WHO/HSC/SAB/99.11.

13

Acceptance, Mindfulness, and Change in Couple Therapy

Andrew Christensen, Mia Sevier,
Lorelei E. Simpson, *and* Krista S. Gattis

Pat and Sam are both unhappy in their relationship. Pat complains that Sam does not give much in the relationship, is uncommunicative, and withdrawn. Pat claims, "Sam just isn't ever there for me." Sam counters that Pat is constantly criticizing and accusing, and is always on Sam's case. Sam claims, "I tune Pat out because it's all the same. In Pat's eyes, I do nothing right. So why even try?"

Pat and Sam have repeated arguments that consist, literally and figuratively, of some variation of the following interaction:

PAT: I need more from you.

SAM: I am trying to please you.

PAT: You are not doing a very good job.

SAM: Yes, I am.

PAT: No, you are not.

SAM: OK, well then, I won't even try.

PAT: Now, you are really doing a bad job.

SAM: I don't care. I quit.

PAT: You don't love me.

SAM: You don't appreciate me.

These complaints are familiar to couple therapists. We have created Pat and Sam from the stories of many couples and given them unisex names so as to avoid both gender stereotyping and a heterosexist bias. One can easily imagine them as a gay couple, a lesbian couple, or a heterosexual couple, in which either partner might be the male or the female.

We use Pat and Sam as our example couple as we try to explain the therapeutic approach of integrative behavioral couple therapy (IBCT). Developed by Andrew Christensen and the late Neil S. Jacobson (Christensen & Jacobson, 2000; Jacobson & Christensen, 1998), IBCT is one of the new behavior therapies. Like other therapies discussed in this book, it emphasizes acceptance and mindfulness, but it does so within the context of a close relationship. To understand IBCT and what is new about it, it is useful to compare it to what we call traditional behavioral couple therapy (TBCT—often referred to as behavioral marital therapy or behavioral couple therapy in earlier writings; Jacobson & Margolin, 1979). At times, we also compare IBCT to traditional cognitive-behavioral couple therapy[1] (CBCT; Baucom & Epstein, 1990). As we discuss the differences between IBCT and TBCT, we use Pat and Sam as our example couple, showing how they might be treated with the different approaches. No matter how intriguing the differences in the conceptualization of a couple's problems, the changes that it seeks in the couple, and the methods for inducing change, however, the most important issue is whether the two treatments lead to different outcomes. Thus, we look briefly at some of the empirical data on these treatments.

CONCEPTUALIZATION OF COUPLE PROBLEMS

TBCT conceptualizes a couple's problems in terms of specific, target behaviors. Often, partners come into therapy with vague complaints about each other, such as "She is selfish," "He is not supportive," and "She can't communicate well." The TBCT therapist tries to pinpoint the specific behaviors that each partner would like changed. By turning vague, general complaints into specific target behaviors, the therapist helps the couple define its problems clearly. These definitions then pave the way for behavior change efforts that follow. For example, a TBCT therapist working with Pat and Sam would try to make Pat's general complaint that "Sam isn't there for

---

[1] There is a newer, "enhanced" version of cognitive-behavioral couple therapy (see Epstein & Baucom, 2002) that overcomes some of the limitations of traditional CBCT that we describe.

me" and Sam's complaint that "Pat is always on my case" more specific and behavioral. In working with Pat's complaint, the therapist might discover that Pat means, in part, that Sam does not initiate conversation with Pat, such as asking about his or her day. Sam's complaint may mean, in part, that Pat criticizes Sam frequently about not making the relationship a priority.

A therapist who is more cognitively oriented might also attempt to identify some problematic cognitions associated with the problematic behaviors. For example, such a therapist would note the overgeneralized, "all-or-nothing" thinking that characterizes Pat, as in Pat's claim that Sam is "never there for me." A cognitively oriented therapist might suggest that Sam maintains the erroneous cognition that "avoidance solves problems."

IBCT focuses on a broader unit of analysis than TBCT or CBCT. Although it also seeks specific examples, it looks for the broad response class that characterizes each partner's complaints. For example, many of Pat's complaints concern the amount of closeness Pat gets from Sam, such as Sam's attention to Pat, interest in doing things with Pat, and responsiveness to Pat's desires. The term "closeness" could be the broader response class in which most of Pat's complaints fall. Furthermore, IBCT identifies the broad relationship theme in the struggle that characterizes a particular couple. This theme usually centers around a difference between partners on some fundamental dimension of relationship functioning. For example, Pat is extroverted and emotional, while Sam is shy and reticent. Pat does indeed want Sam to initiate more conversation, but Pat also wants Sam to initiate physical affection and sex, and to be more responsive when Pat initiates conversation, affection, or sex. In general, Pat wants an animated, emotional, energetic connection with Sam. On the other hand, Sam wants more time alone, more contact with friends, and more privacy. Although Sam does indeed also want fewer criticisms from Pat, this request seems like a reaction to their current struggle. In considering the broad response class of what each partner wants, the IBCT therapist might decide that the theme of "closeness versus independence" characterizes Pat and Sam's struggle. Pat wants a fundamentally closer relationship than Sam, who wants more individual independence than Pat.

Not only do TBCT and IBCT differ in the level of analysis with which they conceptualize the presenting problems of a couple but they also differ in how they conceptualize the reasons for the couple's struggle. TBCT may focus on the reciprocal interplay between problem behaviors, the way in which one problem behavior elicits another. For example, the TBCT therapist might suggest that Sam gets criticized because he or she does not ask about Pat's day, but Sam does not ask about Pat's day because he or she gets criticized so often. The TBCT therapist might further suggest that each partner is in a similar position of "I won't give because I am not being given to." A CBCT therapist would additionally propose that faulty thinking leads to these offending behaviors. Pat criticizes Sam so much, because Pat sees Sam in an extreme, all-or-nothing way ("Sam never shows any interest in me"). Similarly, Sam rarely initiates conversation, because Sam also sees Pat in overgeneralized terms ("Pat is always on my case").

In contrast, IBCT focuses on a broader, multilayered contextual framework for understanding interpersonal problems. IBCT looks at partners' individual histories, as well as their interactional history with each other, that may make them vulnerable to differences from their partner. Relevant history usually includes experiences in their family of origin, particularly relationships with their parents, and romantic history in previous close relationships. For example, Pat, an only child, was doted on by well-to-do parents, was used to lots of attention, and easily felt neglected if little attention was forthcoming. In contrast, Sam was from a lower socioeconomic class family with three children, in which both parents worked hard just to make ends meet. Because his or her siblings tended to do better in school, Sam often felt "less than" them. In fact, Sam generally felt inferior to others and was sensitive to criticism. A painful breakup with a partner that was more educated also contributed to Sam's sense of inferiority. Thus, Pat's history led him or her to be sensitive to any indication of neglect by Sam. On the other hand, Sam's history led him or her to be sensitive to comments, such as criticism, from Pat that might make him or her feel inferior.

In attempting to understand couples, IBCT therapists also focus on what attracts partners to each other. Sometimes these features are related to the very qualities that later lead to problems. Early in their relationship, Pat's and Sam's differences provided a positive connection between them. Pat's effusive style was great for Sam: It made Sam feel admired and appreciated in ways that Sam had never felt before. Also, Pat could be center stage with Sam, who was quite happy to give Pat plenty of attention and accommodate Pat's many needs and desires. At best, Pat was the "life of the party," a delightfully "over-the-top" person. On the other hand, Sam was reserved and quiet, but basked in Pat's reflected light and effusive praise. Pat could bring Sam out somewhat; Sam could meet Pat's needs.

As Pat and Sam each got involved with work and raising their two children, Sam became less attentive to Pat and less accommodating to Pat's needs. Pat became less praising of Sam. To cope with the loss of attention from Sam, Pat became critical and demanding of Sam. Pat told Sam what was wrong and what would make it right, but often in very angry and attacking ways. When threatened, Pat felt defensive and went on the attack. To cope with the loss of praise and increase in criticism from Pat, Sam became withdrawn. Withdrawal would at least end the criticism temporarily. When threatened, Sam retreated. Although, early on in the relationship, Pat provided the kind of positive reinforcement and validation that Sam sorely needed, now Pat provided the kind of criticism that raised Sam's old fears of being inferior. Although, early on, Sam had provided the kind of attention that Pat needed, now Sam withdrew in ways that made the relationship seem empty to Pat. Each of their ways of coping with the changes in their relationship stimulated even more of those negative changes. The more Sam withdrew, the more Pat criticized and demanded; the more Pat criticized and demanded, the more Sam withdrew. They were in a common but vicious cycle of demand–withdraw interaction (Eldridge & Christensen, 2002), and they both felt frustrated and hopeless to alter it.

This conceptualization of a couple's problems—a formulation in IBCT—consists of several components. First, there is the central theme of the couple's struggle—the difference or seeming incompatibility between partners. In the case of Pat and Sam, that theme is closeness–independence. Second, vulnerabilities in one or both partners that arise from some combination of their genes and history provide emotional fuel for their current differences. Pat's sensitivity to inattention and neglect, and Sam's sensitivity to criticism are examples. Third, each partner tries to cope with these differences in ways that seem reasonable to him or her but often unintentionally exacerbates the stress and polarizes their differences. Sam's effort to withdraw from Pat in order to achieve a level of desired independence increases Pat's anxiety, so that Pat pursues, criticizes, and makes demands on Sam, who then withdraws further from Pat. A vicious cycle of withdrawing and demanding then develops between the two of them. As they become polarized in their conflicting positions, each begins to vilify the other in his or her thinking—believing the other does not really love him or her, concluding that the other is "always" this (something bad) or "never" that (something good). Finally, the two may experience a variety of negative emotions that lead them to feeling "stuck" and "trapped." The harder they try, the worse the problem gets. They feel desperate but hopeless to change the situation.

In the first three sessions, IBCT therapists gather information necessary to create a formulation by interviewing the partners together (first session) and each partner alone (second and third sessions). In the fourth session of IBCT, the feedback session, the therapist shares the formulation with the couple. This sharing is done in a collaborative way, so that the partners can elaborate the formulation, amplify parts of the formulation, or alter parts that seem incorrect. If the therapist has really listened to both partners and incorporated their experience into the formulation, the couple usually accepts it as an accurate "story" about their problem.

The formulation guides the subsequent treatment sessions. The content of the treatment usually concerns recent, emotionally salient incidents, both positive and negative, that are reflective of the formulation. A example of a positive incident would be an occasion where Sam was able to respond to Pat's need for attention; a negative incident would be an occasion where Sam felt particularly hurt because of criticism by Pat and withdrew. Upcoming events that are of concern or broader issues of current concern are also common topics. An upcoming weekend away where Pat is concerned that Sam will get involved with shopping and be inattentive would be worthy of discussion, as would some general discussion of their differing expectations of how they spend the weekend together. Each of these incidents and issues is good material for therapy, because it is directly or indirectly related to the formulation. An effort is made to avoid dealing with tangential problems that may arise in the course of treatment. If, for example, Pat and Sam came late to a session, annoyed at each other because of some miscommunication about where they were to meet beforehand, the therapist might give limited focus to that event, if it seemed largely irrelevant to their ongoing problematic concerns—that is to say, the formulation. However, the formulation is not a static conceptual framework for viewing the couple. As the therapist and the couple work together and get increasingly greater understanding of their issues, they may alter and enrich their formulation or the "story" of their concerns.

In IBCT, the formulation is a kind of conceptual scaffold upon which greater relationship mindfulness can be built. During the course of treatment, the couple becomes more aware of the interconnection between seemingly disparate events. Pat's harsh accusation that Sam has a "dwarf libido," and Pat's vigorous entreaty that they spend the day together, may be driven by similar motivations. If treatment is successful in IBCT, partners become attuned to each other's emotional responses. Pat begins to see Sam's withdrawal as defensive—an effort to protect rather than an effort to neglect. They become more mindful of the events in their relationship and the emotional impact of these events, and can thus respond to them differently.

EMOTIONAL ACCEPTANCE, BEHAVIORAL CHANGE, AND COGNITIVE CHANGE AS GOALS IN COUPLE THERAPY

In TBCT, the primary goal of treatment is behavioral change. As documented by extensive research (Weiss & Heyman, 1997), partners in distressed couples display relatively more negative behaviors and fewer positive behaviors toward each other than do their nondistressed counterparts. TBCT tries to alter that balance by increasing the frequency, duration, and intensity of positive behaviors and reducing the frequency, duration, and intensity of negative behaviors. If Pat makes statements that "Sam never listens to me" or "always withdraws during a disagreement," TBCT might teach Pat to use a more modulated style of description and avoid extreme terms such as "always" and "never." The assumption in TBCT is that a change in behaviors will lead to a change in cognitions and emotions.

In traditional CBCT, the focus is less on changing behavior than on changing or "restructuring" cognitions that may drive behavior. CBCT therapists focus on cognitive processing, such as selective attention and "all-or-nothing" thinking, and cognitive factors such as attributions, which refer to partners' explanations of events in their relationship, and assumptions, which refer to partners' beliefs about marriage, men and women, and their partner, such as a belief that disagreement is bad for marriage. In dealing with Pat's "always" and "never" statements, a CBCT therapist might focus on Pat's tendency to attend selectively to Sam's negative behavior and the tendency toward "all-or-nothing" thinking about Sam. The assumption in CBCT is that a change in thinking will lead to changes in behavior and emotion.

In contrast to these approaches, the emphasis in IBCT is on emotional acceptance, the affective response that each partner has to the other. An IBCT therapist would explore each partner's emotional reactions, the conditions that elicit them, and the impact that they have. For example, in dealing with the issue of Pat's use of "always" and "never," the IBCT therapist would explore the conditions that elicit that response in Pat. At times, Pat gets so frustrated with Sam's lack of response that Pat, at the moment, feels like Sam is "never" there when needed. At other times, it is less a response to frustration than an attempt to goad Sam into action. In general, the use of extreme language is part of Pat's characteristic style of presentation: Pat can describe Sam as an "awesome lover" and as "having never really cared" over the course of the same day. In exploring Sam's response to Pat's use of language, the IBCT therapist might discover that, in emotional moments, Sam is angered and hurt by Pat's comments, feeling that nothing will ever please Pat, and vowing not to even try. Often, Sam feels "off center" with Pat, pulled reluctantly into Pat's emotional highs and lows, but sometimes enjoying the ride. IBCT assumes that when these emotional reactions are discussed in a nonjudgemental, empathic way, both partners, over time, become more mindful of each other's reactions and less negatively reactive to them. IBCT further assumes that these discussions create changes in partners' cognitive interpretations of each other's actions and changes in those actions themselves. Over time, Sam may view Pat's actions as less directed at Sam and more a reflection of Pat's mercurial moods. Pat may alter the frequency or intensity with which he or she makes "always" or "never" comments, or both may be able to recover more quickly from an incident in which such a comment disrupts their relationship.

In IBCT, interventions designed to foster emotional acceptance are applicable to a wide array of generally legal and moral behavior, but behavior that is often troublesome and emotionally upsetting. Acceptance interventions are appropriate to everyday behavior that leads to slights, annoyances, and hurts: a partner's outspokenness, a tendency to withdraw when stressed, preoccupation with work, pessimistic views, emotionality, flirtatiousness, and the like. However, dangerous and destructive behavior, such as physical violence and substance abuse, should *not* be the focus of acceptance interventions. Particular instances of these behaviors might be forgiven, but they should never be accepted. However, even within the broad array of behaviors that could be acceptable, IBCT provides no list of what specific behaviors should be accepted. IBCT generally accepts the values of each couple and each partner, as long as they do not promote destructive actions. Therefore, any list of acceptable actions would of necessity be individual. For most couples, sexual infidelity is unacceptable, but other couples find sexual infidelity, under certain conditions, acceptable. Likewise, particular individuals might find unacceptable a relationship with someone who did not want children, someone who was not of a particular religious faith, or a person who smoked. IBCT does, however, seek to lift the curtain of acceptability on a broader array of possible behaviors. When couples end IBCT, they are likely to be more mindful of their partners' actions and reactions, and more accepting of them.

In IBCT, acceptance does not mean submission, nor does it imply a lack of assertion. A focus on acceptance does not mean that IBCT attempts to communicate that partners should or must stay together. With the exception of illegal and destructive behavior, such as violence and substance abuse, IBCT therapists communicate no "should" messages.

At its most fundamental level, IBCT promotes acceptance of the following ideas: Each partner has feelings that are understandable; each partner has a story that makes sense; each partner has hold of some truth about the relationship; and each partner has a position on the problem that is worthy of attention and consideration. When there is little or no acceptance, the feelings may seem outrageous, the story may not make sense—it may seem to contain no truth, and the position itself may inspire ridicule. Out of this fundamental acceptance and the conversations that ensue from it, acceptance of more specific negative behaviors may emerge, such as greater acceptance of a partner's anger, or a greater acceptance of a partner's shyness about initiating sex.

To see the power and the limitations of acceptance, consider the distinction between an "initial problem" and a "reactive problem" (Christensen & Jacobson, 2000). The initial problem is the specific problem that the partners initially face. For example, Pat is more interested in sex than is Sam. The reactive problem emerges from the couple's attempts to deal with the initial problem. Pat and Sam argue about how often they should have sex. Pat accuses Sam of not having a healthy libido. Sam counters that Pat is oversexed. Sam's level of interest in sex is reduced due to the pressure to produce more, and Pat's level of interest in sex is increased because of deprivation. An emotional acceptance by each of the other's level of sexual interest would not solve the initial problem (the difference in sexual interest), but it would reduce all the reactive problems (the arguments, the accusations, and the reactive polarization of interests). Furthermore, acceptance may open up some possibilities for satisfying Pat's sexual needs that the couple did not seriously consider before—such as masturbatory actions by Pat alone, or by Sam for Pat.

There is an important link between the IBCT notion of emotional acceptance of partner and the notion of individual acceptance that is dealt with elsewhere in this book. To accept the experience and behavior of a partner means that one must come to terms with—accept—one's own strong emotional reactions, such as feelings of anger, anxiety, and disappointment. These are the kind of strong feelings that lead one to attack, minimize, ridicule, avoid, or withdraw from the partner. If one accepts these personal feelings rather than acting upon them in these problem-enhancing ways, then one can accept the partner. Thus, acceptance of partner and acceptance of one's own upsetting feelings and thoughts go hand in hand. To truly accept the partner gives little room for experiential avoidance of one's own feelings. Consider, for example, Pat's negative feelings for Sam's mother, Betty. Sam had wanted so much for Pat to share the strong connection that Sam felt with Betty. For Sam to hear Pat's feelings about Betty, and Pat's desire to avoid Betty, arouses strong feelings of anger and disappointment. Sam has urges to attack Pat and to reject Pat just as Pat has rejected Betty, in order to quell Sam's strong emotions. To truly listen to Pat, Sam must accept his or her own feelings. Often, there is no more powerful stimulus for our own emotions than the feelings, experiences, and views of our partner.

METHODS FOR INDUCING CHANGE

Two Types of Change Strategies

The most common way that people deliberately induce behavior change in others is through instruction and training. Instruction usually includes the rationale for the desired behavior and a description of it. Training involves modeling of the desired behavior, practice or rehearsal of it, and corrective feedback. The parent instructs a child to cook on the stove by telling the child about cooking and providing rules about what to do and what not to do. The parent may then model the appropriate behaviors for the child, watch the child practice the behaviors, and provide corrective feedback.

TBCT therapists have adopted these strategies to train couples in better communication and problem solving. The therapist instructs the couple in the purpose and value of specific communication strategies, such as "I statements," "paraphrasing," and "problem definition." The therapist may demonstrate these behaviors for the couple, and then have the partners practice them in the session. Then, the therapist provides corrective feedback about their performance of these skills.

Instruction and training is not required for many behaviors that a therapist may want to induce in clients, because the necessary behaviors are already in their repertoire. Simple requests, encouragement, or demands, perhaps buttressed with appropriate explanations, are all that is necessary. A parent asks the child to cook the dinner tonight, knowing the child has the requisite skills.

TBCT adopted this simple approach of requests and encouragement to elicit positive interaction between partners. In the strategy of behavioral exchange, therapists encourage partners to develop lists of positive actions they could do for each other, then ask them to engage in "caring days" (Jacobson & Margolin, 1979), when they will do a number of these positive acts. In a less formal way, therapists may encourage the couple to have a "date night," to go away on a weekend, or to spend some special time alone with each other every evening. These strategies of direct request are hardly unique to TBCT and find their way into a variety of approaches. Solution-focused therapy (Hoyt, 2002) is almost exclusively based on the identification and encouragement of positive actions by the couple.

These strategies of instruction, training, and direct requests are effective methods of behavior change when the person being changed wants to learn or engage in the behaviors. However, they are not very effective if the person to be changed is not interested, is motivated to do something else, or is disrupted by the presence of strong emotions. For example, telling people the value of eating less food overall and more healthy food in particular has been rather dramatically unsuccessful, even though most people believe in the validity of the message. Despite the public health message, Americans keep putting on weight, simply because unhealthy food is rewarding to eat. Similarly, training people in appropriate exercise regimens has often proven ineffective. Despite widespread information on exercise, most Americans remain physically unfit—because exercise requires consistent effort and is often unrewarding.

Distressed couples present a serious challenge to these methods of inducing behavior change through instruction, training, and direct requests. When talking about an emotional problem, they may be highly motivated to say an accusatory "you" statement, despite their training in "I" statements. Although they may be encouraged to engage in positive activities by the therapist, they may be unwilling to do so when feeling angry and resentful. Even though they have practiced reflective listening, their nonverbal behavior to their partner's provocative communication may indicate anything but understanding. They may summarize their partner's position in a tone that ridicules that position.

To understand the methods of IBCT, and to differentiate them from those of TBCT, a distinction by Skinner (1966) between rule-governed behavior and contingency-shaped behavior is helpful. In the former, behavior is under the control of an explicit rule generated through training or explicit suggestions (e.g., "Do aerobic exercises at least 3 times a week for a half a hour"). Reinforcement occurs because of compliance with the rule.

For example, the exercise trainer rewards the performance of the aerobic exercise or the individual person rewards him- or herself ("It feels good that I did something for my health"). In contrast, contingency-shaped behavior comes about as the natural stimuli and reinforcers in the situation guide relevant behavior. For example, a group begins playing basketball together. They find it enjoyable and join a local league; they end up practicing a couple times a week and playing a game once a week. Their behavior is shaped by the contingencies generated by the group (the pressure to participate and not let the group down, the reinforcement generated when any member plays well, when they win, and when they go for drinks afterward and debrief the game). Their behavior happens to meet the aerobic rule, but only coincidentally; the rule has little or no control over their behavior.

Although rule-governed and contingency-shaped behavior can generate behaviors that look, at first glance, to be virtually identical, they create a different feel. Rule-governed behavior is likely to feel more effortful; contingency-shaped behavior more spontaneous and natural. Contingency-shaped behavior may be more likely to persist, as long as the contingencies remain in place.

With its emphasis on behavior exchange, and communication and problem-solving training, TBCT seeks to induce change through rule-governed behavior. Similarly, traditional cognitive-behavioral approaches seek to alter thinking through rule-governed approaches. The therapist asks clients to track their cognitions about the relationship and trains clients to actively refute any dysfunctional cognitions. For example, if the client identifies a thought that the partner is not loving enough, the client is asked to analyze the evidence for and against that notion, looking in particular for evidence that would constitute an exception to that notion.

In contrast to both TBCT and cognitive approaches, IBCT attempts to induce change through contingency-shaped strategies. Rather than encouraging clients to engage in different behaviors, IBCT therapists call attention to overlooked actions, thoughts, and feelings; they highlight specific actions, thoughts, and feelings that may be glossed over, and they elicit new reactions in each partner. Consider how an IBCT therapist might work with Pat and Sam's pattern of accusation and withdrawal.

PAT: (*to Sam*) I don't know what goes on with you. You just don't engage in the relationship at all. You are completely passive, out to lunch.

THERAPIST: (*to Pat*) You mentioned not knowing what goes on with Sam. You are kind of confused by Sam.

PAT: Yes.

THERAPIST: (*to Sam*) I noticed that when Pat started talking to you, you kind of turned down, and there was a look on your face . . .

SAM: When Pat gets on my case like that, I just tune out.

THERAPIST: For you, it's same old, same old.

SAM: Yes, completely.

PAT: (*agitated*) So you turn off no matter what I say. You can't handle anything I might have to say.

THERAPIST: I think you put your finger on a real bind you are in, Pat. You have something important to say to Sam, something very important, but you don't know if there is any way that you can say it that will get heard. So you end up having no voice in this relationship.

PAT: That's right. And me without a voice is not me. (*smiles; half-chuckles*)

THERAPIST: (*to Sam*) I think that, for very different reasons, you are, oddly enough, in a very similar bind. You have things to say also, but you are so often taken with protecting yourself, taking cover, from what comes across to you as Pat's accusations, that you don't get a chance to focus on what you want to say.

SAM: I hadn't thought of it that way, but it might be true.

In this short exchange, the therapist does not suggest any rules for the couple or correct Pat and Sam for not following rules, such as the rule about "I statements," or the rule about listening by paraphrasing. Instead, the therapist repeatedly refocuses the conversation and highlights less obvious aspects of it. For example, the therapist focuses on the confusion in Pat's accusation (that Pat is confused about what is going on with Sam). The therapist calls attention to Sam's nonverbal withdrawal and reinforces Sam for discussing the withdrawal. It is more productive to discuss withdrawal, which is not withdrawing, than to withdraw. At that point, Pat gets agitated and goes on the attack, but the therapist focuses on the bind Pat is in and suggests that Pat has no voice. Pat smiles at the irony—that a talker such as he or she is would have no voice—but sees the truth in it. Then, the therapist links Pat's predicament to that of Sam. It is a new idea to Sam that neither has any effective voice in the relationship, but Sam considers the notion tentatively. In each of these interventions, the therapist seeks to change the adversarial context of accusing and withdrawing to a more collaborative context, in which each partner has difficulty voicing his or her concerns about the relationship. Also, the therapist may shift Pat's and Sam's views of each other. For Sam, there may be a tiny shift from "Pat is attacking me" to "Pat is attacking me because he or she is confused about what is going on with me." For Pat, there may be a tiny shift from "Sam always withdraws from me" to "Sam withdraws from me but has things to say to me." Certainly, many conversations, much more extended than the one just described, will be required to achieve the kind of contingency-shaped changes that are the goal of IBCT. Yet even in this short exchange, the therapist shapes a new, more productive conversation by shifting the stimuli to which each partner responds and finding ways in which each partner can be reinforced for expressing, or having expressed, his or her experience in the relationship.

Contingency-Shaped Strategies to Promote Acceptance

Having made this essential distinction between two different kinds of change strategies, we can now consider the three specific strategies that IBCT uses to promote acceptance: empathic joining around the problem, unified detachment from the problem, and tolerance building. All three rely on contingency-shaped strategies of change. IBCT does not tell clients that they should be more accepting, or tell them what they should accept. Rather, it tries to create conditions under which partners will naturally increase in their emotional acceptance of each other.

Empathic Joining

In this strategy, IBCT therapists suggest or elicit feelings associated with the couple's problem that are not commonly expressed. These feelings may be unexpressed because they are embarrassing or vulnerable, or because the partner is only dimly aware of them. These emotions, once voiced by one partner, may then elicit more constructive and sympathetic responses in the other. In this way, IBCT therapists attempt to generate an empathic connection between partners around the very issues that drive them apart.

Partners are liable to first discuss their problems by expressing "hard" feelings and thoughts that present the self as strong and point an accusing finger at the other. For example, Pat frequently expresses anger and frustration at Sam and catalogues Sam's inadequacies. These expressions typically lead to defensiveness, counterattack, and withdrawal. IBCT therapists look for the "softer," more vulnerable feelings and thoughts that may also exist alongside the harder feelings and thoughts. IBCT therapists may probe for feelings of disappointment, neglect, and hurt, or feelings that suggest uncertainty, confusion, and doubt. However, even these softer feelings and thoughts may be presented in an accusatory way. Pat may acknowledge feelings of hurt or neglect but voice them as attacks ("You always hurt me"), or admit to confusion and uncertainty about Sam's intentions, but in a manner that leaves little doubt about fault or responsibility ("You would confuse anyone with your lack of response"). So it is a challenge for the therapist to create a therapeutic environment where partners feel safe to express soft feelings and thoughts that portray their raw vulnerability to the other.

Although soft, vulnerable feelings are often the focus in empathic joining, it is important to note that it is the function of the behavior, not its topography, that matters. If one member of a couple commonly expresses soft, vulnerable feelings that the other regularly ignores, IBCT would not target repetitive expression of these feelings as a goal. The therapist would want to find out how these expressions are being received by the ignoring partner, and how the expressing partner reacts to the reception. This exploration might elicit hard feelings and thoughts in the expressing partner that probably exist alongside the frequently voiced but regularly ignored expressions of vulnerability. These are the kind of emotions that, in this case, might command the attention of the partner and elicit a more engaged response.

Similarly, in working with a withdrawn partner such as Sam, the IBCT therapist might try to elicit any response whatsoever, even a hard expression. Any engagement, unless it is actively destructive, may be a good first step for a withdrawn partner and may function to interrupt the engaged partner's domination of air time between them. In the earlier example, the therapist reinforced Sam's initial response that "Pat gets on my case." Of course, the goal is not to turn an "attack–withdraw" pattern into a "mutual attack" pattern, but there are often a number of steps, many of them faltering, in shifting the context between partners from adversaries to sympathetic partners.

Unified Detachment

In contrast to the emotional focus of empathic joining, the emphasis in unified detachment is on creating objective, intellectual distance from the problem. In empathic joining, IBCT therapists alter an ongoing battle between partners by getting them to notice and attend to each other's wounds. In unified detachment, IBCT therapists ask couples to move to a better vantage point, use their binoculars, and observe their ongoing battle.

In unified detachment, IBCT therapists often engage the couple in a descriptive analysis of the sequence of behavior that makes up a particular problematic interaction. For example, suppose Pat and Sam had a difficult evening out at dinner. At the following session, the therapist might enlist the partners' assistance, as relationship detectives, to discover the triggering events that led their interaction astray. Together, they would describe and explore the sequence of events: At first they were doing fine, but the initial triggering event occurred when Pat talked about a problem at work and did not think Sam, examining the menu, was appropriately attentive. Annoyed, Pat made a sarcastic comment about Sam memorizing the menu, which was a triggering event for Sam, who then actively ignored Pat. And the two of them were off and running. The therapist might link this incident to the formulation and characterize it as a case of lack of attention leading to accusation, leading to withdrawal, leading to further accusation.

IBCT therapists also engage couples in comparative analyses of individual incidents. For example, suppose Pat and Sam had another evening out to dinner the following week that went well. The therapist might inquire whether there were any potential problems that they had to navigate. If there were, the therapist would help the partners identify specific actions, however subtle, that each took that enabled him or her to recover. Perhaps Pat, despite annoyance at Sam for inattention, repeated his or her comments, albeit with some tension in his or her voice. Sam suppressed the urge to withdraw from the accusatory tension in Pat's voice, and they were able to recover from a potentially disruptive experience.

Using metaphors, giving problems names, and invoking humor are also ways of creating distance from a problem. For example, depending on their sensibilities, Pat and Sam might respond to names such as "Mount Vesuvius" for Pat and the "cave dweller" for Sam. Mount Vesuvius erupts regularly, but the cave dweller always has available protection. However, the therapist must be careful that the humor does not deride either partner, or that names and metaphors are not used as weapons.

In general, the strategies of unified detachment serve to treat the problem the couple faces as an "it" rather than a "you." Sometimes IBCT therapists use props to objectify the problem and place it outside the relationship. For example, the therapist might suggest that the partners put their problem on an empty chair in the therapist's office and discuss the problem, or express their frustration with it, as "it" is sitting there. The therapist might also suggest that the partners have a chair for the therapist in their home, where they can go to and complain about the problem. Although these particular actions can come across as "gimmicky," their usefulness with a particular couple is judged by whether they achieve their function of detaching the couple from the problem. Because therapists have only limited knowledge of partners' unique histories, there is always some trial and error in finding out which particular types of unified detachment or empathic joining strategies will work.

Promoting emotional acceptance through unified detachment and empathic joining is conceptually distinct. The former is focused on objective analysis of a problem, while the latter is focused on an emotional exploration of the problem. However, in practice, the two strategies are often used together. For example, in debriefing an incident, the IBCT therapist may not only help the partners articulate the important behaviors that unfolded in the sequence of their interaction, and how these behaviors are similar to or different from their usual pattern (unified detachment), but also explore the emotional reactions that each experienced at different points in the sequence (empathic joining). Both strategies lead to what we might call greater "relationship mindfulness," a nonjudgmental awareness of negative relationship roles and interaction patterns, without as much emotional participation in the roles or patterns. That is to say, both strategies make partners more aware of what is happening within themselves and within the other as they go through a problematic sequence of interaction.

As one is more aware of the complex stimuli that constitute a situation, he or she may respond less negatively. One has a greater number of response options to the situation.

Tolerance Building

An important assumption of IBCT is that many important differences between partners, and the problems those differences create, will never be completely erased. Barring major head trauma or psychosurgery, Pat will always be more opinionated, more vocal, and more desirous of attention and contact than Sam. Similarly, Sam will always be more self-conscious, more deliberate, and more desiring of privacy than Pat. So the demons that Pat and Sam have, and the demons that most couples have, can never be destroyed. But they can be tamed. The intensity of a couple's problems can diminish. The power these problems have over the emotional climate of the relationship can be undermined.

Because of this notion that each couple has a perpetual problem with enduring dynamics (Huston, Niehuis, & Smith, 2001), IBCT emphasizes the management of problems rather than their elimination, and emphasizes recovery from problems rather than their prevention. The several strategies of tolerance building assume that problems will reappear but focus on ways to manage them better or recover from them more quickly. Thus, tolerance building is based on an acceptance of the continued existence of a problem.

One important strategy for tolerance building is to have couples enact negative behavior in the session. In this strategy, IBCT therapists instruct partners to deliberately enact clearly defined, negative behaviors that are part of their perpetual problem. For example, a therapist might ask Pat and Sam to enact a typical problematic episode in which Pat is critical and Sam is defensive. The therapist would not do this when Pat is, in fact, feeling critical and Sam is feeling defensive. Rather, it is important to enact the episode when neither partner is feeling the requisite emotions. Why? When the only instigation of a negative episode is the therapist's instructions, the couple will experience the episode very differently. Partners will likely see their own and their partner's behaviors more clearly and thus increase their mindfulness of their problematic pattern. Because the pattern is not provoked, they will probably experience less intense and different emotional reactions than usual. They may see that it is possible to respond in ways other than their usual response. They may experience some desensitization to the usual provocative behavior.

Couples sometimes have a difficult time enacting negative behavior. They may make such a poor attempt at imitating themselves that they smile, giggle, or laugh at the results. This kind of reaction is hardly viewed as a failure. In fact, it provides an excellent occasion for unified detachment. The therapist can join in and promote their view of their problem from a humorous vantage point.

Sometimes individuals can enact negative behavior in such a way that it does trigger emotional reactions in the partner. Most of the time, these emotional reactions are smaller versions of the usual reaction. The therapist can use whatever emotional reactions are generated as an occasion for empathic joining. Because the reactions are not as strong as usual, it may make the exploration and elaboration of emotional responding easier for the therapist to conduct and easier for the partner to empathize with, hear, and understand.

The therapist can follow an enactment of problematic behavior with an enactment of appropriate problem management. For example, the therapist may encourage Pat to enact criticism but encourage Sam to respond to it differently, or ask Sam to respond defensively with Pat and ask Pat to respond differently to Sam's defensiveness. It is, of course, easier to manage difficult behavior when one is not upset, so when the couple is able to manage problematic behavior well in the session, the therapist notes that partners may not be able to do so as easily when their emotions are triggered.

The therapist may also follow the in-session enactment with an assignment to enact a problematic interaction at home, when partners are not actually upset. For example, Pat might be asked to initiate criticism of Sam when he or she is not feeling particularly critical. Pat can therefore observe Sam's reaction more clearly and objectively. Pat is to reveal the ruse immediately, so that a true problematic interaction is not generated by a staged one. Sam is present when the therapist gives the assignment, so Sam's automatic reaction to Pat's criticism may be disrupted. After all, maybe it is not "real."

There are other strategies in tolerance building. The therapist may engage the couple in an analysis of the positive benefits that result from the differences that partners normally experience as negative. At the very least, differences between partners serve a kind of balancing function (e.g., the optimism of one is balanced by the pessimism of the other). Often, the differences are part of a central attraction between the couple. For example, Pat's sociability, particularly his or her generosity with praise, made Sam feel appreciated. Sam's reticence made it easy for Pat to be center stage. Another strategy is to look for alternate sources to fill needs that the partner has difficulty in meeting. Pat certainly needs other friends to fill the need for social contact.

Each of these "tolerance building" interventions communicates to the partners that their problem will reappear but can be managed. These interventions serve a kind of relapse prevention function in couple therapy. They prepare the partners for the inevitable reappearance of some of the problems that brought them to therapy in the first place.

Deliberate Change Strategies in IBCT

Although the focus of IBCT is on building emotional acceptance, with the assumption that emotional acceptance often brings about important behavior changes, IBCT also employs the traditional change strategies of TBCT: behavior exchange, communication training, and problem-solving training. Usually, the IBCT therapist starts out with acceptance strategies, but if a couple's initial presentation suggests that traditional change strategies would solve the problem and that the couple would be responsive to these strategies, then the therapist should start with change. For example, if a couple presents with a specific problem and is not in an adversarial role vis-à-vis each other, then the therapist might begin treatment with problem solving. However, the more frequent sequence is that IBCT begins with acceptance strategies, then shifts to change strategies when partners are more collaborative with each other but need to increase their positive interaction, improve communication, or negotiate differences.

When traditional change strategies are conducted in IBCT, they are usually implemented in a more individualized, less formal, and less rule-governed way. To make the change interventions more individualized, IBCT therapists would use the formulation of the couple's problem to inform behavior exchange, communication training, and problem solving. By using the formulation as a basis for these traditional interventions, the IBCT therapist may increase partners' mindfulness of their common patterns and alternatives to those patterns. For example, based on the formulation for Pat and Sam, the IBCT therapist would know that any initiation of contact by Sam toward Pat would likely be reinforcing for Pat. So behavioral exchange exercises that led to those kind of initiations would be encouraged.

To make change strategies less formal and less rule-governed, IBCT therapists often reduce the number of rules for change strategies, move toward more general principles, and modify rules according to what will help the couple most. For example, rather than teach couples to use specific "I statements" or to use the XYZ formula ("When you do X in situation Y, then I feel Z), the therapist might simply encourage partners to talk more about themselves and their own emotions when discussing problems. For example, the therapist might say to Pat, "Sam needs to hear more about you and your feelings, rather than your thoughts or opinions of him or her." Traditional problem solving is guided by a number of rules, such as "Start off the discussion with a positive statement about your partner relevant to the discussion" and "Don't move on to the solution phase until you have clearly defined the problem." IBCT therapists should only incorporate rules if they are essential to success for a particular couple. For example, if Pat and Sam mix the consideration of solutions with the definition of the problem, but this mix usually does not derail the discussion, then the therapist would be wise to leave the rule in the rule book. Sometimes a consideration of possible solutions helps define what the real problem is.

IBCT therapists are not as optimistic as TBCT therapists that couples can make many changes in their behavior and that these changes will persist. Therefore, IBCT therapists attempt to make only those deliberate changes in behavior that are essential for constructive functioning in a particular couple. Rather than a position of changing as much as can be changed, IBCT therapists change as little as is needed. In that way, IBCT therapists hope that a few important changes may persist.

Finally, IBCT therapists often return to acceptance strategies when change strategies stimulate strong emotions or elicit patterns of polarized interaction. Empathic joining, unified detachment, and tolerance building may therefore be mixed in with the change process. IBCT assumes that both acceptance and change will be required to alter most of the presenting problems that trouble couples. The preference in IBCT is that greater emotional acceptance will lead to unstructured, "spontaneous" change in couples as a result of different experiences of the partners. However, IBCT does incorporate efforts toward deliberate, structured change in therapy, but often these efforts involve an integration of acceptance and change strategies, much like the integration of acceptance and change that is the solution to couples' presenting problems.

EVIDENCE FOR THE EFFECTIVENESS
OF INTEGRATIVE BEHAVIORAL COUPLE THERAPY

IBCT was developed in part because of the limited outcome results from TBCT. There is more evidence on TBCT than on any other couple treatment. TBCT has consistently performed better than control groups, and, by American Psychological Association Division 12 standards, TBCT has reached the highest level of empirical support, that of an "efficacious and specific treatment" (Baucom, Shoham, Meuser, Daiuto, & Stickle, 1998; Chambless & Hollon, 1998). However, despite this positive support, the evidence indicates that only a bare majority of couples make reliable improvements during therapy, and only about one third recover at the end of treatment, that is to say, look more like normal than distressed couples (Jacobson et al., 1984). Furthermore, the evidence indicates poor maintenance over long-term follow-up (Jacobson, Schmaling, & Holtzworth-Munroe, 1987; Snyder, Wills, & Grady-Fletcher, 1991).

Also damaging to TBCT is some of the evidence on therapy process. Although changes in communication are the presumed mechanism for improved satisfaction in TBCT, research has shown that changes in communication are inconsistently related to improvements in satisfaction (e.g.,

Baucom & Mehlman, 1984). Also, couples often do not continue using the skills they learned in therapy (Jacobson et al., 1987).

IBCT was developed with the prediction that it would be at least as powerful as TBCT in the short-term and more powerful than TBCT in the long-term (Jacobson & Christensen, 1998). There have been three studies of IBCT that provide support for that prediction. In a dissertation, Wimberly (1997) showed that an IBCT group treatment for couples was superior to a wait-list control group. In a preliminary study Jacobson, Christensen, Prince, Cordova, and Eldridge (2000) showed that experienced clinicians could deliver both TBCT and IBCT to couples, that TBCT generated levels of reliable improvement consistent with previous research, but that IBCT generated somewhat higher levels of improvement in satisfaction (80% of couples in IBCT and 64% of couples in TBCT demonstrated clinically significant change). A major, two-site clinical trial is currently under way (Christensen et al., 2004) that examines treatment response in a sample of chronically and seriously distressed couples. Immediate posttreatment results indicate that IBCT and TBCT couples showed substantial improvements in relationship satisfaction during treatment, that IBCT couples improved steadily over treatment but that TBCT couples improved more quickly early in treatment but then leveled off later in treatment, and that IBCT couples showed a nonsignificantly higher level of reliable improvement in satisfaction than TBCT couples (71% of couples in IBCT vs. 59% of couples in TBCT). Couples are assessed every 6 months for 2 years following treatment. Although all couples have not yet reached the 2-year follow-up, a majority have. Analysis of the available data indicates that IBCT couples maintain and improve their satisfaction over 2 years significantly more so than do TBCT couples. In addition to this outcome data, studies of the process of change in therapy, not yet completed, will address the mechanisms by which both TBCT and IBCT improve relationship satisfaction. Although there are much more data to come, the evidence so far is extremely promising in its support of IBCT.

CONCLUSIONS

In this chapter, we have described IBCT (Christensen & Jacobson, 2000; Jacobson & Christensen, 1998) by comparing it to TBCT (Jacobson & Margolin, 1979) and to a lesser extent, traditional CBCT (Baucom & Epstein, 1990). IBCT differs from other behavioral couple therapies in its focus on broad response classes versus narrow target behaviors, its focus on emotional acceptance over direct behavioral change, and its emphasis on contingency-shaped versus rule-governed change strategies. IBCT is similar to many of the individual therapies described in this book because of its focus on emotional acceptance and mindfulness, although in IBCT, the focus of acceptance and mindfulness is the relationship. When IBCT is successful, partners become more emotionally accepting of each other, although this acceptance often requires an acceptance of strong emotions within themselves. Similarly, partners become more mindful of the contingencies that exist within their own relationships and are thus able to respond in more diverse, flexible, and constructive ways in their relationships. Currently available data provide promising support for the ability of IBCT to improve functioning in distressed couples.

In the course of this chapter, we followed Pat and Sam as they may have experienced IBCT. At the conclusion of therapy, Pat was effusive in praise of the therapist and therapy, emphasizing, of course, the benefit that both had had on Sam. In contrast, Sam gave a more muted reaction to therapy but did acknowledge that it had been helpful, and gave the therapist a warm handshake at the end.

ACKNOWLEDGMENT

This chapter was supported by Grant No. MH56223 from the National Institute of Mental Health to Andrew Christensen.

REFERENCES

Baucom, D. H., & Epstein, N. (1990). *Cognitive-behavioral marital therapy.* New York: Brunner/Mazel.

Baucom, D. H., & Mehlman, S. K. (1984). Predicting marital status following behavioral marital therapy. In K. Hahlweg & N. S. Jacobson (Eds.), *Marital interaction: Analysis and modification* (pp. 89–104). New York: Guilford Press.

Baucom, D. H., Shoham, V., Meuser, K. T., Daiuto, A. D., & Stickle, T. R. (1998). Empirically supported couple and family interventions for marital distress and adult mental health problems. *Journal of Consulting and Clinical Psychology, 66,* 53–88.

Chambless, D. L., & Hollon, S. D. (1998). Defining empirically supported therapies. *Journal of Consulting and Clinical Psychology, 66,* 7–18.

Christensen, A., & Jacobson, N. S. (2000). *Reconcilable differences.* New York: Guildford Press.

Christensen, A., Atkins, D. C., Berns, S., Wheeler, J., Baucom, D. H., & Simpson, L. E. (2004). Traditional versus integrative behavioral couple therapy for significantly and chronically distressed married couples. *Journal of Consulting and Clinical Psychology, 72,* 176–191.

Eldridge, K. A., & Christensen, A. (2002). Demand-withdraw communication during couple conflict: A review and analysis. In P. Noller & J. A. Feeney (Eds.), *Understanding marriage: Developments in the study of couple interaction* (pp. 289–322). New York: Cambridge University Press.

Epstein, N. B., & Baucom, D. H. (2002). *Enhanced cognitive-behavioral therapy for couples.* Washington, DC: American Psychological Association.

Hoyt, M. F. (2002). Solution-focused couple therapy. In A. S. Gurman & N. S. Jacobson

(Eds.), *Clinical handbook of couple therapy* (3rd ed., pp. 335–369). New York: Guilford Press.

Huston, T. L., Niehuis, S., & Smith, S. E. (2001). The early marital roots of conjugal distress and divorce. *Current Directions in Clinical Science, 10,* 116–119.

Jacobson, N. S., & Christensen, A. (1998). *Acceptance and change in couple therapy: A therapist's guide to transforming relationships.* New York: Norton.

Jacobson, N. S., Christensen, A., Prince, S. E., Cordova, J., & Eldridge, K. (2000). Integrative Behavioral Couple Therapy: An acceptance-based, promising new treatment for couple discord. *Journal of Consulting and Clinical Psychology, 68*(2), 351–355.

Jacobson, N. S., Follette, W. C., Revenstorf, D., Baucom, D. H., Hahlweg, K., & Margolin, G. (1984). Variability in outcome and clinical significance of behavioral marital therapy: A reanalysis of outcome data. *Journal of Consulting and Clinical Psychology, 52,* 497–504.

Jacobson, N. S., & Margolin, G. (1979). *Marital therapy: Strategies based on social learning and behavior exchange principles.* New York: Brunner/Mazel.

Jacobson, N. S., Schmaling, K. B., & Holtzworth-Munroe, A. (1987). Component analysis of behavioral marital therapy: 2-year follow-up and prediction of relapse. *Journal of Marital and Family Therapy, 13,* 187–195.

Skinner, B. F. (1966). An operant analysis of problem solving. In B. Kleinmuntz (Ed.), *Problem solving: Research method teaching* (pp. 225–257). New York: Wiley.

Snyder D. K., Wills, R. M., & Grady-Fletcher, A. (1991). Long-term effectiveness of behavioral versus insight-oriented marital therapy: A 4-year follow-up study. *Journal of Consulting and Clinical Psychology, 59,* 138–141.

Weiss, R. L., & Heyman, R. E. (1997). A clinical-research overview of couples interactions. In W. K. Halford & H. J. Markman (Eds.), *Clinical handbook of marriage and couple intervention* (pp. 13–41). New York: Wiley.

Wimberly, J. D. (1997). An outcome study of integrative couples therapy delivered in a group format [Doctoral dissertation, University of Montana, 1997]. *Dissertation Abstracts International: Section B: The Sciences and Engineering, 58*(12-B), 6832.

Index